# Cytolytic Lymphocytes and Complement: Effectors of the Immune System

## Volume I

Editor

**Eckhard R. Podack, M.D.**
Professor of Microbiology and Immunology
and
Professor of Medicine
New York Medical College
Valhalla, New York

Current address:
Professor
Department of Microbiology and Immunology
University of Miami School of Medicine
Miami, Florida

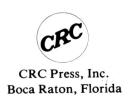

CRC Press, Inc.
Boca Raton, Florida

**Library of Congress Cataloging-in-Publication Data**

Cytolytic lymphocytes and complement

  Includes bibliographies and index.
  1. T cells.  2. Killer cells.  3. Complement
(Immunology)  I. Podack, Eckhard R.  [DNLM: 1. Complement
--immunology.  2. Cytotoxicity, Immunologic.  3. Killer
Cells, Natural--immunology.  4. T Lymphocytes,
Cytotoxic--immunology.  QW 568 C997]
QR185.8.T2C98  1988      616.07'9      87-22431

ISBN 0-8493-6968-1 (v. 1)
ISBN 0-8493-6969-X (v. 2)

This book represents information obtained from authentic and highly regarded sources. Reprinted material is quoted with permission, and sources are indicated. A wide variety of references are listed. Every reasonable effort has been made to give reliable data and information, but the author and the publisher cannot assume responsibility for the validity of all materials or for the consequences of their use.

Direct all inquiries to CRC Press, Inc., 2000 Corporate Blvd., N.W., Boca Raton, Florida, 33431.

International Standard Book Number 0-8493-6968-1 (Volume I)
International Standard Book Number 0-8493-6969-X (Volume II)
Library of Congress Card Number 87-22431
Printed in the United States

*Dedication*

To my father, Dr. med. Waldemar W. Podack,
in gratitude for stimulating my interest in science.

# INTRODUCTION

These volumes, *Cytolytic Lymphocytes and Complement: Effectors of the Immune System,* originate from the realization that pathways of recognition and killing of foreign targets follow similar routes in the humoral and cellular part of the immune system. In particular, the homology of immunoglobulins with the T-cell-MHC-antigen receptor at the beginning of the recognition sequence and the homology of complement component C9 with lymphocyte perforin 1 (P1) as pore formers at the end of the effector sequence are striking examples.

From my own point of view, the catalyst for suspecting mechanistically similar pathways in the effector systems of complement and cytolytic lymphocytes derived from the discovery of the polymerization of C9 to the circular structure of poly C9 (see Figure 1), which is responsible for the well-known ultrastructural complement lesions described originally in 1964. This simple finding immediately clarified conceptually the mechanisms for the formation of transmembrane pores both by complement and by cytolytic T- and NK-cells.

The motivation to assemble these volumes through the contributions of outstanding investigators in complement and lymphocyte research thus was, and is, to increase the awareness that mechanisms and molecular models studied in one system may well be of relevance to the other. Since complement has been studied in detail in all of its aspects, including activation, host protection, cytolysis, and repair mechanisms, it can serve as a guiding model system for the investigator of cellular mechanisms.

Effector cells, on the other hand, have the facility to interact with targets through surface membrane receptors allowing them an additional degree of complexity compared to humoral systems. This complexity, combined with the subcellular organization of cells (for example, the sequestration of cytolytic proteins in granules), offers alternatives for the mediation and regulation of cellular pathways that can be quite different from the humoral pathway.

Owing to these differences, the approaches to the use of the two effector systems for immune therapy are quite distinct. However, both are being explored at this time, and only future work will tell which combination of immune therapy will be most effective.

It is one of the most fascinating aspects of research to experience the development of common concepts with the attendant simplifications and understanding at the molecular level of previously poorly understood phenomena. It is hoped that this book will contribute to this process.

**E. R. Podack**

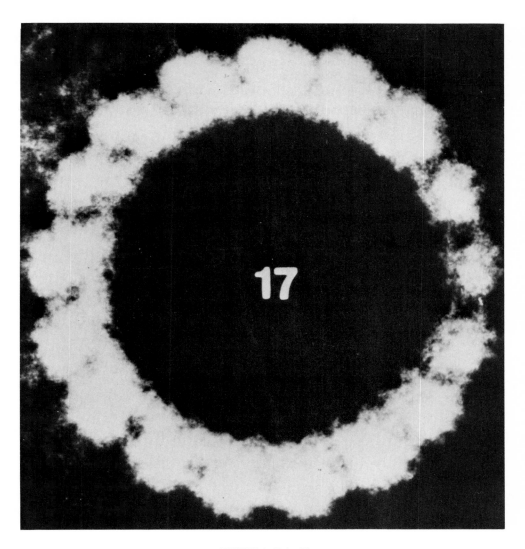

FIGURE 1. Poly C9.

# THE EDITOR

**Eckhard R. Podack, M. D.,** was appointed Full Professor of Microbiology and Immunology at the University of Miami School of Medicine in 1987. Prior to this appointment, he had been Professor of Medicine, Microbiology, and Immunology at the New York Medical College in Valhalla, New York, since 1984. From 1974 to 1984, he was associated with the Department of Immunology at the Research Institute of Scripps Clinic in La Jolla, California.

Dr. Podack holds the M.D. from Johann-Wolfgang-Goethe University in Frankfurt, Germany, and wrote his dissertation in Biochemistry at the Georg August University of Göttingen in Germany. His research thesis was honored with the Annual Award by the German Diabetes Society in 1973. Post-doctoral fellowship training was completed in the Department of Biochemistry at the University of Göttingen before he moved to this country in 1974. In biochemistry and immunology, Dr. Podack is internationally recognized and is a frequent invited lecturer to universities in Europe and the United States.

After collaborating with Hans Müller-Eberhard at the Scripps Research Foundation from 1974 to 1978 on complement components and activation, he spent the next six to eight years studying independently the molecular biology of molecules that cytotoxic lymphocytes use to kill their targets.

Dr. Podack is the recipient of two National Institutes of Health grants, an American Cancer Society grant, two Fellowship grants for his Post-Doctoral fellows, and a proposal of studies from private industry.

Dr. Podack is Associate Editor of the *Journal of Immunology* and Ad Hoc Reviewer for nine additional scientific journals. He reviews grant applications for the Veterans Administration, the National Science Foundation, the Fogarty International Fellowship Center, and the National Institutes of Health.

# CONTRIBUTORS, VOLUME I

**M. Amin Arnaout**
Department of Pediatrics
Children's Hospital
Boston, Massachusetts

**Barbara A. Benson**
Research Service
VA Medical Center
Minneapolis, Minnesota

**Gideon Berke**
Department of Cell Biology
Weizmann Institute of Science
Rehovot, Israel

**Steven J. Burakoff**
Department of Pediatrics
Dana-Farber Cancer Institute
Boston, Massachusetts

**David F. Carney**
Department of Pathology
University of Maryland
Baltimore, Maryland

**Zanvil A. Cohn**
The Rockefeller University
New York, New York

**Neil R. Cooper**
Department of Molecular Immunology
Scripps Clinic and Research Foundation
La Jolla, Callifornia

**Agustin P. Dalmasso**
Laboratory Service
VA Medical Center
Minneapolis, Minnesota

**Gunther Dennert**
Department of Microbiology
University of Southern California
Los Angeles, California

**Julia L. Greenstein**
Department of Pediatric Oncology
Dana-Farber Cancer Institute
Boston, Massachusetts

**Zvi Keren**
Department of Cell Biology
Weizmann Institute of Science
Rehovot, Israel

**M. Edward Medof**
Department of Pathology and Medicine
Case Western Reserve University
Cleveland, Ohio

**Steven J. Mentzer**
Department of Pediatric Oncology
Dana-Farber Cancer Institute
Boston, Massachusetts

**Michael K. Pangburn**
Department of Biochemistry
University of Texas Health Center
Tyler, Texas

**Eckhard R. Podack**
Department of Microbiology
 and Immunology
University of Miami
 School of Medicine
Miami, Florida

**David H. Raulet**
Center for Cancer Research and
 Department of Biology
Massachusetts Institute of Technology
Cambridge, Massachusetts

**Verne N. Schumaker**
Molecular Biology Institute
University of California, Los Angeles
Los Angeles, California

**Moon L. Shin**
Department of Pathology
University of Maryland
Baltimore, Maryland

**Jürg Tschopp**
Institute of Biochemistry
University of Lausanne
Epalinges-sur-Lausanne, Switzerland

**John Ding-E. Young**
Cell Physiology and Immunology
  Laboratory
Rockefeller University
New York, New York

**Robert J. Ziccardi**
Department of Molecular Immunology
Scripps Clinic and Research Foundation
La Jolla, California

## CONTRIBUTORS, VOLUME II

**Bharat B. Aggarwal**
Department of Molecular Biology
  and Immunology
Genentech, Inc.
South San Francisco, California

**Ramani A. Aiyer**
Department of Molecular Biology
  and Immunology
Genentech, Inc.
South San Francisco, California

**Michael J. Bevan**
Department of Immunology
Scripps Clinic and Research Foundation
La Jolla, California

**Benjamin Bonavida**
Department of Microbiology and
  Immunology
School of Medicine
University of California, Los Angeles
Los Angeles, California

**Thomas J. Braciale**
Department of Pathology
Washington University School of
  Medicine
St. Louis, Missouri

**Vivian Lam Braciale**
Department of Pathology
Washington University
  School of Medicine
St. Louis, Missouri

**Jen W. Chiao**
Department of Medicine
New York Medical College
Valhalla, New York

**John J. Cohen**
Department of Microbiology and
  Immunology
University of Colorado Medical School
Denver, Colorado

**Zanvil A. Cohn**
The Rockefeller University
New York, New York

**Gunther Dennert**
Department of Microbiology
University of Southern California
Los Angeles, California

**Richard C. Duke**
Department of Microbiology
  and Immunology
University of Colorado Medical School
Denver, Colorado

**Brett T. Gemlo**
Department of Surgery
University of California
San Francisco, California

**Elizabeth Ann Grimm**
Departments of Tumor Biology
  and General Surgery
University of Texas System Cancer
  Center
M. D. Anderson Hospital
Houston, Texas

**Hans Hengartner**
Department of Experimental Pathology
Institute of Pathology
Zurich, Switzerland

**Frederick C. Kull, Jr.**
Wellcome Research Laboratories
Research Triangle Park
North Carolina

**Lewis L. Lanier**
Research and Development Department
B.D. Monoclonal Center
Mountain View, California

**Leo Lefrancois**
Department of Immunology
Scripps Clinic and Research Foundation
La Jolla, California

**Ben-Yao Lin**
Department of Microbiology
New York Medical College
Valhalla, New York

**Aron Lukacher**
Department of Pathology
Washington University School of
 Medicine
St. Louis, Missouri

**Abraham Mittelman**
Division of Neoplastic Disease
New York Medical College
Valhalla, New York

**Warren W. Myers**
Department of Research
Becton Dickinson
Mt. View, California

**Carl F. Nathan**
Cornell Medical College
New York Hospital
New York, New York

**Kristin Penichet**
Department of Microbiology and
 Immunology
New York Medical College
Valhalla, New York

**Joseph H. Phillips**
Department of Research and Development
Becton Dickinson
Mt. View, California

**Eckhard R. Podack**
Department of Microbiology
 and Immunology
University of Miami
 School of Medicine
Miami, Florida

**Anthony A. Rayner**
Department of Surgery
University of California
San Francisco, California

**Nancy H. Ruddle**
Department of Epidemiology
 and Public Health
Yale University Medical School
New Haven, Connecticut

**Donald Scott Schmid**
Division of Viral Diseases
Centers for Disease Control
Atlanta, Georgia

**Uwe D. Staerz**
Basel Institute for Immunology
Basel Switzerland

**Marianne T. Sweetser**
Department of Pathology
Washington University School of
 Medicine
St. Louis, Missouri

**Carl-Wilhelm Vogel**
Department of Biochemistry and
 Medicine, and Vincent T. Lombardi
 Cancer Center
Georgetown University
Washington, D.C.

**Susan C. Wright**
Department of Microbiology and
 Immunology
UCLA School of Medicine
Los Angeles, California

**John Ding-E. Young**
Cell Physiology and Immunology
 Laboratory
Rockefeller University
New York, New York

# TABLE OF CONTENTS, VOLUME I

## TABLE OF CONTENTS, VOLUME II

**Section II.B: Cytolytic Mechanism — Killer Lymphocytes**

**Section II.C: Soluble Cytotoxic Factors Produced by Lymphocytes**

# Section I.A: Recognition — Complement

Chapter 1

# C1 STRUCTURE AND ANTIBODY RECOGNITION

**Verne N. Schumaker**

## TABLE OF CONTENTS

## I. INTRODUCTION

This chapter will focus upon the remarkable structure of the first component of complement, C1, and upon its interactions with C1-inhibitor and with antibody. A comprehensive review of C1 has just appeared;[17] therefore, we will concentrate on experimental studies published after the writing of that review and a hypothetical, but particularly satisfying, model for the structure of C1, variants of which have been proposed by three different laboratories.

Reviews which discuss the early components of the classical pathway, especially C1 and C1q, have been written by Cooper,[17] Lachmann and Hughes-Jones,[44] Colomb et al.,[15,16] Ziccardi,[94] Reid,[66] Loos,[47] and Porter and Reid,[61,67] among others.

The destruction and elimination of bacteria, virus, and toxins by the humoral arm of the immune system involves antibody molecules, phagocytic cells, and the alternate and classical pathways as well as the membrane attack complex of complement.[43,50] Activation of either complement pathway results in the release of anaphylatoxic peptides causing increased vascular permeability, smooth muscle contraction, release of histamine from mast cells, and chemotaxis of phagocytes to the site of infection;[34,35] as well as the deposition of potent opsonins such as C3b[54,99] and activation of the terminal components which assemble to mount a direct attack on the membrane of the invader[7,51] (and see Chapter 10, this volume).

Immune complexes composed of IgM and IgG as well as certain bacterial and viral cell wall materials, are included among the strong activators of the classical pathway. Individuals deficient in the early components of the classical pathway, C1q, C1r, C2 and C4, are only occasionally more vulnerable to bacterial and viral infection;[1] presumably, the alternate pathway can usually provide the critical defense effector functions, as it must prior to the development of effective levels of antibody in a naive host. Deficient individuals appear to be susceptible to immune-complex-associated renal diseases;[12,26,80] thus, the early components may play an important role in the solubilization and elimination of immune complexes.

The key role of immune complex recognition and initiation of the classical pathway is the principle function of the first component of complement. We will begin with an overview to illustrate the probable structures of the macromolecules involved, the names of some of their component parts, and what is meant by the "recognition" and "initiation" processes.

## II. MULTIVALENT ATTACHMENT OF C1 TO A CLUSTER OF ANTIBODY Fc INITIATES THE CLASSICAL COMPLEMENT PATHWAY

Immune complex recognition is accomplished by the binding of C1 to a cluster of antibody Fc, as schematically illustrated in Figure 1, and its subsequent activation[71,98] C1 is a complex composed of five protein subcomponents: one C1q, two C1r and two C1s.[89] The C1q subcomponent is a fascinating macromolecule, consisting of a central "stem" with six branching "arms", each arm terminating in a globular C1q "head".[61] The heads bind to complementary regions on the Fc domains of IgG and IgM. Since the binding of a single head to a single Fc is weak, tight binding of C1q to an immune complex requires multivalent attachment to a cluster of Fc, as illustrated in Figure 1.[98,106]

Binding of C1 to immune complexes is usually followed by a slower activation step in which most of the bound C1 becomes proteolytically active. Activation involves the other subcomponents; the two C1r and two C1s subcomponents are shown in Figure 1 as a string of balls wound among the C1q arms. C1r and C1s are proenzymes, and activation involves proteolytic cleavage of the C1r polypeptide. The activated C1r then cleaves C1s which, in turn, cleaves the next components in the classical pathway, C4 and C2, to initiate the classical component cascade.[86]

Not only can C1 activate by binding multivalently to an immune complex, but also C1

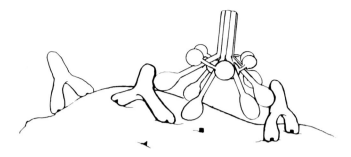

FIGURE 1.    The first component of complement is shown attached multivalently through the C1q heads to antibody binding sites located on the Fc piece of IgG anitbody bound to antigenic groups on a bacterial surface. The $C1r_2Cs_2$ tetramer is illustrated in this cartoon as the chain of subcomponents wound among the collagenous arms of C1q. (From Schumaker et al., *Molec. Immunol.*, 23, 557, 1986. With permission.)

can activate spontaneously in solution at 37°C, with a half-life of about 4 min. Spontaneous activation is greatly slowed by C1-inhibitor, a protein which may form a reversible complex with unactivated C1, as well as very tight complexes with activated C1r and C1s.[92;93]

## III. STRUCTURE OF C1q

C1q has a molecular weight of 459,300 g/mole,[66] a radius of gyration of 12.8 nm,[57] and a sedimentation coefficient of 10.2 Svedbergs.[45,64,71] Assuming a partial specific volume of 0.756 mℓ/g,[58] a Stokes radius of 9.6 nm and a frictional ratio of 1.87 may be calculated.

Amino acid sequences have been determined for the 224 residues of the A and 226 residues of the B chains and for the first 110 residues of the C chain;[63,68] the B chain has been cloned;[69,70] intrachain disulfides have been established;[65] and the ultrastructure is known from electron microscope studies.[9,41,72,74] C1q is a glycoprotein containing approximately 8.0% carbohydrate, of which two-thirds is glucosylgalactosyl disaccharide units linked to hydroxylsine in the collagenous regions,[63] and the remainder is composed of six asparagine-linked carbohydrates located on the C1q heads.[68,97]

Figure 2 illustrates the basic design of this remarkable molecule, which is constructed from 18 polypeptide chains. As indicated at the top of the figure, each polypeptide chain has typical collagen amino acid sequence along one-half of its length; then the sequence becomes similar to that of more conventional globular proteins. Three chains, one of each type, A, B, and C, assemble to form a regular collagen triple helix with a globular region at the C-terminal end; this structure will form a portion of the C1q stem, an arm, and one of the C1q heads. The chains are disulfide bonded, A to B, close to the N-terminus, and a second disulfide bond near the N-terminus links C chains in two adjacent triple helices, to form a structural unit composed of two helices and two heads. Three such structural units are assembled to form the C1q "bouquet", composed of a central stem, six radiating arms, and six globular heads.[61]

One curious feature of the C1q molecule is the sharp bend in the triple helix where the C1q arms branch away from the stem. This bend coincides with an interruption of the regular collagen sequence at that location: there is an alanine in place of a glycine at residue 36 of the C chain, and an insertion of a threonine between two gly-X-Y triplets at residue 39 in the A chain.

Recently, a space-filling model of C1q was constructed in the form of a collagen triple helix, using the known amino acid sequences for the collagenous portions of the A, B, and C chains of C1q.[37] This space-filling model was used to assign atomic coordinates which

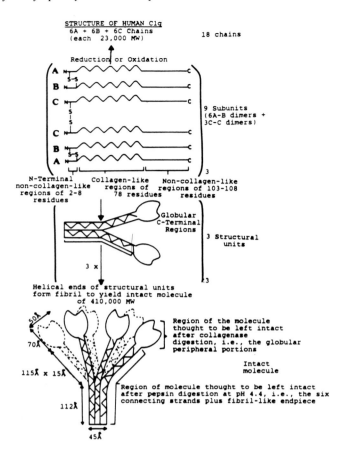

FIGURE 2.    This excellent illustration shows how 18 polypeptide chains assemble to form the six C1q heads and collagenous arms and stem. A detailed explanation is provided in the text. (From Porter, R. R. and Reid, K. B. M., *Adv. Prot. Chem.*, 33, 1, 1979. With permission.)

were then improved by energy minimization refinement: changing bond lengths, angles, torsional angles, and van der Waals distances to minimize conformational energy of the whole molecule. From this model, the "kink" in the triple helix arose naturally; the authors state that the formation of the characteristic collagen back-bone hydrogen bonds in the kink region was easily possible when a kink of about 60° relative to the helix axis was introduced.

To complete the model, six identical collagen helices were then assembled, positioning the kink so that the collagenous arms bent away from the central axis, as visualized with the electron microscope. The model maintains six-fold symmetry when the hydrophobic interaction edges are brought together, and an interesting feature is the symmetrical inter-C-chain disulfide structure at the N-terminal end of the stem. The six cysteinyl residues which contribute the three disulfide bonds connecting C chains in adjacent triple helices are symmetrically located. Thus, the disulfide bonds could be reformed to connect the alternate adjacent pairs without disturbing the hydrophobic contacts forming the stem. This results in "a sixfold cyclic symmetry . . . Other modes of disulphide bridging are only possible when the $C_6$ symmetry is reduced to $C_3$".[37] The model also shows that hydrophobic interactions between sidechains play a dominant role in the stabilization of the microfibrillar endpiece. A number of attractive electrostatic interactions between side chains of opposite charge also contribute.

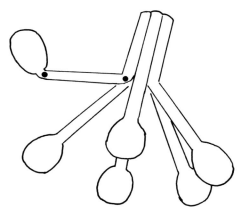

FIGURE 3.   Two different locations of flexible joints on C1q. A semi-flexible joint, located at the kink where the arms branch away from the head, is visualized in many different angular conformations with the electron microscope. The existence of the other flexible joint, located where the arm joins the C1q head, is inferred from time-resolved fluorescence depolarization measurements on intact C1q and on C1q stalks.

Flexibility of C1q has often been suggested, and the location of a semi-flexible joint at the kink was proposed from an electron microscopic study of the different conformations which C1q can assume.[72] The distribution of angles was found to peak "sharply at 50°, although clearly resolved images in which the angles are calculated to be as small as 20° or as large as 85° are seen occasionally." Flexibility in the kink region is *not* predicted from the refined, space-filling model for C1q described above; the authors state that only limited flexibility is expected, which should not be much different from that of normal straight collagen triple helices. However, regular collagen triple helices exhibit considerable flexibility, leading to a distribution of cone angle which compares well with the width of the distribution actually found.[37]

Flexibility of C1q has been examined by time-resolved fluorescence polarization techniques, and both rapid (25ns) and slow (>1000ns) correlation times were detected. The rapid component is compatible with "wobbling motions of the C1q heads about arm-head junctions".[37] The slow correlation time is compatible with wagging motion of the arm head units about the semi-flexible joint, as well as global tumbling motions of the entire C1q molecule (Figure 3).

Flexibility of C1q at the kink may be biologically relevant if C1q is to bind to a randomly arranged cluster of antibody Fc on the surface of an immune complex. In addition, "Rapid wobbling or twisting motions of the C1q heads would likely facilitate proper alignment of the binding sites on the heads with complementary sites on the Fc regions of antigen-bound antibodies".[27] Moreover, flexibility is probably required in the assembly and disassembly of C1 from C1q and $C1r_2C1s_2$. Finally, flexibility may be involved in the mechanism of activation of C1.[73,87]

## IV. STRUCTURES OF C1r AND C1s

Prior to activation, C1r and C1s are each composed of single, glycosylated polypeptide chains with a molecular weight of about 85,000, of which 7.4% is estimated to be carbohydrate. In the presence of EDTA, C1s is found as a 4.3 ± 0.3S monomer, it dimerizes in the presence of calcium ions. In contrast, C1r is found as a 6.7 ± 0.4S dimer in the presence and absence of calcium[81,83,84] In the absence of calcium, $C1r_2$ spontaneously autoactivates in a process which involves a structural change which can be detected by intrinsic

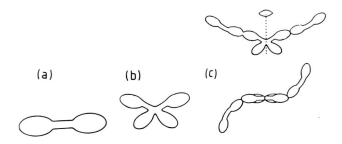

FIGURE 4. Schematic illustrations of the ultrastructures of C1s, C1r$_2$, and two orientations of the C1r$_2$C1s$_2$ tetramer c and d. (From the electron microscopic study of Weiss *et al.*, *J. Molec. Biol.*, 189, 573, 1986. With permission.)

fluorescence, circular dichroism and monoclonal antibodies.[85] Below pH 5, C1r reversibly dissociates to form monomers.[2]

Enzymatic activity is induced by the cleavage of a single argile peptide bond[4] to produce the N-terminal A or heavy chain ($M_r$ = 58,000 for C1r, $M_r$ = 56,000 for C1s) which is linked by a disulfide bond to the C-terminal B chain ($M_r$ = 32,000 for C1r, $M_r$ = 27,000 for C1s).[75] The B chain has been completely sequenced for C1r[3] and partially sequenced for C1s.[11] For C1r, the B chain contains 242 residues (27,096) and shows a strong sequence homology with other mammalian serine proteases. The histidyl, aspartyl, and seryl residues which form the catalytic site have been identified at positions 39, 94, and 191, respectively. Sequence has been determined for about 75% of the residues of the B chain of C1s; "somewhat surprisingly" it is about 59% different from C1r. Similar sequence differences with C1r are found for other mammalian serine proteases (56 to 71%).[11]

Additional proteolysis of activated C1r and C1s showed these proteins are each composed of two globular domains joined by an interconnecting strand domain to give a dumbbell-like structure.[86] Autoproteolysis of C1r allowed the heavy or A chain to be separated into three parts, alpha, beta, and gamma. Alpha represents the N-terminal half of the A chain (195-196 amino acids in C1r) and forms a single globular domain (the alpha domain) responsible for calcium binding and the C1r-C1s interaction. Beta forms the interconnecting strand (68 residues in C1r) and gamma (167 amino acids in C1r) is the carboxyterminal portion of the A chain, which is located on the other globular domain (the gamma-B domain) and disulfide bonded to the B chain (242 amino acids).[5,24] The gamma-B domains of autolysed, activated C1r$_2$ retain their dimeric structure and catalytic activity after controlled proteolysis.

C1s is cleaved into four chains by plasmin, the first two of which, alpha 1 and alpha 2, form a globular domain corresponding to the alpha domain of C1r, and responsible for the C1s-C1r interaction. C1s beta represents interconnecting strand. C1s gamma forms a portion of the other domain and is disulfide bonded to the B chain.[86]

The ultrastructures of C1s and C1r$_2$ have been studied by electron microscopy, and "C1s monomers are visualized as dumbbells with globular domains of about equal size (average diameter 5 ± 1 nm) with a center to center distance of 11 ± 1 nm" joined by a flexible interconnecting rod (Figure 4a). C1r$_2$ dimers were visualized, and "Particles with the shape of an asymmetric X were observed. These are interpreted as being composed of two dumbbells, with similar dimensions as those derived from C1s monomers." (Figure 4b) "C1r . . . apparently dimerizes by interactions near the junction between the rod and one of its globular domains".[87]

## V. STRUCTURES OF $C1r_2C1s_2$

When equivalent quantities of purified $C1r_2$ and $C1s$ are mixed together in the presence of calcium, they spontaneously associate to form a long, flexible tetrameric structure composed of two C1r and two C1s. The tetramer has a sedimentation coefficient of 8.1 S, and a translational frictional coefficient of 2.0; electron microscopy shows flexible structures about 500nm long.[79,81] The ordering of the subunits along the chain is C1s-C1r-C1r-C1s; this ordering was first suggested from the marked stability of the $C1r_2$ dimer[81] and subsequently confirmed using biotin-labeled C1s and ferritin-labeled avidin, to locate the C1s at the ends of the chain.[87] A schematic illustration of the tetramer is shown in Figure 4c.

The tetramer appears to possess twofold symmetry; thus, it frequently appears in electron micrographs as an inverted S-shaped chain lying on the carbon support. This may be readily explained if each half of the molecule is curved, if one side has a greater affinity for the support than the other, and if the two halves are related by a twofold symmetry axis.[81]

Since the domains responsible for the C1r-C1r interaction also contain the catalytic sites, this places the C1r catalytic sites on the two central domains of the tetramer. Since the domains responsible for the C1r-C1s interactions do not contain the catalytic sites, this places the C1s catalytic sites at the two ends of the tetramer.[86]

## VI. STRUCTURE OF C1

In the presence of calcium ions, one molecule of tetramer and a single C1q spontaneously assemble to form the first component of complement, C1.[89] This interaction is reversible and dependent upon both temperature and salt concentration. At 4°C and physiological ionic strength, the dissociation constant for the binding of unactivated tetramer to C1q is $K_d = 15$ n$M$; upon activation, the interaction becomes weaker, with $K_d = 141$ n$M$.[100] If the ionic strength is dropped or if the temperature is raised to 37°C, the complex becomes much stronger.[96,101]

After stabilization by crosslinking, C1 has been visualized with the electron microscope.[59,79] The gallery shown in Figure 5 displays images viewed both from the side and from the top, and the tetramer appears to be folded into a compact structure located centrally on the C1q molecule in the region between the kink and the C1q heads; the tetramer does not appear to touch the C1q heads, for in many images about one-half of the length of the arms is still visible.

Several models proposing a more detailed ultrastructure for C1 have been advanced.[15-17,58,59,73,87] In the last of these, the C1r ultrastructure described by Weiss et al.[87] was folded into the configuration described by Poon et al.;[59] this structure is presented in Figures 6A and 6B. The rationale for this design is based upon both symmetry and function:

1.  Macromolecular structures which assemble spontaneously usually take advantage of symmetry to maximize the number of identical contact sites. C1 has sixfold symmetry, and the tetramer has twofold symmetry. In order to maximize the number of identical contact sites, it is necessary to bring the sixfold symmetry axis of the C1q and the twofold symmetry axis of the $C1r_2C1s_2$ tetramer into coincidence. This automatically places the tetramer in the center of the cone formed by the spreading collagenous arms of the C1q. The two protruding ends of the tetramer may then be wrapped around the cone, as shown in Figure 6A.

2.  To be functionally acceptable, the tetramer should be folded on the C1q to bring the terminal C1s domains into coincidence with the central C1r domains; thus, the C1s substrate should be brought into contact with the potential catalytic sites on C1r. We believe the only way identical contacts can be formed between the two pairs of domains

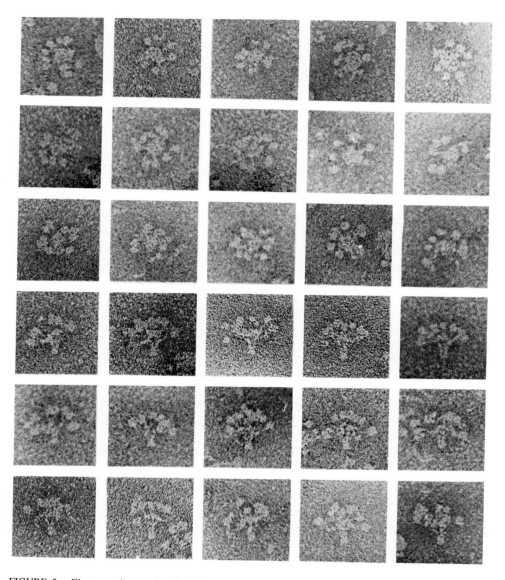

FIGURE 5.    Electron micrographs of C1 chemically cross-linked with a water-soluble carbodiimide, show both "top views" (first three rows) and "side views" (second three rows). The extra mass, presumably the $C1r_2C1s_2$ tetramer, appears to be located centrally when viewed from the top, and adjacent to the kink among the C1q arms when viewed from the side (From Poon, et al., *J. Mol. Biol.*, 168, 563, 1983. With permission.)

is to fold the tetramer into a figure "8", as shown in Figure 6B. When a scale model is constructed, it is found that the terminal domains of C1s may be brought into contact with the central domains of C1r. Thus, all four of the domains which contain the potential catalytic sites are brought into contact. The symmetrical model for C1 shown in Figure 6B fulfills the structural requirement of maximizing the number of identical contact sites, and it also fulfills the functional requirement of bringing the C1s substrate domains into contact with the C1r proenzyme domains which eventually will cleave them to produce the active C1s enzymes.[15,16,73,87]

It has been observed that the rate of dissociation of tetramer from the C1q subcomponent

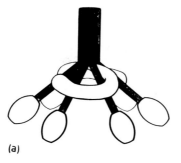

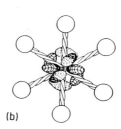

(a)

(b)

FIGURE 6. Models for C1 suggested by Poon et al.[59] and by Weiss et al.[87] In (a) the tetramer is centered between the C1q arms, and the protruding ends wrap around the outside of the cone. In (b) the catalytic domains of the C1r$_2$ portion of the tetramer are centered between the C1q arms, the protruding ends wrap around the cone, and the catalytic domains of C1s are brought back inside of the cone. (Figure 6a from Poon et al., *J. Mol. Biol.*, 168, 563, 1983; with permission. Figure 6b from Weiss et al., *J. Mol. Biol.*, 189, 573, 1986; with permission.)

was very slow when C1 became bound to immune complexes;[76] if the model for C1 shown in Figure 6 is correct, the tetramer probably became trapped among the C1q arms when the heads became attached to the immune complex.

## VII. STRUCTURE OF C1-INHIBITOR

Activated C1 is rapidly inactivated by a proteolytic inhibitor found in normal serum, called C1-inhibitor.[91] This molecule is a glycoprotein of about 104,000 molecular weight, of which 35% is carbohydrate; its sedimentation coefficient is 3.7S and its partial specific volume is 0.667 m$\ell$/g.[30] These data are compatible with a cylindrical molecule having a diameter of 1.5 nm and a length of 64 nm, assuming 20% hydration. The size and shape of C1-inhibitor also have been determined by electron microscopy. Odermatt et al.[53] found a long, thin structure, somewhat resembling a match; "A simplified model . . . consists of a globular structure having a diameter of 4 nm and a rod-like domain of length 33 nm and diameter 2 nm" (Figure 7).

C1-inhibitor forms SDS-resistant bonds with activated C1r and C1s. It also inactivates kallikrein and plasmin[62] and factors XIa and XIIa;[23] other proteolytic inhibitors found in serum are more potent inactivators of kallikrein and plasmin, but only C1-inhibitor reacts with activated C1.[29] Four molecules of C1-inhibitor react with, and cause disassembly of the activated C1; the products are one molecule of C1q and two enzymatically inactive, tetrameric complexes which presumably have the linear structure, (C1-inh)-C1r-C1s-(C1-inh).[90]

Recently it has been suggested that C1-inhibitor forms a reversible complex with unactivated C1, preventing spontaneous activation; this important regulatory role will be discussed later.

## VIII. ANTIBODY RECOGNITION BY C1q AND C1

Immunoglobulins IgM and IgG, but not IgA, IgD, or IgE, will bind to C1.[6] Binding occurs through the C1q heads[32,56,66] and the C$\nu$2 region of IgG[14] and the C$\mu$4 region of IgM.[102,103] X-ray studies show that IgG has a two-fold axis of symmetry. Therefore, the C$\nu$2 region probably possesses two distinct binding sites for C1q heads. The precise location of the C1q sites on the C$\nu$2 domains is not known; however, three different locations have been proposed and are discussed in detail by Burton;[10] ionic strength studies suggest that

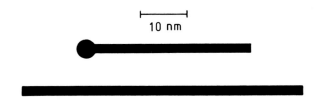

FIGURE 7.    Model for C1 inhibitor resembles a match, as seen with the electron microscope (at top), and a long rod, as determined from hydrodynamic studies (bottom). (From Odermatt *et al., FEBS Lett.*, 131, 283, 1981. With permission)

this binding is predominantly electrostatic in nature, but a hydrophobic component also appears to be present.

In solution C1q binds weakly to monomeric IgG. Thus, binding between a single $IgG_3$ and C1q head was estimated as 34 $\mu M$ in direct binding experiments using the analytical ultracentrifuge, and the other subclasses bound a little less well, with dissociation constants measured at 20° of 85, 157, and 299 $\mu M$ for $IgG_1$, $IgG_2$, and $IgG_4$, respectively.[71] Since normal immunoglobulin concentrations are in excess of 100 $\mu M$ in human plasma, and since the $IgG_1$ predominates, the C1q heads appear to be at least half saturated under physiological conditions, that is, an average of about 3 IgG molecules are reversibly bound to each C1q. This raises the interesting question of why the C1 does not immediately activate in plasma. Indeed, in vitro, in the absence of C1 inhibitor, high concentrations of monomeric IgG did appear to promote the activation of C1,[82] although it is always difficult in such studies to provide absolutely convincing evidence that activation is not due to small amounts of contaminating dimers and trimers. In plasma at 37°, however, C1 appears very stable in the presence of very high concentrations of monomeric immunoglobulins; this is likely to be due to the presence of C1-inhibitor, as will be discussed later.

Immune complexes composed of clustered IgG bound to antigen are strong activators of C1, probably because they present a cluster of Fc to which C1 can bind multivalently. Metzger[48,49] defined the associative model for complement activation by antigen, " . . . polymerization of the antibody by a multideterminant antigen would be the critical and perhaps sufficient role played by antigen''. Several recent studies support the associative model: thus, Hughes-Jones et al.[33] showed that two different monoclonal antibodies to the same antigen act synergistically in activating C1. Circolo et al.[13] found that IgG antibody bound to red cells coupled with complexes of hapten-labelled protein showed a sharp increase in its ability to activate complement when compared to the same density of hapten distributed at random over the cell surface. Kazatchkine et al.[36] showed that univalent antibody, and Watts et al.[88] showed that the Fabc fragment, formed by cleavage and removal of one of the two Fab pieces from IgG antibody, will activate complement just as effectively as intact antibody when bound at the same density. Hanson and Schumaker[28] show that IgG immunoglobulin bound to C1q in solution, retains most of its segmental flexibility; thus, the immunoglobulin hinge does not appear to be locked in place when the Fc piece binds to the C1q head. Liberti et al.[46] have showed that the activation of C1 is independent of the degree of filling of the antibody combining site. Johnson and Hoffmann[104] demonstrated that reduction and alkylation of the hinge disulfide of either antibody or normal rabbit IgG equally well reduced their abilities to activate complement and to bind complement; they conclude that impairment in C1 activation results from an effect on the C1 binding site itself rather than on a defect in the ability of the reduced and alkylated antibody to transmit a putative conformational signal from the antigen binding site to the C1 binding site. Thus, multivalent binding of C1 to several Fc bound to the same surface appears to be a critical feature for C1 activation, and neither distortion of the angle between the Fab arms nor allosteric signal transmission from the Fab to the Fc appears to be required for complement activation by immune complexes.

Activation by IgG clearly does not require the presence of antigen; for example, Tschopp *et al.*[82] have shown that chemically cross-linked IgG dimers, trimers, and tetramers activate in the absence of antigen, and activation is increasingly effective with complex size. Although in the presence of plasma or C1-inhibitor, binding appears to be essential for activation, it has been realized for many years[8] that binding and activation are two separate events; binding occurs first but does not invariably result in activation. Glutaraldehyde-aggregated IgG and chemically cross-linked Fc bind C1 but do not activate C1.[19,22] In this regard, it is interesting that binding of C1q to antibody which, in turn, is bound to lipid haptens incorporated into vesicles, is the same whether the lipid is in a fluid or a solid state;[52] activation of C1, however, follows C1 binding and is enhanced in the fluid state.[20,55]

IgM antibody molecules present an interesting contrast to IgG antibody, because IgM is a cluster of IgG-like subunits, called IgMs, disulfide-bonded together, with J-chain,[42] to form a disk fringed with Fabs. The binding between C1q and IgM in solution at physiological ionic strength was found to be very weak ($K_d$ = $10^{-4}$ $M$) but increased markedly as the ionic strength was lowered to one-half physiological ($K_d$ = $10^{-6}$ $M$). The slope of a log K vs. log ionic strength plot over this range was straight, and was interpreted that 6 ions are released when C1q binds to IgM. Scatchard and Hill plots showed that IgM possesses two independent binding sites for C1q, and electron microscope studies with cross-linked complexes showed that these two sites are located upon opposite sides of the IgM disk.[60]

Rather surprisingly, C1 bound much tighter than C1q to IgM at physiological ionic strength.[95] Binding in solution of C1 to IgM did not appear to result in activation of the C1.

The weight of the evidence suggests that IgG does not undergo substantial conformational change when bound to antigen; clustering of IgG may be sufficient to cause activation of C1. For IgM, however, another explanation is required, for single molecules of IgM antibody bound to red blood cells initiate complement-induced lysis.[105,106] Since single molecules of IgM already represent a cluster of IgG-like subunits, an additional conformational change upon binding would seem to be required. Both a distortive model[21] and an allosteric model[18] have been suggested. The conformational change could uncover cryptic C1q binding sites or enhance the affinity of sites already exposed.

## IX. A HYPOTHETICAL MODEL FOR THE COMPLEX FORMED BETWEEN C1 AND C1-INHIBITOR AND ITS POSSIBLE ROLE IN THE ACTIVATION OF COMPLEMENT

In the absence of C1-inhibitor, C1 activates spontaneously in solution with a half-life of 4 min at 37°C.[92,93] In the presence of physiological concentrations of C1-inhibitor, however, the rate of spontaneous activation is decreased by about three orders of magnitude. (Bianchino, et al., unpublished experiments). A complex between unactivated C1 and C1-inhibitor has been observed in ultracentrifuge studies;[95] it seems reasonable to suggest that spontaneous activation of C1 does not occur when inhibitor binds to C1. Figure 8 is a schematic illustration of a hypothetical complex formed between two molecules of C1-inhibitor and the two C1r proenzyme domains on C1. Since C1-inhibitor is a long, asymmetric molecule, the rod-like portion of the inhibitor would protrude well beyond the end of the C1 cone.

Before discussing the functional significance of this model, it is of interest to note one experimental observation which suggests that two molecules of inhibitor are required to prevent spontaneous activation of C1, as shown in Figure 8. At physiological concentrations, there are seven molecules of inhibitor for each molecule of C1. If the concentration of C1 is kept constant while experimentally diluting the concentration of inhibitor, there is an

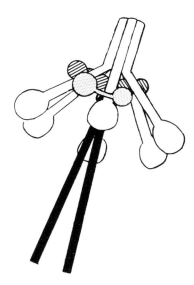

FIGURE 8.   Model of a postulated complex formed between C1 and two molecules of C1-inhibitor, in which the inhibitor is suggested to bind to the catalytic domains of the $C1r_2$ subcomponent, which is located centrally inside the cone formed by the spreading C1q arms. The protruding arms of the inhibitor would sterically block binding by multiple heads to an immune complex. Conversely, once C1 is bound by multiple heads to a cluster of IgG, the $C1r_2$ would be protected from the inhibitor by the cage formed by the surrounding arms and the surface to which the antibody is attached. (From Schumaker et al., *Molec. Immunol.*, 23, 557, 1986. With permission.)

abrupt increase in the rate of activation when the inhibitor is diluted by a factor of four.[78,92,93] Dilution by a factor of four reduces the ratio of inhibitor to C1 to less than 2, and, thus, there would be insufficient inhibitor to block all of the prosites on C1. Rapid activation would be expected, as observed, if two molecules of inhibitor are required to prevent spontaneous activation of C1 at 37°C.

The functional significance of the model shown in Figure 8, is that the protruding ends of the C1-inhibitor sterically block the direct approach of the C1 to an immune complex. Conversely, once C1 binds to an immune complex, then the C1r would be protected from C1-inhibitor by the spreading arms of C1q, and spontaneous activation could occur. Thus, activation of C1 by immune complexes may involve the release of C1 from an inhibition. This release requires that the interaction between unactivated C1 and C1-inhibitor be reversible, and it also requires a cluster of Fc bound to the same surface. The details of the activation mechanism, how C1r cleaves C1r and then C1s, are not addressed by this model, but it is suggested that they are similar to the spontaneous activation which occurs when C1 is studied in solution in the absence of C1 inhibitor. In that case, activation is rapid with a half-life of about 4 min.[92,93]

Monoclonal antibodies to C1q have been employed to probe the activation mechanism[25,31,77] In order to test the model just described, Kilchherr et al.[38-40] used a monoclonal antibody directed against C1q, 1H11, its (Fab)₂ fragments, and its monovalent Fab to activate C1 in the presence of C1 inhibitor. Both the intact antibody and the bivalent (Fab)₂ activated completely and stoichiometrically, at a ratio of one antibody combining site to 1 C1q head. The univalent Fab of 1H11 bound well to C1q, but it showed no detectable activation of C1. From these experiments, Kilchherr et al[40] conclude that bivalent antibody is required for activation, but the Fc piece is not essential in this system. The complexes formed between the intact antibody or its F(ab)₂ and C1q were studied further by electron microscopy and analytical ultracentrifugation, and found to be dimers composed of two C1q held together

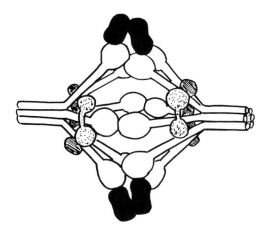

FIGURE 9. Two C1 molecules are schematically illustrated forming a ''head-to-head'' dimer held together by several $(Fab)_2$ which cross-link C1q heads to create the dimer. It is suggested that C1-inhibitor would be too long to fit inside the cage, and would be excluded, allowing the C1 to activate spontaneously. (From Kilchherr, et al., *J. Immunol.*, 137, 255, 1986. With permission.)

by multiple antibody molecules. ''A model for C1 activation is proposed in which two C1q subcomponents are joined by multiple $F(ab)_2$ bridging C1q heads. The model is analogous to touching opposing finger tips, the two hands representing the two C1q, forming a cage. C1-inhibitor, which probably binds to C1r through the open end of the C1 cone, is too asymmetric to be included within this cage. Thus, the C1 dimers are released from the inhibitory action of C1-inhibitor, and activation proceeds spontaneously at 37°C.''[39] The proposed model for the C1 dimer which excludes inhibitor and activates spontaneously is shown in Figure 9.

## X. SUMMARY

The primary structure and the ultrastructure of C1q are well understood from amino acid sequence and electron microscope studies. A plausible model for the secondary and tertiary structure of the collagenous portion of C1q has been proposed, by fitting the known amino acid sequences into the collagen triple helix, refining the atomic coordinates with an energy minimization program, and assembling six helices into the C1q bouquet. The ultrastructure of the $C1r_2C1s_2$ tetramer has been determined, and the locations of the catalytic domains established. C1q and the tetramer have been assembled to yield a model for C1 which satisfies the electron microscope observations as well as symmetry and functional requirements; variants of this model have been proposed by three different laboratories.

Using the model developed for C1 and the known ultrastructure of C1-inhibitor, a model for the complex formed between C1 and its inhibitor is now proposed. This model suggests that immune complexes compete with C1-inhibitor for C1, and that once C1 is bound to the immune complex, inhibitor is excluded. Activation may then proceed, either spontaneously or through additional interactions between C1 and the immune complex. Finally, some experiments with monoclonal antibodies directed against C1q which support this model, are discussed.

## XI. ACKNOWLEDGMENTS

The author is pleased to acknowledge the generous support of our researches by the National Science Foundation PCM-8215394, and by the National Institutes of Health, GM-13914.

# REFERENCES

1. **Alper, C. A. and Rosen, F. S.,** Inherited deficiencies of complement proteins in man, *Spring. Sem. Immunopathol.,* 7, 251, 1984.
2. **Arlaud, G. J., Chesne, S., Villiers, C. L., and Colomb, M. G.,** A study on the structure and interactions of the C1 subcomponents C1r and C1s in the fluid phase, *Biochim. Biophys. Acta,* 616, 105, 1980.
3. **Arlaud, G. J. and Gagnon, J.,** Complete amino acid sequence of the catalytic chain of human complement subcomponent C1r, *Biochemistry,* 22, 1758, 1983.
4. **Arlaud, G. J. and Gagnon, J.,** Identification of the peptide bond cleaved during activation of human C1r, *FEBS Lett.,* 180, 234, 1985.
5. **Arlaud, G. J. and Gagnon, J.,** Primary structure of human C1r: Identification of beta-hydroxyaspartic acid and complete sequence, *Complement,* 2, 4 (Abstr. 5), 1985.
6. **Augener, W., Grey, H. M., Cooper, N. R., and Muller-Eberhard, H. J.,** The reaction of monomeric and aggregated immunoglobulins with C1, *Immunochemistry,* 8, 1011, 1971.
7. **Bhakdi, S. and Tranum-Jensen, J.,** Membrane Damage by Complement, *Biochim. Biophys. Acta,* 737, 343, 1983.
8. **Borsos, T., Rapp, H. J., and Walz, V. L.,** Activation of the first component of complement. Activation of C′1 to C′1a in the hemolytic system, *J. Immunol.,* 92, 108, 1964.
9. **Brodsky-Doyle, B., Leonard, K. R., and Reid, K. B. M.,** Circular dichroism and electron microscopy studies of human subcomponent C1q before and after limited proteolysis by pepsin, *Biochem. J.,* 159, 279, 1976.
10. **Burton, D. R.,** Immunoglobulin G: Functional sites, *Molec. Immunol.,* 22, 161, 1985.
11. **Carter, P. E., Dunbar, B., Fothergil, J. E.,** The serine proteinase chain of human complement component C1s, *Biochem. J.,* 215, 565, 1983.
12. **Chapuis, R. M., Hauptmann, G., Grosshans, E., and Isliker, H.,** Structural and functional studies in C1q deficiency, *J. Immunol.,* 129, 1509, 1982.
13. **Circolo, A., Battista, P., and Borsos, T.,** Efficiency of activation by anti-hapten antibodies at the red cell surface: effect of patchy vs. random distribution of hapten, *Molec. Immunol.,* 22, 207, 1985.
14. **Colomb, M. G. and Porter, R. R.,** Characterization of a plasmin digest fragment of rabbit immunoglobulin gamma that binds antigen and complements, *Biochem. J.,* 145, 177, 1975.
15. **Colomb, M. G., Arlaud, G. J., and Villiers, C. L.,** Activation of C1, *Phil. Trans. R. Soc. Lond. B,* 306, 283, 1984.
16. **Colomb, M. G., Arlaud, G. J., and Villiers, C. L.,** Structure and activation of C1: Current concepts, *Complement,* 1, 69, 1984.
17. **Cooper, N. R.,** The classical complement pathway: Activation and regulation of the first complement component, *Adv. Immunol.,* 37, 151, 1985.
18. **Crossland, K. D. and Koshland, M. E.,** Expression of Fc effector function in homogeneous murine anti-ars IgM, in *Protein Conformation as an Immunological Signal,* Celada, F., Schumaker, V. N., and Sercarz, E. E., Eds., Plenum Publishing, New York, 1983, 59.
19. **Curd, J. and Cooper, N. R.,** C1 binding to complexes consisting of crosslinked Fc molecules from human immunoglobulin G, *J. Immunol.,* 120, 1796, 1978.
20. **Esser, A. F., Bartholomew, R. H., Parce, J. W., and McConnell, H. M.,** The physical state of membrane lipids modulates the activation of the first component of complement, *J. Biol. Chem.,* 254, 1768, 1979.
21. **Feinstein, A., Richardson, N. E., Gorick, B. D., and Hughes-Jones, N. C.,** Immunoglobulin M conformational change is a signal for complement activation, in *Protein Conformation as an Immunological Signal,* Celada, F., Schumaker, V. N., and Sercarz, E. E., Eds., Plenum Publishing, New York, 1983, 47.
22. **Folkerd, E. J., Gardner, B., and Hughes-Jones, N. C.,** The relationship between the binding ability and the rate of activation of the complement component C1, *Immunology,* 41, 179, 1980.
23. **Forbes, C. D., Pensky, J., and Ratnoff, O. D.,** Inhibition of activated Hageman factor and activated plasma thromboplastin antecedent by purified serum C1 inactivator, *J. Lab. Clin. Med.,* 76, 809, 1970.
24. **Gagnon, J. and Arlaud, G. J.,** Primary structure of the A chain of human complement classical pathway enzyme C1r: N-terminal sequences and alignment of autolytic fragments and CNBr cleavage peptides, *Biochem. J.,* 225, 135, 1985.
25. **Golan, M. D., Burger, R., and Loos, M.,** Conformational changes in C1q after binding to immune complexes: Detection of neoantigens with monoclonal antibodies, *J. Immunol.,* 129, 445, 1982.
26. **Hannema, A. J., Kluin-Nelemans, H. C., Hack, C. E., Mallee, C., Van Helden, H. P. T., and Erenber-Belmer, A. J. M.,** A functional deficiency of C1q in 3 family members, *Molec. Immunol.,* 19, 1373, 1982.
27. **Hanson, D. C., Siegel, R. C., and Schumaker, V. N.,** Segmental flexibility of the C1q subcomponent of human complement and its possible role in the immune response, *J. Biol. Chem.,* 260, 3576, 1985.

28. **Hanson, D. C. and Schumaker, V. N.,** Immunoglobulin G antibody bound to the C1q subcomponent of human complement exhibits segmental flexibility, *J. Mol. Biol.,* 183, 377, 1985.
29. **Harpel, P. C. and Cooper, N. R.,** Studies of human plasma C1-inactivator-enzyme interactions. 1. Mechanisms of interaction with C1s, plasmin and trypsin, *J. Clin. Invest.,* 55, 593, 1975.
30. **Haupt, H., Heimburger, N., Kranz, T., and Schurick, H. G.,** Ein Beitrag zur Isolierung und Charakterisierung des C1-Inaktivators aus Humanplasma, *Eur. J. Biochem.,* 17, 254, 1970.
31. **Heinz, H. P., Burger, R., Golan, M. D., and Loos, M.,** Activation of the first component of complement, C1, by a monoclonal antibody recognizing the C chain of C1q, *J. Immunol.,* 132, 804, 1984.
32. **Hughes-Jones, N. C. and Gardener, B.,** Reaction between the isolated globular subunits of the complement component C1q and IgG-complexes, *Molec. Immunol.,* 16, 697, 1979.
33. **Hughes-Jones, N. C., Gorick, B. D., and Howard, J. C.,** The mechanism of synergistic complement-mediated lysis of rat red blood cells by monoclonal IgG antibodies, *Eur. J. Immunol.,* 13, 635, 1983.
34. **Hugli, T. E.,** Structure and function of the anaphylatoxins, *Springer Sem. Immunopathol.,* 7, 193, 1984.
35. **Hugli, T. E. and Muller-Eberhard, H. J.,** Anaphylatoxins: C3a and C5a, *Adv. Immunol.,* 26, 1, 1978.
36. **Kazatchkine, M. D., Couderc, J., Ventura, M., Maillet, F., Duc, H. T., and Liacopoulas, P.,** Activation of the classical complement pathway by a monoclonal hybrid gamma 1-gamma 2a mouse monovalent anti-TNP antibody bound to TNP-conjugated cells, *Immunobiology,* 164, 262, 1983.
37. **Kilchherr, E., Hofmann, H., Steigemann, W., and Engel, J.,** A structural model of the collagen-like region of C1q comprising the kink region and the fibre-like packing of the six triple helices, *J. Mol. Biol.,* 186, 403, 1987.
38. **Kilchherr, E., Schumaker, V. N., and Curtiss, L. K.,** Activation of C1 by Monoclonal Antibodies Directed Against C1q, *Biochem. Biophys. Res. Com.,* 126, 785, 1985.
39. **Kilchherr, E., Schumaker, V., and Curtiss, L. K.,** C1 activation by a monoclonal antibody, *Complement,* 2, 42 (Abstr. 119), 1985.
40. **Kilchherr, E., Schumaker, V. N., Phillips, M. L., and Curtiss, L. K.,** Activation of the first component of human complement, C1, by monoclonal antibodies directed against different domains of subcomponent C1q, *J. Immunol.,* 137, 255, 1986.
41. **Knobel, H. R., Villiger, W., and Isliker, H.,** Chemical analysis and electron microscope studies of human C1q prepared by different methods, *Eur. J. Immunol.,* 5, 78, 1975.
42. **Koshland, M. E.,** Structure and function of J chain, *Adv. Immunol.,* 20, 41, 1975.
43. **Lachmann, P. J.,** Complement, in *The Antigens,* Vol. 5, Sela, M., Ed., Academic Press, New York, 1979, 283.
44. **Lachmann, P. J. and Hughes-Jones, N. C.,** Initiation of complement activation, *Springer Sem. Immunopathol.,* 7, 143, 1984.
45. **Liberti, P. A. and Paul, S. M.,** Gross conformation of C1q: a subcomponent of the first component of complement, *Biochemistry,* 17, 1952, 1978.
46. **Liberti, P. A., Bauschand, B. M., and Schoenberg, L. M.,** On the mechanism of C1q binding to antibody I. Aggregation and/or distortion of IgG vs. combining site transmitted effects, *Molec. Immunol.,* 19, 143, 1982.
47. **Loos, M.,** The classical complement pathway: Mechanism of activation of the first component by antigen-antibody complexes, *Prog. Allergy,* 30, 135, 1982.
48. **Metzger, H.,** Effect of antigen binding upon the properties of antibodies, *Adv. Immunol.,* 18, 169, 1974.
49. **Metzger, H.,** The effects of antigen on antibodies: Recent studies, *Contemp. Topics Molec. Immunol.,* 7, 119, 1978.
50. **Muller-Eberhard, H. J.,** Complement, *Ann. Rev. Biochem.,* 44, 697, 1975.
51. **Muller-Eberhard, H. J.,** The Membrane Attack Complex, *Spring. Sem. Immunopathol.,* 7, 93, 1984.
52. **McConnell, H. M.,** *Harvey Lectures,* 72, 231, 1978.
53. **Odermatt, E., Berger, H., and Sano, Y.,** Size and shape of human C1-inhibitor, *FEBS Lett.,* 31, 283, 1981.
54. **Pangburn, M. K. and Muller-Eberhard, H. J.,** The Alternative Pathway of Complement, *Springer Sem. Immunopathol.,* 7, 163, 1984.
55. **Parce, J. W., Kelley, D., and Heinzelman, K.,** Measurements of antibody-dependent binding, proteolysis, and turnover of C1s on liposomal antigen localizes the fluidity-dependent step in C1, *Biochim. Biophys. Acta.,* 736, 92, 1983.
56. **Paques, E. P., Huber, R., Priess, H., and Wright, J. D.,** Isolation of the globular region of the subcomponent q of the C1 component of complement, *Hoppe-Seyler's Z. Physiol. Chem.,* 360, 177, 1979.
57. **Perkins, S. J., Villiers, C. L., Arlaud, G. J., Boyd, J., Burton, D. R., Colomb, M. G., and Dwek, R. A.,** Neutron scattering studies of subcomponent C1q of first component C1 of human complement and its association with subunit $C1r_2$-$C1s_2$ within C1, *J. Mol. Biol.,* 179, 547, 1984.
58. **Perkins, S. J.,** Molecular modelling of human complement subcomponent C1q and its complex with $C1r_2C1s_2$ derived from neutron-scattering curves and hydrodynamic properties, *Biochem. J.,* 228, 13, 1985.

59. **Poon, P. H., Schumaker, V. N., Phillips, M. L., and Strang, C. J.,** Conformation and restricted segmental flexibility of C1, the first component of human complement, *J. Mol. Biol.,* 168, 563, 1983.

60. **Poon, P. H., Phillips, M. L., and Schumaker, V. N.,** Immunoglobulin M possesses two binding sites for complement subcomponent C1q, and soluble 1:1 and 2:1 complexes are formed in solution at reduced ionic strength, *J. Biol. Chem.,* 260, 9357, 1985.

61. **Porter, R. R. and Reid, K. B. M.,** Activation of the complement system by anitbody-antigen complexes: The classical pathway, *Adv. Prot. Chem.,* 33, 1, 1979.

62. **Ratnoff, O. D., Pensky, J., Ogston, D., and Naff, G. B.,** The inhibition of plasmin, plasma kallikrein, plasma permeability factor, and the C1r subunit of the first component of human complement by serum C'1 esterase inhibitor, *J. Exp. Med.,* 129, 315, 1969.

63. **Reid, K. B. M.,** Complete amino acid sequences of the three collagen-like regions present in subcomponent C1q of the first component of human complement, *Biochem. J.,* 179, 367, 1979.

64. **Reid, K. B. M., Lowe, D. M., and Porter, R. R.,** Isolation and characterization of C1q, a subcomponent of the first component of complement, from human and rabbit sera, *Biochem. J.,* 130, 749, 1972.

65. **Reid, K. B. M. and Porter, R. R.,** Subunit composition and structure of subcomponent C1q of the first component of human complement, *Biochem. J.,* 155, 19, 1976.

66. **Reid, K. B. M.,** Proteins involved in the activation and control of the two pathways of human complement, *Biochem. Soc. Trans.,* 11, 1, 1983.

67. **Reid, K. B. M. and Porter, R. R.,** The proteolytic activation systems of complement, *Ann. Rev. Biochem.,* 50, 433, 1981.

68. **Reid, K. B. M., Gagnon, J., and Frampton, J.,** Completion of the amino acid sequences of the A and B chains of subcomponent C1q of the first component of human complement, *Biochem. J.,* 203, 559, 1982.

69. **Reid, K. B. M., Bentley, D. R., and Wood, K. J.,** Cloning and characterization of the complementary DNA for the B chain of normal human serum C1q, *Phil. Trans. R. Soc. B,* 306, 345, 1985.

70. **Reid, K. B. M., Bentley, D. R., and Wood, K. J.,** Application of molecular cloning to studies on the complement system, *Immunology,* 55, 185, 1985.

71. **Schumaker, V. N., Calcott, M. A., Spiegelberg, H. L., and Muller-Eberhard, H. J.,** Ultracentrifuge studies of the binding of IgG of different subclasses to the C1q subunit of the first component of complement, *Biochemistry,* 15, 5175, 1976.

72. **Schumaker, V. N., Poon, P. H., Seegan, G. W., and Smith, C. A.,** A semi-flexible joint in the C1q subunit of the first component of human complement, *J. Mol. Biol.,* 148, 191, 1981.

73. **Schumaker, V. N., Hanson, D. C., Kilchherr, E., Phillips, M. L., and Poon, P. H.,** A molecular mechanism for the activation of the first component of complement by immune complexes, *Molec. Immunol.,* 23, 557, 1986.

74. **Shelton, E., Yonemasu, K., and Stroud, R. M.,** Ultrastructure of the human complement component, C1q, *Proc. Natl. Acad. Sci. USA,* 69, 65, 1972.

75. **Sim, R. B., Porter, R. R., Reid, K. B. M., and Gigli, I.,** The structure and enzymatic activities of the C1r and C1s subcomponents of C1, the first component of human serum complement, *Biochem. J.,* 163, 219, 1977.

76. **Sim, R. B., Arlaud, G. J., and Colomb, M. G.,** C1 inhibitor-dependent dissociation of human complement component C1 bound to immune complexes, *Biochem. J.,* 179, 449, 1979.

77. **Solomon, E. and Jones, E. A.,** in *Monoclonal Antibodies,* Kennett, R. H., McKearn, T. J., and Bechtol, K. B., Eds., Plenum Press, New York, 1980, 75.

78. **Spath, P. J., Wuthrich, B., and Butler, R.,** Quantification of C1-inhibitor functional activities by immunodiffusion assay in plasma of patients with hereditary angioedema — evidence of a functionally critical level of C1-inhibitor concentration, *Complement,* 1, 147, 1984.

79. **Strang, C. J., Siegel, R. C., Phillips, M. L., Poon, P. H., and Schumaker, V. N.,** Ultrastructure of the first component of human complement: electron microscopy of the crosslinked complex, *Proc. Nat. Acad. Sci. USA,* 79, 586, 1982.

80. **Thompson, R-A., Haeney, M., Reed, K. B. M., Davis, J. G., White, R. H., and Cameron, A. H.,** A genetic defect of the C1q subcomponent of complement associated with childhood (immune complex) nephritis, *N. Engl. J. Med.,* 303, 22, 1980.

81. **Tschopp, J., Villiger, W., Fuchs, H., Kilchherr, E., and Engel, J.,** Assembly of subcomponents C1r and C1s of the first component of complement: electron microscope and ultracentrifugal studies, *Proc. Nat. Acad. Sci. USA,* 77, 7014, 1980.

82. **Tschopp, J., Schulthess, R., Engel, J., and Jaton, J-C.,** Antigen-independent activation of the first component of complement C1 by chemically crosslinked rabbit IgG oligomers, *FEBS Lett.,* 112, 152, 1980.

83. **Valet, G and Cooper, N. R.,** Isolation and characterization of the proenzyme form of the C1r subunit of the first complement component, *J. Immunol.,* 112, 1667, 1974.

84. **Valet, G. and Cooper, N. R.,** Isolation and characterization of the proenzyme form of subunit C1s of the first complement component, *J. Immunol.,* 112, 339, 1974.

85. **Villiers, C. L., Arlaud, G. J., and Colomb, M. G.,** Autoactivation of human subcomponent C1r involves structural changes reflected in modifications of intrinsic fluorescence, circular dichroism and reactivity with monoclonal antibodies, *Biochem. J.,* 215, 369, 1984.
86. **Villiers, C. L., Arlaud, G. J., and Colomb, M. G.,** Domain structure and associated functions of subcomponents C1r and C1s of the first component of human complement, *Proc. Nat. Acad. Sci. USA,* 82, 4477, 1985.
87. **Weiss, V., Fauser, C., Engel, J.,** Functional model of subcomponent C1 of human complement, *J. Mol. Biol.,* 189, 573, 1986.
88. **Watts, H. F., Anderson, V. A., Cole, V. M., and Stevenson, G. T.,** Activation of complement pathways by univalent antibody derivatives with intact Fc zones, *Mol. Immunol.,* 22, 803, 1985.
89. **Ziccardi, R. J. and Cooper, N. R.,** The subunit composition and sedimentation properties of human C1, *J. Immunol.,* 118, 2047, 1977.
90. **Ziccardi, R. J. and Cooper, N. R.,** Active disassembly of the first component of complement, C1, by C1-inactivator, *J. Immunol.,* 123, 788, 1979.
91. **Ziccardi, R. J.** Activation of the early components of the classical complement pathway under physiologic conditions, *J. Immunol.,* 126, 1769, 1981.
92. **Ziccardi, R. J.,** Spontaneous activation of the first component of human complement (C1) by an intramolecular catalytic activity, *J. Immunol.,* 128, 2500, 1982.
93. **Ziccardi, R. J.,** A new role for C1-inhibitor in homeostasis: Control of activation of the first component of human complement, *J. Immunol.,* 128, 2505, 1982.
94. **Ziccardi, R. J.,** The first component of human complement (C1): Activation and control, *Springer Sem. Immunopathol.,* 6, 213, 1983.
95. **Ziccardi, R. J.,** Demonstration of the interaction of native C1 with monomeric immunoglobulins and C1-inhibitor, *J. Immunol.,* 134, 2559, 1985.
96. **Ziccardi, R. J.,** Nature of the interaction between the C1q and C1r$_2$C1s$_2$ subunits of the first component of human complement, *Molec. Immunol.,* 22, 489, 1985.
97. **Mizuochi, T., Yonemasu, K., Yamashita, K., and Kobata, A.,** The Asparagine-Linked Sugar Chains of Subcomponent C1q of the First Component of Human Complement, *J. Biol. Chem.,* 253, 7404, 1979.
98. **Dower, S. K. and Segal, D. M.,** C1q Binding to Antibody Coated Cells — Predictions from a Single Multivalent Binding Model, *Mol. Immunol.,* 18, 823, 1981.
99. **Ross, G. D. and Medhof, M. E.,** Membrane complement receptors specific for bound fragments of C3, *Adv. Immunol.,* 217, 1985.
100. **Siegel, R. C. and Schumaker, V. N.,** Measurement of the association constants of the complexes formed between intact C1q or pepsin-treated C1q stalks and the unactivated or activated C1r$_2$C1s$_2$ tetramers, *Molec. Immunol.,* 20, 53, 1983.
101. **Ziccardi, R. J.,** The role of immune complexes in the activation of the first component of human complement, *J. Immunol.,* 132, 283, 1984.
102. **Hurst, M. M.., Volanakis, J. E., Hester, R. B., Stroud, R. M., and Bennett, J. C.,** The structural basis for binding of complement by immunoglobulin M., *J. Exp. Med.,* 140, 1117, 1974.
103. **Plaut, A. G., Cohen, S., and Tomasi, T. B., Jr.,** Immunoglobulin M: Fixation of human complement by the Fc fragment, *Science,* 176, 55, 1972.
104. **Johnson, B. A. and Hoffmann, L. G.,** The effect of reduction and alkylation on structure and function of rabbit IgG antibody. 2. Effects of classical pathway C-3 convertase formation, *Molec. Immunol.,* 21, 77, 1984.
105. **Borsos, T., Chapuis, R. M., and Langone, J. J.,** Distinction between fixation of C1 and the activation of complement by natural IgM antihapten antibody: Effect of cell surface hapten density, *Molec. Immunol.,* 18, 863, 1981.
106. **Borsos, T. and Rapp, H. T.,** Complement fixation at cell surfaces by 19S and 7S antibodies, *Science,* 150, 505, 1965.

Chapter 2

# ACTIVATION OF C1 AND THE CLASSICAL PATHWAY OF COMPLEMENT*

**Robert J. Ziccardi and Neil R. Cooper**

## TABLE OF CONTENTS

*   This is publication number 4220-IMM from the Research Institute of Scripps Clinic. This work was supported by United States Public Health Service Grant AI 14502 and AI 17354.

## I. INTRODUCTION

Complement is a group of serum proteins that play a vital role in host defense against infection. Activation of the complement system triggers sequential biochemical reactions, which are accompanied by the generation of numerous biologically active mediators of inflammation, ultimately leading to the destruction and clearance of invading organisms. The classical pathway of complement is initiated by the first complement component (C1).[*] After an activating substance, such as an immune complex, binds and activates C1, C1 then activates the second (C2) and fourth (C4) complement components thereby triggering the complement cascade. The purpose of this report is to summarize the known molecular principles involved in C1 activation and its physiologic control, while emphasizing contemporary aspects. Other recent reviews dealing with C1 are by Cooper,[1] Lachmann and Hughes-Jones,[2] Colomb et al.,[3] and Schumaker.[4] C1 is of interest not only because of its importance as the initiator of the classical complement pathway, but also since it is the most readily defined and easily studied mediator of immunoglobulin function. Furthermore, C1 in itself is an intriguing biochemical model involving specific protein-protein interactions, induced conformational changes and activation by limited proteolysis (Figure 1).

## II. MACROMOLECULAR NATURE OF C1

C1 is a 16S glycoprotein composed of 22 polypeptide chains and having a molecular weight of 750,000.[5-7] Under physiologic conditions, C1 consists of two subunits, C1q and $C1r_2s_2$. The association constant for $C1q + C1r_2s_2 \rightleftharpoons C1qr_2s_2$ is 3.6 to 6.7 $\times$ $10^7 M^{-1}$.[8,9] Since the concentration of C1 in normal human serum (NHS) is $1.8 \times 10^{-7} M$,[7] approximately 30% of the C1 in NHS is calculated to be present as free subunits. This value may vary in NHS if other serum factors influence the equilibrium constant. Of related interest is that Laurell et al.[10] observed free $C1r_2s_2$ in normal and pathologic human sera, as ascertained by crossed immunoelectrophoresis. Thus, under physiologic conditions, C1 should be regarded as two weakly interacting proteins — C1q and $C1r_2s_2$. C1 concentration dependent dissociation must be considered when studying C1. It has been shown, for example, that the kinetics of C1 activation are affected by C1 dissociation with dilution.[11,12]

### A. The C1q Subunit of C1

The binding site(s) for immune complexes is located in the C1q subunit of C1;[13] an affinity constant of approximately $10^8 M^{-1}$ has been calculated for the interaction.[14,15] C1q is an 11S glycoprotein with a molecular weight of 410,000,[16] being composed of three distinct polypeptide chains termed A, B, and C. One C1q molecule contains six copies of each chain.[17] For a serum protein, C1q has a most unusual chemical and morphologic structure. Calcott and Müller-Eberhard[16] first reported that C1q is similar to such structural proteins as collagen, because of its high content of glycine, hydroxylysine and hydroxyproline, in addition to equimolar amounts of glucose and galactose. Sequencing analysis has confirmed these findings, since the amino terminal end of each polypeptide chain contains the repeating triplet gly-X-Y with glucosyl-galactosyl disaccharide bound to many of the hydroxylysine residues in the repeated triplet.[17,18] Additional carbohydrate (linked through asparagine residues) is located in the A chains.[19]

When visualized by electron microscopy, C1q appears to be six globular domains held together by fibril-like connecting strands,[20] that are somewhat flexible.[21] Neutron small-angle scattering analysis has demonstrated that C1q in solution assumes an open conformation "in readiness for interaction with other proteins".[22] The globular heads of C1q contain the

[*]    See List of Abbreviations at end of this chapter.

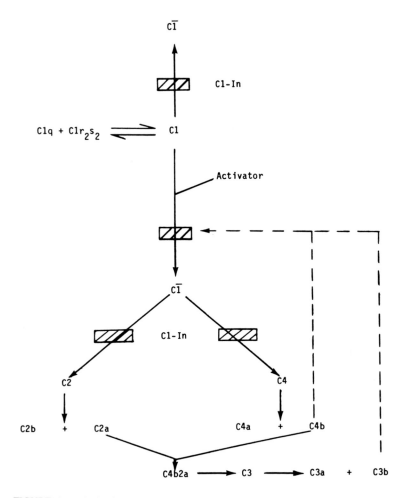

FIGURE 1. Activation and control of the first component of complement. In this scheme, points of inhibition are indicated by the shaded rectangles. While the fluid phase activation of C1 is inhibited by C1-inhibitor (C1-In), activator-induced C1 activation is not. However, the latter is inhibited by nascent C3b and C4b. Finally activated C1 (i.e., $\overline{\text{C1}}$) is rapidly inactivated by C1-In, thereby limiting C2 and C4 activation. These regulatory mechanisms prevent excessive complement activation that would be detrimental to the host.

carboxyl terminal regions of each polypeptide chain, whereas the fibril-like strands form a helical configuration from association of the amino terminal collagen-like portions of each chain.[17] These globular heads interact with immunoglobulin[23] and the fibril-like structure interacts with $C1r_2s_2$.[9,24]

## B. The $C1r_2s_2$ Subunit of C1

The enzymatic potential of C1 is located in the $C1r_2s_2$ subunit, which comprises two antigenically and functionally distinct polypeptide chains termed C1r ($M_r$ 85,000)[6] and C1s ($M_r$ 85,000).[6] Each $C1r_2s_2$ molecule contains two C1r polypeptide chains and two C1s polypeptide chains.[7] In the presence of EDTA, $C1r_2s_2$ dissociates into one noncovalently linked $C1r_2$ dimer and two C1s monomers.[6,25,26] This $C1r_2$ dimer can be dissociated in the presence of detergent or low pH.[25,27] Metal ions such as calcium are required for the assembly of the 340,000 Dalton tetrameric $C1r_2s_2$, which appears as a linear array of six to eight globular domains when visualized by electron microscopy.[6,28] The assignment of functions to the different domains in $C1r_2s_2$ has been recently achieved by Villiers et al.[29]

The ultrastructural appearance of macromolecular C1 is dominated by the C1q features.[28] $C1r_2s_2$ has been assigned to the regions between the C1q heads and the fibril-like central portion. Only after chemically cross-linking $C1r_2s_2$ to C1q, which prevents C1 dissociation,[28] can one use electron microscopy to visualize macromolecular C1. The ultrastructural, biophysical and functional properties of C1 and its subunits have been considered in the formulation of models proposed by numerous groups to describe the molecular architecture of macromolecular C1.[1,3,4,30-32]

## C. Nature of the C1 Metal Ion Requirement

Lepow and colleagues[33,34] have demonstrated that calcium is required for C1 function and maintenance of its macromolecular structure. Each $C1r_2s_2$ molecule binds four calcium ions ($K_d = 15$ $\mu M$), whereas C1q binds three ions with a lower affinity ($k_d = 76$ $\mu M$.[35] Furthermore, the native structure of $C1r_2s_2$ is metal ion dependent,[6] but the structure of C1q is unaffected by metal ions.[36] During the analysis of the primary structure of C1r, Arlaud and Gagnon[38] identified a beta-hydroxyaspartic acid residue, an amino acid associated with calcium binding potential.

According to a recent report,[37] other metal ions can replace calcium in C1. In fact, each of the divalent cations tested from the first transition period of the periodic table (i.e., $Ca^{2+}$, $Mn^{2+}$, $Co^{2+}$, $Ni^{2+}$, and $Zn^{2+}$) as well as $Cd^{2+}$ and $Tb^{3+}$ effectively mediate the formation of 16S activatable C1, which can initiate the classical complement pathway in NHS treated with immune complexes. $Mg^{2+}$ and $Ba^{2+}$ are not effective cofactors of C1. All of the active metal ions have the same apparent binding affinity for this activation promoting site(s) on C1. These functional affinity constants are consistent with the affinity constant reported for $^{45}Ca$ binding to $C1r_2s_2$ (i.e., $6.7 \times 10^4 M^{-1}$).[35] At high metal ion concentrations, ion binding to distinct lower affinity site(s) inhibit C1 assembly and function. The further to the right in the periodic table, the better the inhibitor the metal ion.

Since the serum concentration of calcium is far greater than that of any other active metal ion, calcium is the probable physiologic cofactor of C1. However, the significance of C1 inhibition by the binding of metal ions to a second site(s) remains to be determined. Furthermore, since a number of these metal ions are paramagnetic or fluorescent, they should prove useful in vitro in conjunction with sophisticated spectroscopic techniques to facilitate studying the mechanism of C1 activation and the role played by metal ions in that activation process.

## III. C1 ACTIVATION

C1 circulates in a precursor state, and only after "activation" does it acquire functional activity, i.e., the ability to initiate the classical complement pathway. The most apparent physicochemical change in C1 upon activation is the cleavage of each 85,000 Dalton C1r and C1s polypeptide chain into two disulfide held chains of approximately 57,000 and 28,000 Daltons.[39-41] Accompanying this limited proteolysis is the conversion of C1r and C1s from proenzymes to active serine proteases.[25,42,43] C1r sequencing analysis by Arlaud et al.[44] has allowed assignment of locations for three active residues (i.e., His, Asp, Ser) common to all serine proteases and comprising the "charge relay" site. Further analyses have shown that C1r lacks a "histidine loop" disulfide bond present in all other serine proteases.[44,45]

The natural substrate of activated C1r is C1s,[25,46] while activated C1s cleaves C2 and C4.[47,48] They are highly specific proteases and their enzymatic activities are modulated by their interaction with C1q as well as by their substrates C2 and C4.[49-51] Activated C1r and

C1s cleave various synthetic substrates, with thiolester peptides, in particular, being good substrates.[52]

## A. Molecular Mechanism of C1 Activation

The following model has been proposed to describe the intramolecular activation of C1:[41] Each polypeptide chain of $C1r_2$ has the potential to cleave and thereby activate the other, but cannot do so in $C1r_2s_2$ due to spatial constraints. However, the reciprocal cleavage of each C1r chain does occur after $C1r_2s_2$ molecular rearrangement induced, for example, by binding to immune-complex bound C1q. After this $C1r_2$ autoactivation, $C1s_2$ is activated by activated $C1r_2$ thereby completing the intramolecular activation process. This hypothesis is consistent with those subsequently proposed by others.[1-4,17,53-56] Experimental evidence favoring this intramolecualr mechanism includes the fact that $C1r_2$ autoactivates[41] and that activated $C1r_2$ activates $C1s_2$.[25,46] Purified $C1r_2$ spontaneously autoactivates at 37°C by an intramolecular mechanism when partially denatured by removal with EDTA from $C1r_2s_2$, which itself is stable.[12,27,41] The integrity of the $C1r_2$ dimer is required for this autoactivation.[27] Furthermore, native $C1r_2s_2$ can be activated by dinitrophenyl-polylysine, apparently by induced conformational changes.[57] An intermediary form of C1r containing a complete active site has been described.[58]

One would expect that conformational changes should accompany C1 activation, which involves the cleavage of four polypeptide chains, and in fact such changes have been detected by the following techniques: (1) circular dichroism spectroscopy,[55,59] (2) fluorescence spectroscopy with the fluorophore 7-(p-methoxybenzylamino)-4-nitrobenz-2-oxa 1,3 diazole,[60] (3) differential protein iodination,[61,62] and (4) production of monoclonal antibodies to neoantigens on activator-bound C1q.[63] Finally, the temperature dependent sensitivity of the interaction of C1q with $C1r_2s_2$ has been interpreted to reflect conformational changes within one of the subunits that are similar to those occurring during C1 activation.[64]

## B. C1 Activation Induced by Immune Complexes

C1 is activated by interaction with certain antigen-antibody complexes. Human IgG and IgM bind C1, but IgA, IgD, and IgE do not.[65] Furthermore, subclass specificity is a factor, with IgG3 the most reactive and IgG4 the least reactive of the four subclasses of IgG.[65,66] The C1 binding site has been assigned to the $C\gamma2$ domain of the Fc portion of IgG[67] and $C\mu4$ region of the IgM Fc.[68,69] Recently, the IgG binding site has been localized to the last two β strands of $C\gamma2$, which starts at gly (316) and ends at Lys (340).[70,71] However, synthethic peptides, tailored to resemble the "C1q binding site" and shown to inhibit C1q-IgG interaction, are not derived from this region of IgG.[72,73] The reason for this contradiction is unclear. Perhaps peptide inhibition is nonspecific or the active amino acid sequence is not unique. It may not even be restricted to $C\gamma1$, as Isenman and colleagues demonstrated that $C\gamma3$ also contains C1q binding regions that are buried in native IgG.[74]

Metzger has proposed that the binding of antigen to antibody either induces a conformational change in the antibody's Fc portion, thereby facilitating C1 activation (allosteric model), or merely aggregates or clusters the Fc portion of the molecules, thereby enhancing the affinity for the multivalent C1q (associative model).[75] Recent evidence favors the associative model. Tschopp and colleagues used chemically cross-linked oligomers of specific IgG in the presence and absence of bound monovalent nonasaccharide antigen to demonstrate the C1 activation is independent of antigen binding.[76] Hughes-Jones et al. demonstrated that the synergy between antibody molecules in activating C1 is due to their allowing C1q to bind bivalently to the immune complex.[77] Studies of Liberti et al. are also inconsistent with an allosteric model, since the occupancy of antigen combining sites does not correlate with the interaction of C1q with immune complexes.[78]

The mere binding of C1 to a substance does not necessarily result in C1 activation. Allan

**Table I**

**KINETICS OF C1 ACTIVATION: DEPENDENCE ON THE STRENGTH OF INTERACTION BETWEEN C1q AND $C1r_2s_2$**

| C1 | Ionic strength (M) | C1 activation (rate constant)[a] $(min^{-1})$ | C1 association Constant[b] $(M^{-1})$ |
|---|---|---|---|
| Fluid phase | 0.08 | 0.69 | $23 \times 10^7$ |
| Fluid phase | 0.11 | 0.20 | $12 \times 10^7$ |
| Fluid phase | 0.15 | 0.13 | $8 \times 10^7$ |
| Fluid phase | 0.21 | 0.05 | $1 \times 10^7$ |
| Immune complex-bound | 0.15 | 0.86 | $26 \times 10^7$ |

[a]   First order rate constants were calculated from kinetic curves.
[b]   Association constant is defined for $C1q + C1r_2s_2 \rightleftharpoons C1$, for fluid phase C1; and immune complex-C1q + $C1r_2s_2 \rightleftharpoons$ immune complex-C1, for immune complex-bound C1.

From Ziccardi, R. J., *J. Immunol.*, 132, 283, 1984. With permission.

and Isliker first demonstrated this by showing that tryptophan-modified IgG had the same affinity for C1 as native IgG, but lost its ability to activate C1[79] Furthermore, the rate of C1 activation does not correlate with the activator's affinity for C1.[80] On the other hand, the strength of interaction between C1q and $C1r_2s_2$ increases with C1 binding to an activator. This phenomenon, which Reid et al.[24] were the first to observe, was recently quantified by Hughes-Jones and Gorick,[8] and supported by data from several other groups.[9,81]

To establish the contribution of immune complexes in activating complement, a critical comparison of spontaneous (see Section III.D below) and immune complex-induced C1 activation was undertaken.[82] Kinetic analyses revealed that immune complex-bound C1 activated seven times faster than fluid phase C1 spontaneously activated. The rate of spontaneous C1 activation increased after decreasing the solution ionic strength. In fact at one-half physiologic ionic strength (i.e., 0.08 *M*), the kinetics of spontaneous C1 activation were indistinguishable from the kinetics of activation of immune complex-bound C1 at physiologic ionic strength (Table I). The enhanced fluid phase C1 activation at low ionic strength resulted neither from C1 nor C1q aggregation, nor from selective effects on the $C1r_2s_2$ subunit; however, at the reduced ionic strength, the C1 association constant (defined for $C1q + C1r_2s_2 \rightleftharpoons C1qr_2s_2$) did increase to $2.3 \times 10^8\ M^{-1}$, which is equal to that for C1 bound to an immune complex at physiologic ionic strength (Table I). Therefore, C1 can spontaneously activate in the fluid phase as rapidly as C1 on an immune complex when the strength of interaction between C1q and $C1r_2s_2$ is the same in both systems. Thus, immune complexes enhance the intrinsic C1 autoactivation process by strengthening the association of C1q with $C1r_2s_2$.[82]

## C. C1 Activation Induced by Nonimmune Substances

In addition to being activated by antibody, C1 is activated by numerous nonimmune substances including viruses,[83] bacteria,[84] C-reactive protein,[85,86] carbohydrate,[87] cytoskeletal filaments,[88] heart mitochondrial membranes,[89,90] myelin membranes,[91,92] endotoxin,[93,94] monosodium urate crystals,[95] and cardiolipin.[96] Although antibody independent complement activation is advantageous to the host by allowing immediate responses to invasive organisms, it may also be involved in pathogenic mechanisms as some of the examples described above would suggest. Because of recent evidence that the control protein C1-inhibitor (C1-In) can block certain C1 activation induced by nonimmune substances,[97] the activation potential of such substances should be assessed in the presence of C1-In before being characterized as physiologically relevant.

Bartholomew and Esser have studied the mechanism of antibody independent C1 activation by murine leukemia virus.[98] C1 activation by this virus required not only the interaction of C1q with the virus membrane protein P15(E), but interestingly also the interaction of C1s with p15(E). Tenner et al.[99] have also recently demonstrated that the C1 activator E. Coli J-5 has binding sites for not only C1q, but also C1s. However, the antibody independent activation of C1 by anti-venom polysaccharide does not require a similar interaction with C1r or C1s.[87] Furthermore, an interaction between C1r and C1s and immune complexes has not been demonstrated, although this matter has not yet been investigated thoroughly.

## D. Spontaneous C1 Activation

The ability of C1 to spontaneously activate was first observed in 1958, as partially purified C1 became activated when incubated at 37°C.[100] This observation was confirmed in 1980 when using C1 reconstituted from highly purified C1q, C1r and C1s.[101] Recent studies proved that C1 spontaneously autoactivates by an intramolecular autocatalytic mechanism.[12] Spontaneous activation follows concentration independent first order kinetics (half-life = 4 min and rate constant = 0.173 min$^{-1}$ at 37°C).[12] The percent of activatable C1 decreases with dilution due to C1 dissociation (i.e., $C1qr_2s_2 \rightleftharpoons C1q + C1r_2s_2$). Spontaneous C1 activation at 37°C is approximately five times slower than that induced by immune complexes.[12,102]

Since "spontaneous C1 autoactivation" is a conceptually as well as physiologically significant phenomenon, it is important to demonstrate that it is a property of native C1 and not caused by protease contamination in protein preparations, nor by activated C1, nor by protein denaturation during preparation. The involvement of contaminating proteases in spontaneous C1 activation is ruled out by the following:[12]

1.  Activation follows concentration independent first order kinetics.
2.  It is unaffected by the general protease inhibitor, phenylmethylsulfonyl fluoride, but reversibly blocked by a known inhibitor of C1 activation, nitrophenylguanidinobenzoate.
3.  Although proteases yield multiple cleavages of C1r and C1s,[103] only the characteristic single polypeptide chain cleavage accompanies spontaneous C1 activation.
4.  Only C1 present in the macromolecular form spontaneously activates, i.e., the dissociated $C1r_2s_2$ does not;[12] on the other hand, proteases cleave $C1r_2s_2$ independent of its incorporation into macromolecular C1.[103]
5.  The qualitative and quantitative nature of the metal ion requirements for spontaneous C1 activation are the same as for immune complex-induced C1 activation.[37]
6.  Finally, all preparations of C1 spontaneously activate at comparable rates. Inasmuch as each subunit used to reconstitute C1 was purified by at least two different established methods, it is unlikely that spontaneous C1 autoactivation could be attributed to contamination by proteases.

The first order kinetics as well as the lack of any effect by added activated C1 rule out the possibility that activated C1 is responsible for activating native C1.[12] Considering that little C1 activation is observed in NHS incubated at 37°C, it is essential to exclude the possibility of protein denaturation during isolation or radiolabeling. That spontaneous autoactivation is in fact a property of native C1 is indicated by the following:

1.  Spontaneous activation of purified radiolabeled C1 is inhibited when this C1 is added to NHS.[12] The regulatory protein C1-In is the serum factor responsible for controlling spontaneous C1 activation (see discussion below).[97]

2.   C1 spontaneously activates in NHS pretreated with plicatic acid, which inactivates C1-In.[104]
3.   Each C1 subunit was purified by numerous different published methods, and all these preparations activated at comparable rates. One method completely excluded EDTA and thereby produced $C1r_2s_2$ that had not been dissociated.

Thus, native C1 spontaneously autoactivates by an intramolecular mechanism. This fact allows one to study the mechanism of C1 activation at the molecular level more easily than before by using biophysical techniques that are more readily applied in the absence of complicating activator. Furthermore, a critical comparison of spontaneous and activator-induced C1 activation has shed some light on the role of activators in the intrinsic C1 activation process (see Section III.B above).

## IV. INITIATION OF THE CLASSICAL PATHWAY BY ACTIVATED C1

The C1s subunit of activated C1 is a serine protease that specifically cleaves the second (C2) and fourth (C4) complement components, thereby leading to their activation and the initiation of the complement cascade.[47,48] Each protein is cleaved into two fragments with the larger fragments (i.e., C2a and C4b) associating in the presence of magnesium to form an equimolar complex.[105,106] This protein complex now expresses a new enzymatic activity, i.e., the ability to cleave and activate the third component of complement, C3.[107] The catalytic site of this C3 convertase resides in the C2a subunit.[107]

## V. CONTROL OF C1 FUNCTION

The glycoprotein C1-In controls the functions of C1 in human serum.[108] The molecular weight of C1-In is 104,000, sedimentation coefficient 3.7S and carbohydrate content 35%.[109] Bound sialic acid is not important for C1-In function, but does affect its catabolism.[110] Preliminary protein sequence data has been reported for C1-In[111] as well as some sequence analysis of cDNA clones.[112] These authors described sequence homology between C1-In and antithrombin III and alpha-1-antitrypsin.[112]

An inhibitor of C1q hemolytic activity has been purified from human serum and has been identified as a chondroitin 4-sulfate proteoglycan.[113] Although the physiologic significance of this molecule has yet to be established, Ghebrehiwet et al.[114,115] have proposed that it may be related to a lymphocyte receptor for C1q.

### A. C1-In Control of C1 Enzymatic Activity

C1-In firmly binds to activated C1r and C1s, blocking their enzymatic activities[25,41,116] and, thereby, preventing the activation of C2 and C4. A 1:1 complex is formed between C1-In and activated C1r or C1s;[41,116] an ester bond between the active site serine of the enzyme and C1-In has been proposed, since the complexes are dissociated by hydroxyl-amine.[117] Other experiments indicate that a lysine residue of C1-In is involved in this interaction as well.[118]

C1-In is the only serum factor controlling the function of activated C1. [125]I labeled activated C1r and C1s bind only C1-In in plasma.[119] Furthermore, the early classical complement pathway has been reconstituted from purified C1q, C1r, C1s, C1-In, C2 and C4, all at physiologic concentrations. When treated with aggregated IgG, this purified component mixture and NHS are indistinguishable with respect to C2 and C4 consumption when equal amounts of C1 are activated.[102] C1-In is extraordinarily efficient considering that in its presence, activated C1 has a half-life of only 13 sec under physiologic conditions.[102] This rapid inactivation of activated C1 minimizes damage to host tissue during complement activation.

## B. C1-In Disassembly of Activated C1

A second role for C1-In in C1 control was described in 1979 by Ziccardi and Cooper[120] and Sim et al.[121] In NHS or a purified protein mixture, Cl-In efficiently disassembles immune complex-bound activated C1. Two molecules of C1rC1s (C1-In)$_2$ are released into the fluid phase for every molecule of activated C1.[120] C1rC1s (C1-In)$_2$ has a molecular weight of 380,000 and sedimentation coefficient of 9S.[120] This active disassembly accounts for the appearance of activated C1 dissociation products in pathologic human sera.[122] Furthermore, the antigenic nature of the activated C1r subunit is drastically changed in this C1-In complex.[123,124] This alteration is the basis for an immunoassay that detects C1 activation in human serum,[123,125,126] and also an assay that measures C1-In function in human serum,[126,127] a test that is a diagnostic indicator of the disease hereditary angioedema.

Although activated C1r and C1s are released from an activating immune complex by C1-In, most C1q appears to remain bound to the activator.[121] Since C1q, free of C1r$_2$s$_2$, performs functions not possible when in macromolecular C1 (see below), activated C1 disassembly by C1-In could be a physiologically significant process.

## C. C1-In Control of the Activation of C1

The most recently discerned function of C1-In is that of controlling the C1 activation process itself.[97] As an example, purified C1 can activate spontaneously, but does not in NHS,[12] due to the presence of C1-In.[97] Not only does C1-In block spontaneous C1 activation but also C1 activation induced by such nonimmune substances as DNA and heparin.[97] Thus, C1-In functions earlier in the complement sequence than initially thought. However, C1 activation induced by immune complexes (antibody sensitized erythrocytes and tetanus-antitetanus) is not significantly affected by C1-In.[97,128]

In controlling C1 activation, C1-In prevents the proteolysis of C1r as well as C1s.[97] Therefore, C1-In is thought to interact with a form of C1 that is in an intermediate or transitional state, conformationally distinct from native C1 but not yet proteolyzed to activated C1.[97] This hypothesis contrasts with that of Lepow et al.,[129] who proposed that C1-In binding to activated C1 prevented spontaneous autoactivation. However, consistent with our theory is the model of Porter and Reid depicting a reversible interaction between activator-bound C1 and nitrophenylguanidinobenzoate.[17] Recent ultracentrifugal studies have demonstrated that unactivated C1 is, in fact, associated with C1-inhibitor under physiological conditions.[130] $^{125}$I-C1-In was mixed with an excess of native C1 and was centrifuged through a sucrose density gradient containing 100 $\mu M$ nitrophenylguanidinobenzoate (NPGB) throughout, which was present to prevent C1 activation during centrifugation. As can be seen in Figure 2A, one-third of the C1-In co-sedimented with native C1 with an S-rate of 16S. $^{125}$I-C1-In alone sedimented as a single 4S boundary (Figure 2B). When NPGB was omitted (Figure 2C) or activated C1 was used (not shown), the S-rate of $^{125}$I-C1-In was only 12S. This lower S-rate was due to the release of C1rC1s(C1-In)$_2$ from activated C1. Thus under physiological conditions, native C1 is reversibly bound to C1-In.[130]

The mechanism by which immune complexes escape control by C1-In is unclear, although it may be related to the inherently faster C1 activation rate induced by immune complexes than by other stimuli, since at reduced temperatures even immune complex induced C1 activation is blocked by C1-In.[97] Furthermore, C1-In does have a minor effect on C1 activation induced by heat aggregated IgG,[131] which is a heterogeneous mixture of IgG oligomers, and the rate of this C1 activation is dependent on the oligomer's size.[76,132] The report of Folkerd et al.[80] that C1-In has a significant effect on the activation C1 by rabbit IgG-sheep antirabbit IgG immune complexes may indicate that only activators meeting specific (but unknown) requirements escape C1-In control. It is important to emphasize that C1-In control of C1 activation depends on the nature of the activator, but once activated, active C1 is efficiently controlled by C1-In regardless of the activator.[102]

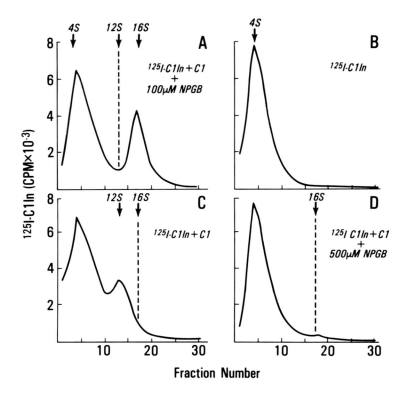

FIGURE 2.    Interaction of C1-In with native C1: demonstration by ultra-centrifugation. $^{125}$I-C1-In was mixed with an excess of native C1 ($0.5 \times 10^{-8}$ $M$ vs. $50 \times 10^{-8}$ $M$, respectively) in 50 $\mu\ell$ of Tris-buffered saline, pH 7.5, ionic strength 0.14 $M$, containing 1.5 m$M$ calcium. Samples were centrifuged through sucrose density gradients in the same buffer containing 100 $\mu M$ NPGB (panel A), 500 $\mu M$ NPGB (panel D), or no NPBG (panel C). When included throughout gradients, NPGB at the same concentration was also present in the applied sample. The sedimentation of $^{125}$I-C1-In alone is depicted in panel B. In the presence of native C1, one-third of the C1-In co-sedimented with C1 at 16S (panel A). (From Ziccardi, R. J., *J. Immunol.*, 134, 2559, 1985. With permission.)

The apparent selectivity by C1-In for allowing immune in preference to nonimmune C1 activation is important to the host, because the easily activatable C1 is prevented from spontaneously activating and from activating through interaction with such host substances as cellular debris. However, C1 can still respond to invasive agents tagged with antibody. Thus, C1-In plays a physiologic role in homeostasis by preventing nonspecific C1 activation.[97]

## D. Mechanism of Complement Activation in Hereditary Angioedema

A congenital deficiency of C1-inhibitor function is associated with the disease hereditary angioedema (HAE).[133,134] This disorder is characterized by transient but recurrent, nonpruritic swelling of tissues throughout the body, with the symptomatology depending on the organs involved. For example, intestinal attacks lead to a diversity of symptoms including pain, cramps, vomiting and diarrhea. The most frequent cause of death is airway obstruction secondary to laryngeal edema. Of the two forms this disease takes,[135] the more common includes a reduced level of C1-In protein (5 to 30% of normal), and the variant form manifests as normal or elevated levels of nonfunctional C1-In.[135,136] Both forms of HAE are inherited as an autosomal-dominant trait.[135,137] In addition, acquired deficiency of C1-In with resulting angioedema has been observed in association with various other diseases.[138] Treatment with androgens reduces the attacks and increases the circulating levels of functional C1-In.[139]

How decreased C1-In function contributes to the pathogenesis of the disease is unclear. Evidence has been presented implicating a kinin-like fragment of C2 generated by the combined actions of the complement and fibrinolytic systems.[140] However, recent studies suggest that bradykinin may also be a mediator of edema in HAE.[141,142]

Activated C1, C2 and C4 are detectable in plasma from patients with HAE,[143] generally without significant activation of complement components beyond these three. As yet, the mechanism by which C1 becomes activated in HAE serum is unknown. Serum proteases such as plasmin and Hageman factor, proposed to be poorly controlled when C1-In levels are low, have been implicated.[144] Nevertheless, their role seems unlikely in light of the recently discovered human antiplasmin, a highly potent plasmin inhibitor,[145] and the relative inefficiency of protease induced C1 activation.[103] Another suggested mechanism for the abundance of activated C1 in the sera of patients with HAE is spontaneous C1 autoactivation due to low C1-In levels.[97,146] In vitro experiments support this hypothesis.[97] The concentration of C1-In necessary for controlling spontaneous C1 autoactivation has been established as ranging from 0.35 to 2.0 times physiologic. These amounts effectively block the spontaneous autoactivation of physiologic concentrations of C1;[97] however, C1-In concentrations of 0.25 times physiologic and lower are ineffective. This is consistent with the fact that the sera of affected patients with HAE contain only 0.05 to 0.30 times physiologic concentrations of C1-In.[135] Furthermore, the ability to control spontaneous C1 autoactivation with an only moderate increase in C1-In concentration in vitro[97] is also consistent with recent studies by Spath et al.[147] who found that a certain critical level of functional C1-In was necessary to keep the patients asymptomatic. Thus, an overabundance of spontaneous C1 autoactivation, due to insufficient levels of C1-In, may underlie the classical pathway activation detected in the sera of such patients.

### E. Inhibition of C1 Activation by Nascent C3b and C4b

Different mechanisms of C1 turnover by a single complement fixing site on an immune complex can be envisioned. For example, an entire molecule of activated C1 could be displaced from the immune complex by a molecule of native C1, which would then be activated and subsequently also displaced. Alternatively immune-complex bound C1q could turn over $C1r_2s_2$. The known properties of C1 are consistent with these mechanisms.[11,148,149] The turnover of C1 by immune complexes has recently been confirmed.[150] This was readily demonstrated in a system of purified proteins but not normal human serum. The following results indicated that C3 and C4 were the serum factors responsible for the inhibition of C1 turnover by immune complexes.[150]

1.  In a purified protein system composed of C1 and C1-In at pH 7.5, ionic strength 0.14$M$, doses of immune complexes that activated all the C1 in 60 min at 37°C, yielded no detectable C1 activation when C2, C3, and C4 were also present (Figure 3). Activation was quantified by SDS-PAGE analysis and hemolytic titration.
2.  NHS was treated with methylamine in order to inactivate C3 and C4 without affecting C1, C2 and C1-In. Doses of immune complexes that consumed no C1 in NHS, consumed all the C1 in methylamine-treated NHS.
3.  Reconstitution of methylamine-treated NHS with C3 and C4 rendered the serum again resistant to excessive C1 consumption by immune complexes.

Immune complexes used in these studies included EA-IgG, EA-IgM, tetanus-human antitetanus, and aggregated human IgG. Thus in NHS there is a mechanism of feedback inhibition by which nascent C3b and C4b inhibit C1 turnover by immune complexes.[150] These recent studies[150] confirm observations made by Lachmann in 1966.[151] This mechanism of control might be physiologically important for the prevention of excessive complement activation by low concentrations of immune complexes (Figure 1).

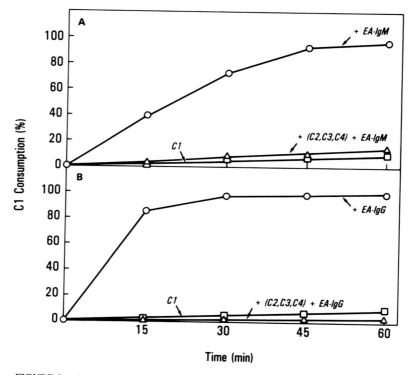

FIGURE 3. Immune complex induced consumption of C1: inhibition by C2 + C3 + C4. Physiological concentrations of purified C1 and C1-In in buffer at pH 7.5 and ionic strength 0.14 *M* were incubated at 37°C in the presence and absence of 7 × 10⁸ EA-IgM/m$\ell$ (panel A) or 3 × 10⁸ EA-IgG/m$\ell$ (panel B), and the resulting C1 consumption was measured as a function of time by hemolytic titration. In both cases, the immune complexes consumed all of the C1 by 60 min. C1 turnover was occurring, since the mixtures contained 50 to 100 times fewer molecules of antibody than C1. The addition of physiological concentrations of C2, C3, and C4 inhibited the immune complex induced C1 consumption. (This figure was reproduced from Reference 150.) (From Ziccardi, R. J., *J. Immunol.*, 136, 3378, 1986. With permission.)

## VI. C1 FUNCTIONS UNRELATED TO THE COMPLEMENT CASCADE

Recent reports indicate that C1 may have physiologic functions in addition to initiation of the classical pathway. For example, human peripheral blood leukocytes have a receptor for C1q.[115,152-155] This C1q receptor has been purified and partially characterized.[115] Significantly, the collagen-like portion of C1q, which binds to the receptor, is inaccessible in macromolecular C1.[152,154] However, after disassembly of activated C1 by C1-In, immune complex-bound C1q is free to react with C1q receptors, potentially serving as a bridge between immune complexes and effector cells.[120,156] Thus, C1q may play a direct role in the destruction and clearance of classical pathway activators. This hypothesis is supported by reports of C1q-dependent mechanism of cellular cytotoxicity[157] and C1q-dependent stimulation of an oxidative response by human polymorphonuclear leukocytes.[158]

C1q binds to the opsonic protein fibronectin.[159-161] As is true for C1q receptors, the C1q binding site for fibronectin is inaccessible in macromolecular C1,[161] but becomes exposed after C1-In disassembly of activated C1.[161] Thus, C1q may also mediate the clearance of complement activators in conjunction with fibronectin. Furthermore, Bohnsack et al.[162] have recently demonstrated that C1q binds through its collagen-like tail to laminin. They have suggested that this may be a mechanism of deposition of immune complexes in basement membranes.

Other functions described for C1q include that of a macrophage receptor for Fc or polyanions,[163] and that of a modulator for the aggregation of human platelets and their adhesion to collagen.[164] Finally, the interrelationships between complement and other effector systems are just beginning to be appreciated. For example, the addition of activated Hageman factor fragment to NHS results in C1 activation.[165] Additionally, mouse submandibular gland nerve growth factor can substitute for C1 in initiating the classical pathway and may be relevant in the host reaction to tissue damage.[166]

## VII. SUMMARY

The first component of human complement (C1) is a 750,000 Dalton glycoprotein that requires calcium or other specific metal ions to maintain its native structure and function. Under physiologic conditions, C1 comprises two weakly interacting subunits, C1q and $C1r_2s_2$, with C1q containing the binding site(s) for activators and $C1r_2s_2$ possessing enzymatic potential. C1 circulates in a precursor state and only after "activation" does it acquire functional activity, manifested as enzymatic activity specific for its natural substrates C2 and C4. C1 activation, which is accompanied by limited proteolysis and conformational changes, can be induced by immune complexes or certain nonimmune substances. C1 also spontaneously activates at 37°C by an intramolecular autocatalytic mechanism although at a slower rate than that induced by activators. Immune complexes enhance the intrinsic C1 autoactivation process by strengthening the association of C1q with $C1r_2s_2$.

C1 functions are controlled by the serum glycoprotein C1-inhibitor (C1-In) which blocks the enzymatic activities of activated C1. Under physiologic conditions, activated C1 has a half-life of only 13 sec in the presence of C1-In. Activated C1 is efficiently disassembled by C1-In, thereby releasing two inactive $C1rC1s(C1-In)_2$ complexes per C1 molecule, leaving C1q activator-bound with biologically reactive sites uncovered that are not expressed in macromolecular C1. The most recently recognized function of C1-In is that of controlling the C1 activation process itself. While having only limited effect on immune complex-induced C1 activation, C1-In effectively controls certain nonimmune-induced as well as spontaneous C1 activation. Under physiological conditions, native C1 is reversibly bound to C1-In. Thus, C1-In plays an important role in regulating nonspecific complement activation. This is relevant for the understanding of the human disease hereditary angioedema. An overabundance of spontaneous C1 autoactivation, due to low C1-In levels, might underlie the abnormal activation of complement via the classical pathway detected in the sera of these patients. Furthermore, a mechanism of feedback inhibition has been recently described whereby nascent C3b and C4b inhibit C1 turnover by immune complexes. This control is important in preventing the otherwise excessive activation of complement by low concentrations of immune complexes. Finally, recent studies indicate that C1 may have other important biological functions in addition to initiating the complement cascade.

## VIII. LIST OF ABBREVIATIONS

C1 or $C1qr_2s_2$, first component of complement; C1-In, C1-inhibitor; C2, second component of complement; C3, third component of complement; C4, fourth component of complement; EA-IgG, sheep erythrocytes sensitized with rabbit IgG antibodies; EA-IgM, sheep erythrocytes sensitized with rabbit IgM antibodies; EDTA, ethylenediaminetetraacetic acid; HAE, hereditary angioedema; $M_r$, molecular weight; NHS, normal human serum; NPGB, nitrophenylguanidinobenzoate; SDS PAGE, polyacrylamide gel electrophoresis in the presence of sodium dodecyl sulfate.

# REFERENCES

1. **Cooper, N. R.,** The classical complement pathway: Activation and regulation of the first complement component, *Adv. Immunol.,* 37, 151, 1985.
2. **Lachmann, P. J. and Hughes-Jones, N. C.,** Initiation of complement activation, *Springer Semin. Immunopathol.,* 7, 143, 1984.
3. **Colomb, M. G., Arlaud, G. J., and Villiers, C. L.,** Structure and activation of C1: Current concepts, *Complement,* 1, 69, 1984.
4. **Schumaker, V. N.,** Structure of C1 and antibody recognition (in these volumes).
5. **Siegel, R. C., Schumaker, V. N., and Poon, P. K.,** Stoichiometry and sedimentation properties of the complex formed between C1q and C1r$_2$s$_2$ subcomponent of the first component of complement, *J. Immunol.,* 127, 2447, 1981.
6. **Tschopp, J., Villiger, W., Fuchs, H., Kilchherr, E., and Engel, J.,** Assembly of subcomponents C1r and C1s of first component of complement: electron microscopic and ultracentrifugal studies, *Proc. Nat. Acad. Sci. USA,* 77, 7014, 1980.
7. **Ziccardi, R. J. and Cooper, N. R.,** The subunit composition and sedimentation properties of human C1, *J. Immunol.,* 118, 2047, 1977.
8. **Hughes-Jones, N. C. and Gorick, B. D.,** The binding and activation of the C1r-C1s subunit of the first component of human complement, *Mol. Immunol.,* 19, 1105, 1982.
9. **Siegel, R. C. and Schumaker, V. N.,** Measurement of the association constants of the complexes formed between intact C1q or pepsin-treated C1q stalks and the unactivated or activated C1r$_2$s$_2$ tetramers, *Mol. Immunol.,* 20, 53, 1983.
10. **Laurell, A-B, Martensson, U., and Sjoholm, A. G.,** C1 subcomponent complexes in normal and pathological sera studied by crossed immunoelectrophoresis, *Acta Pathol. Microbiol. Scand. (C),* 84, 455, 1976.
11. **Kilchherr, E., Fuchs, H., Tschopp, J., and Engel, J.,** Dissociation of C1 and concentration dependence of its activation kinetics, *Mol. Immunol.,* 19, 683, 1982.
12. **Ziccardi, R. J.,** Spontaneous activation of the first component of human complement (C1) by an intramolecular autocatalytic mechanism, *J. Immunol.,* 128, 2500, 1982.
13. **Müller-Eberhard, H. J.,** Complement, *Annu. Rev. Biochem.,* 44, 697, 1975.
14. **Hughes-Jones, N. C.,** Functional affinity constants of the reaction between $^{125}$I-labelled C1q and C1q binders and their use in the measurement of plasma C1q concentrations, *Immunology,* 32, 191, 1977.
15. **Lin, T.-Y. and Fletcher, D. S.,** Interaction of human C1q with insoluble immunoglobulin aggregates, *Immunochemistry,* 15, 107, 1978.
16. **Calcott, M. A. and Müller-Eberhard, H. J.,** C1q protein of human complement, *Biochemistry,* 11, 3443, 1972.
17. **Porter, R. P. and Reid, K. B. M.,** The biochemistry of complement, *Nature,* 275, 699, 1978.
18. **Reid, K. B. M., Gagnon, J., and Frampton, J.,** Completion of the amino acid sequences of the A and B chains subcomponent C1q of the first component of human complement, *Biochem. J.,* 203, 559, 1982.
19. **Mizuochi, T., Yonemasu, K., Yamashita, K., and Kobata, A.,** The asparagine linked sugar chains of subcomponent C1q of the first component of human complement, *J. Biol. Chem.,* 253, 7404, 1978.
20. **Shelton, E., Yonemasu, K., and Stroud, R. M.,** Ultrastructure of the human complement component, C1q, *Proc. Nat. Acad. Sci. USA,* 69, 65, 1972.
21. **Schumaker, V. N., Poon, P. H., Seegan, G. W., and Smith, C. S.,** Semi-flexible joint in the C1q subunit of the first component of human complement, *J. Mol. Biol.,* 148, 191, 1981.
22. **Gilmour, S., Randall, J. T., William, K. J., Dwek, R. A., and Tarbet, J.,** The conformation of subcomponent C1q of the first component of human complement, *Nature,* 285, 512, 1980.
23. **Knobel, H. R., Heusser, C., Rodrick, M. L., and Isliker, H.,** Enzymatic digestion of the first component of human complement (C1q), *J. Immunol.,* 112, 2094, 1974.
24. **Reid, K. B. M., Sim, R. B., and Faiers, A. P.,** Inhibition of the reconstitution of the hemolytic activity of the first component of human complement by a pepsin-derived fragment of subcomponent C1q, *Biochem. J.,* 161, 239, 1977.
25. **Ziccardi, R. J. and Cooper, N. R.,** Physicochemical and functional characterization of the C1r subunit of the first complement component, *J. Immunol.,* 116, 496, 1976.
26. **Ziccardi, R. J. and Cooper, N. R.,** Direct demonstration and quantitation of the first complement component in human serum, *Science,* 199, 1080, 1978.
27. **Arlaud, G. J., Villiers, C. L., Chesne, S., and Colomb, M.,** Purified proenzyme C1r. Some characteristics of its activation and subsequent proteolytic cleavage, *Biochim. Biophys. Acta,* 616, 116, 1980.
28. **Strang, C. J., Siegel, R. C., Phillips, M. L., Poon, P. H., and Schumaker, V. N.,** Ultrastructure of the first component of human complement: electron microscopy of the crosslinked complex, *Proc. Nat. Acad. Sci. USA,* 79, 586, 1982.

29. **Villiers, C. L., Arlaud, G. J., and Colomb, M. G.,** Domain structure and associated functions of subcomponents C1r and C1s of the first component of human complement, *Proc. Nat. Acad. Sci.,* 82, 4477, 1985.

30. **Poon, P. H., Schumaker, V. N., Phillips, M. L., and Strang, C. J.,** Conformation and restricted segmental flexibility of C1 to first component of human complement, *J. Mol. Biol.,* 168, 563, 1983.

31. **Colomb, M. G., Arlaud, G. J., and Villiers, C. L.,** Activation of C1, *Phil. Trans. R. Soc.,* London, B, 306, 283, 1984.

32. **Perkins, S. J.,** Molecular modelling of human subcomponent C1q and its complex with C1r$_2$s$_2$ derived from neutron scattering curves and hydrodynamic properties, *Biochem. J.,* 228, 13, 1985.

33. **Lepow, I. H., Wurz, L., Ratnoff, O. D., and Pillemer, L.,** Studies on the mechanism of inactivation of human complement by plasmin and by antigen-antibody aggregates. I. The requirement for a factor resembling C1 and the role of Ca + +, *J. Immunol.,* 73, 146, 1954.

34. **Lepow, I. H., Naff, G. B., Todd, E. W., Pensky, J., and Hinz, C. F.,** Chromatographic resolution of the first component of human complement into three activities, *J. Exp. Med.,* 117, 983, 1963.

35. **Villiers, C. L., Arlaud, G. J., Painter, R. H., and Colomb, M. G.,** Calcium binding properties of the C1 subcomponents C1q, C1r and C1s, *FEBS Lett.,* 117, 289, 1980.

36. **Liberti, P. A. and Paul, S. M.,** Gross conformation of C1q: a subcomponent of the first component of complement, *Biochemistry,* 17, 1952, 1978.

37. **Ziccardi, R. J.,** Nature of the metal ion requirement for assembly and function of the first component of human complement (C1), *J. Biol. Chem.,* 258, 6187, 1983.

38. **Arlaud, G. J. and Gagnon, J.,** Primary structure of human C1r: identification of Beta-hydroxyaspartic acid and complete sequence, *Complement,* 2, 4, 1985.

39. **Sakai, K. and Stroud, R. M.,** Purification, molecular properties and activation of C1 proesterase, C1s, *J. Immunol.,* 110, 1010, 1973.

40. **Sim, P. B., Porter, R. B., Reid, K. B. M., and Gigli, I.,** The structure and enzymatic activities of the C1r and C1s subcomponents of C1, the first component of human serum complement, *Biochem. J.,* 163, 219, 1977.

41. **Ziccardi, R. J. and Cooper, N. R.,** Activation of C1r by proteolytic cleavage, *J. Immunol.,* 116, 504, 1976.

42. **Barkas, T., Scott, G. K., and Fothergill, J. E.,** Purification, characterization and active site-studies on human serum complement subcomponent C1s, *Biochem. Soc. Trans.,* 1, 1219, 1973.

43. **Reid, K. B. M. and Porter, R. R.,** The proteolytic activation systems of complement, *Annu. Rev. Biochem.,* 50, 433, 1981.

44. **Arlaud, G. J., Gagnon, J., and Porter, R. R.,** The catalytic chain of human complement subcomponent C1r, *Biochem. J.,* 201, 49, 1982.

45. **Gagnon, J. and Arlaud, G. J.,** Primary structure of the A chain of human complement classical pathway enzyme C1r, *Biochem. J.,* 225, 135, 1985.

46. **Naff, G. B. and Ratnoff, O. P.,** The enzymatic nature of C1r. Conversion of C1s to C1 esterase and digestion of amino acid esters by C1r, *J. Exp. Med.,* 128, 571, 1968.

47. **Cooper, N. R. and Ziccardi, R. J.,** The nature and reactions of complement enzymes, in *Proteolysis and Physiological Regulation,* Vol. 11, Ribbons, D. W. and Brew, K., Eds., Miami Winter Symposium, Academic Press, New York, 1976, 167.

48. **Haines, A. L. and Lepow, I. H.,** Studies on human C1 esterase. I. purification and enzymatic properties, *J. Immunol.,* 92, 456, 1964.

49. **Gigli, I. and Austen, K. F.,** Fluid phase destruction of C2 by C1. II. Unmasking by C4i of C1 specificity for C1, *J. Exp. Med.,* 130, 833, 1969.

50. **Strunk, R. and Colten, H. R.,** The first component of human complement (C1): kinetics of reaction with its natural substrate, *J. Immunol.,* 112, 905, 1974.

51. **Thielens, N. M., Villiers, M-B., Reboul, A., Villiers, C. L., and Colomb, M. G.,** Human complement subcomponent C2: purification and proteolytic cleavage in fluid phase by C1s, C1r$_2$-C1s$_2$ and C1, *FEBS Lett.,* 141, 19, 1982.

52. **McRae, B. J., Lin, T-Y., and Powers, J. C.,** Mapping the substrate binding site of human C1r and C1s with peptide thioesters, *J. Biol. Chem.,* 256, 12362, 1981.

53. **Dodds, A. W., Sim, P. B., Porter, R. R., and Kerr, M. A.,** Activation of the first component of human complement (C1) by antibody-antigen aggregates, *Biochem. J.,* 175, 383, 1978.

54. **Loos, M.,** The classical complement pathway: Mechanism of activation of the first component by antigen-antibody complexes, *Prog. Allergy,* 30, 135, 1982.

55. **Tschopp, J.,** Kinetics of activation of the first component of complement (C1) by IgG oligomers, *Mol. Immunol.,* 19, 651, 1982.

56. **Villiers, C. L., Duplaa, A-M., Arlaud, G. J., and Colomb, M. G.,** Fluid phase activation of proenzymic C1r purified by affinity chromatography, *Biochim. Biophys. Acta,* 700, 118, 1982.

57. **Goers, J. W.., Ziccardi, R. J., Schumaker, V. N., and Glovsky, M. M.,** The mechanism of activation of the first component of human complement by a univalent hapten-IgG antibody complex, *J. Immunol.,* 118, 2182, 1977.
58. **Niinube, M., Veno, Y., Hitomi, Y., and Fujii, S.,** Detection of intermediary C1r well complete active site, using a synthetic proteinase inhibitor, *FEBS Lett.,* 172, 159, 1984.
59. **Villiers, C. L., Arlaud, G. J., and Colomb, M. G.,** Autoactivation of C1r involves structural changes reflected in modifications of intrinsic fluorescence, circular dichroism, and reactivity with monoclonal antibodies, *Biochem. J.,* 215, 369, 1983.
60. **Kasahara, Y., Takahashi, K., Nagasawa, S., and Koyama, J.,** Formation of a conformationally changed C1r, a subcomponent of the first component of human complement, as an intermediate of its autoactivation reaction, *FEBS Lett.,* 141, 128, 1982.
61. **Bauer, J. and Valet, G.,** Conformational changes of the subunits C1q, C1r and C1s of human complement component C1 demonstrated by $^{125}$I-labelling, *Biochim. Biophys. Acta,* 670, 129, 1981.
62. **Villiers, C. L., Chesne, S., Lacroix, M. B., Arlaud, G. J., and Colomb, M. G.,** Structural features of the first component of human complement, C1, as revealed by surface iodination, *Biochem. J.,* 203, 185, 1982.
63. **Golan, M. D., Burger, R., and Loos, M.,** Conformational changes in C1q after binding to immune complexes: detection of neoantigens with monoclonal antibodies, *J. Immunol.,* 129, 445, 1982.
64. **Ziccardi, R. J.,** Nature of the interactions between the C1q and C1r₂s₂ subunits of C1, *Mol. Immunol.,* 22, 489, 1985.
65. **Augener, W., Grey, H. M., Cooper, N. R., and Müller-Eberhard, H. J.,** The reaction of monomeric and aggregated immunoglobulins with C1, *Immunochemistry,* 8, 1011, 1971.
66. **Schumaker, V. N., Calcott, M. A., Spiegelberg, H. L., and Müller-Eberhard, H. J.,** Ultracentrifuge studies of the binding of IgG of different subclasses to the C1q subunit of the first component of complement, *Biochemistry,* 15, 5175, 1976.
67. **Colomb, M. and Porter, R. R.,** Characterization of a plasmin-digest fragment of rabbit immunoglobulin gamma that binds antigen and complement, *Biochem. J.,* 145, 177, 1975.
68. **Hurt, M. M., Volanakis, J. E., Hester, R. B., Stroud, R. M., and Bennett, J. C.,** The structural basis for binding of complement by immunoglobulin M, *J. Exp. Med.,* 140, 1117, 1974.
69. **Plaut, A. G., Cohen, S., and Tomasi, T. B., Jr.,** Immunoglobulin M: Fixation of human complement by the Fc fragment, *Science,* 176, 55, 1972.
70. **Burton, D. R., Boyd, J., Brampton, A. D., Easterbrook-Smith, S. B., Emanuel, E. J., Novotony, J., Rademacher, T. W., van Schravendijk, M. R., Sternberg, M. J. E., and Dwek, R. A.,** The C1q receptor site on immunoglobulin G., *Nature,* 288, 338, 1980.
71. **Emanuel, E. J., Brampton, A. D., Burton, D. R., and Dwek, R. A.,** Formation of complement subcomponent C1q-immunoglobulin G complex, *Biochem. J.,* 205, 361, 1982.
72. **Boackle, R. J., Johnson, B. J., and Caughman, G. B.,** An IgG primary sequence exposure theory for complement activation using synthetic peptides, *Nature,* 282, 742, 1979.
73. **Lucas, T. J., Munoz, H., and Erickson, B. W.,** Inhibition of C1-mediated immune hemolysis by monomeric and dimeric peptides from the second constant domain immunoglobulin G, *J. Immunol.,* 127, 2555, 1981.
74. **Isenman, D. E., Ellerson, J. R., Painter, R. H., and Dorrington, K. J.,** Correlation between the exposure of aromatic chromophores at the surface of the Fc domains of immunoglobulin G and their ability to bind complement, *Biochemistry,* 16, 233, 1977.
75. **Metzger, H.,** The effect of antigen on antibodies: Recent studies, *Contemp. Top. Mol. Immunol.,* 7, 119, 1978.
76. **Tschopp, J., Schulthess, T., Engel, J., and Jaton, J-C.,** Antigen-dependent activation of the first component of complement C1 by chemically crosslinked rabbit IgG-oligomers, *FEBS Lett.,* 112, 152, 1980.
77. **Hughes-Jones, N. C., Gorick, B. D., Miller, N. G. A., and Howard, J. C.,** IgG pair formation on one antigenic molecule is the main mechanism of synergy between antibodies in complement mediated lysis, *Eur. J. Immunol.,* 14, 974, 1984.
78. **Liberti, P. A., Bausch, P. M., and Schoenberg, L. M.,** On the mechanism of C1q binding to antibody-I. Aggregation and/or distortion of IgG vs. combing site transmitted effects, *Mol. Immunol.,* 19, 143, 1982.
79. **Allan, R. and Isliker, R.,** Studies on the complement binding site of rabbit IgG. II. The reaction of rabbit IgG and its fragments with C1q, *Immunochemistry,* 11, 243, 1974.
80. **Folkerd, E. J., Gardner, B., and Hughes-Jones, N. C.,** The relationship between the binding ability and the rate of activation of the complement component C1, *Immunology,* 41, 179, 1980.
81. **Ziccardi, R. J. and Tschopp, J.,** The dissociation properties of native C1, *Biochem. Biophys. Res. Commun.,* 107, 618, 1982.
82. **Ziccardi, R. J.,** The role of immune complexes in the activation of C1, *J. Immunol.,* 132, 283, 1984.

83. **Cooper, N. R., Jensen, F. C., Welsh, Jr. R. M., and Oldstone, M. B. A.,** Lysis of RNA tumor viruses by human serum: direct antibody independent triggering of the classical complement pathway, *J. Exp. Med.,* 144, 970, 1976.

84. **Betz, S. J. and Isliker, H.,** Antibody independent interaction between Escherichia coli J5 and human complement components, *J. Immunol.,* 127, 1748, 1981.

85. **Claus, D. R., Siegel, J., Petras, K., Osmand, A. P., and Gewurz, H.,** Interactions of C-reactive protein with the first component of human complement, *J. Immunol.,* 119, 187, 1977.

86. **Kaplan, M. H. and Volanakis, J. E.,** Interaction of C-reactive protein complexes with the complement system. I. Consumption of human complement associated with the reaction of C-reactive protein with pneumococcal C-polysaccharide and with the choline phosphatides, lecithin, and sphingomyelin, *J. Immunol.,* 112, 2135, 1974.

87. **Schultz, D. R. and Arnold, P. I.,** The first component of human complement: on the mechanism of activation by some carbohydrates, *J. Immunol.,* 126, 1994, 1981.

88. **Linder, E., Lehto, V-P., and Stenman, S.,** Activation of complement C cytoskeletal intermediate filaments, *Nature,* 278, 176, 1979.

89. **Giclas, P. C., Pinckard, R. N., and Olson, M. S.,** In vitro activation of complement by isolated human heart subcellular membranes, *J. Immunol.,* 122, 146, 1979.

90. **Storrs, S. B., Kolb, W. P., Pinckard, R. N., and Olson, M. S.,** Characterization of the binding of purified human C1q to heart mitochrondrial membranes, *J. Biol. Chem.,* 256, 10924, 1981.

91. **Cyong, J-C., Witkin, S. S., Rieger, B., Barbarese, E., Good, R. A., and Day, N. K.,** Antibody independent complement activation by myelin via the classical complement pathway, *J. Exp. Med.,* 155, 587, 1982.

92. **Vanguri, P., Koski, C. L., Silverman, B., and Shin, M. L.,** Complement activation by isolated myelin: Activation of the classical pathway in the absence of myelin specific antibodies, *Proc. Nat. Acad. Sci. USA,* 79, 3290, 1982.

93. **Cooper, N. R. and Morrison, D. C.,** Binding and activation of the first component of human complement by the lipid A region of lipopolysaccharides, *J. Immunol.,* 120, 1862, 1978.

94. **Loos, M., Bitter-Suermann, D., and Dierich, M.,** Interaction of the first (C1), the second (C2), and the fourth (C4) component of complement with different preparations of bacterial lipopolysaccharides and with lipid A, *J. Immunol.,* 112, 935, 1974.

95. **Giclas, P. C., Ginsberg, M. H., and Cooper, N. R.,** Immunoglobulin G independent activation of classical complement pathway by monosodium urate crystals, *J. Clin. Invest.,* 63, 759, 1979.

96. **Kovacsovics, T., Tschopp, J., Kress, A., and Isliker, H.,** Antibody independent activation of C1, the first component of complement, by Cardiolipin, *J. Immunol.,* 135, 2695, 1985.

97. **Ziccardi, R. J.,** A new role for C1-inhibitor in homeostasis: Control of activation of the first component of human complement, *J. Immunol.,* 128, 2505, 1982.

98. **Bartholemew, R. M. and Esser, A. F.,** Mechanism of antibody-independent activation of the first component of complement (C1) on retrovirus membranes, *Biochemistry,* 19, 2847, 1980.

99. **Tenner, A. J., Ziccardi, R. J., and Cooper, N. R.,** Antibody independent C1 activation by E. coli, *J. Immunol.,* 133, 886, 1984.

100. **Lepow, I. H., Ratnoff, O. D., and Levy, L. R.,** Studies on the activation of a proesterase associated with partially purified first component of human complement, *J. Exp. Med.,* 107, 451, 1958.

101. **Lin, T-Y. and Fletcher, D. S.,** Activation of a complex of C1r and C1s subcomponents of human complement C1 by the third subcomponent C1q, *J. Biol. Chem.,* 255, 7756, 1980.

102. **Ziccardi, R. J.,** Activation of the early components of the classical complement pathway under physiologic conditions, *J. Immunol.,* 126, 1769, 1981.

103. **Cooper, N. R.,** unpublished data, 1983.

104. **Giclas, P. C.,** Effect of plicatic acid on human serum complement includes interference with C1 inhibitor function, *J. Immunol.,* 129, 168, 1982.

105. **Nagasawa, S. and Stroud, R. M.,** Cleavage of C2 by C1s into the amligenically distinct fragments C2a and C2b: Demonstration of binding of C2b to C4b, *Proc. Nat. Acad. Sci. USA,* 74, 2998, 1977.

106. **Schreiber, R. D. and Müller-Eberhard, H. J.,** Fourth component of human complement: description of a three chain structure, *J. Exp. Med.,* 140, 1324, 1974.

107. **Kerr, M. A.,** The human complement system: assembly of the classical pathway C3 convertase, *Biochem. J.,* 189, 173, 1980.

108. **Pensky, J., Levy, L. R., and Lepow, I. H.,** Partial purification of a serum inhibitor of C1 esterase, *J. Biol. Chem.,* 236, 1674, 1961.

109. **Haupt, H., Heimburger, N., Kranz, T., and Schwick, H. G.,** Ein beitrag zur isolierung und charakterisierung des C1-Inaktivators aus humanplasma, *Eur. J. Biochem.,* 17, 254, 1970.

110. **Minta, J. O.,** The role of sialic acid in the functional activity and the hepatic clearance of C1-Inh, *J. Immunol.,* 126, 245, 1981.

111. **Harrison, R. A.,** Human C1-inhibitor: improved isolation and preliminary structural characterization, *Biochemistry,* 22, 5001, 1983.
112. **Davis, A. E., Whitehead, A. S., Harrison, R. A., and Rosen, F. S.,** Isolation and characterization of cDNA clones for human C1 inhibitor, *Complement,* 2, 20, 1985.
113. **Silvestri, L., Baker, J. R., Roden, L., and Stroud, R. M.,** The C1q inhibitor in serum is a chondroitin 4-sulfate proteoglycan, *J. Biol. Chem.,* 256, 7383, 1981.
114. **Ghebrehiwet, B. and Hamburger, M.,** Purification and partial characterization of a C1q inhibitor from the membranes of human peripheral blood lymphocytes, *J. Immunol.,* 129, 157, 1982.
115. **Ghebrehiwet, B., Silvestri, L., and McDevitt, C.,** Identification of the Raji cell membrane-derived C1q inhibitor as a receptor for human C1q, *J. Exp. Med.,* 160, 1375, 1984.
116. **Harpel, P. C. and Cooper, N. R.,** Studies on human plasma C1-inactivator-enzyme interactions, *J. Clin. Invest.,* 55, 593, 1975.
117. **Chesne, S., Villiers, C. L., Arlaud, G. J., Lacroix, M. B., and Colomb, M. G.,** Fluid phase interaction of C1 inhibitor (C1-Inh) and the subcomponents C1r and C1s of the first component of complement, C1, *Biochem. J.,* 201, 61, 1982.
118. **Minta, J. U. and Aziz, E.,** Analysis of the reactive site peptide bond in C1-inhibitor by chemical modification of tyrosyl, lysyl and arginyl residues: The essential role of lysyl residues in the functional activity of C1-Inh, *J. Immunol.,* 126, 250, 1981.
119. **Sim, R. B., Reboul, A., Arlaud, G. J., Villiers, C. L., and Colomb, M. G.,** Interaction of 125I-labelled complement subcomponents C1r and C1s with protease inhibitors in plasma, *FEBS Lett.,* 97, 111, 1979.
120. **Ziccardi, R. J. and Cooper, N. R.,** Active disassembly of the first complement component, C1, by C1-Inactivator, *J. Immunol.,* 123, 788, 1979.
121. **Sim, R. B., Arlaud, G. J., and Colomb, M. G.,** C1-Inhibitor dependent dissociation of human complement C1 bound to immune complexes, *Biochem. J.,* 179, 449, 1979.
122. **Laurell, A-B., Johnson, U., Martensson, U., and Sjoholm, A. G.,** Formation of complexes composed of C1r, C1s and C1 inactivator in human serum on activation of C1, *Acta Pathol. Microbiol. Scand.(C),* 86, 299, 1978.
123. **Ziccardi, R. J. and Cooper, N. R.,** Demonstration and quantitation of activation of the first component of complement in human serum, *J. Exp. Med.,* 147, 385, 1978.
124. **Ziccardi, R. J. and Cooper, N. R.,** Modulation of the antigenicity of C1r and C1s by C1 inactivator, *J. Immunol.,* 121, 2148, 1978.
125. **Yan, D., Gu, X., Wang, D., and Yang, S.,** Studies on immunopathogenesis in epidemic hemorrhagic fever: sequential observations on activation of the first complement component in sera from patients with epidemic hemorrhagic fever, *J. Immunol.,* 127, 1064, 1981.
126. **Ziccardi, R. J.,** Specific C1 dissociation immunoassay as an indicator for classical pathway activation of complement and C1-Inactivator function, Laboratory Research Methods, *Biol. Med.,* 4, 433, 1980.
127. **Ziccardi, R. J. and Cooper, N. R.,** Development of an immunochemical test to assess C1-Inactivator function in human serum and its use for the diagnosis of herediatry angioedema, *Clin. Immunol., Immunopathol.,* 15, 465, 1980.
128. **Medicus, R. G. and Chapuis, R. M.,** The physiological mechanism of C1 activation, *Hoppe-Seyler's Z. Physiol. Chem.,* 362, 17, 1981.
129. **Lepow, I. H., Naff, G. B., and Pensky, J.,** Mechanisms of activation of C1 and inhibition of C1 esterase, in *CIBA Foundation Symposium: Complement,* Churchill, London, 1965, 74.
130. **Ziccardi, R. J.,** Demonstration of the interaction of Native C1 with monomeric immunoglobulins and C1 inhibitor, *J. Immunol.,* 134, 2559, 1985.
131. **Ziccardi, R. J.,** Initiation of the classical complement pathway: control of activator mediated and spontaneous C1 activation, *Mol Immunol.,* 19, 1413, 1982.
132. **Doekes, G., Van Es, L. A., and Daha, M. R.,** Influence of aggregate size on the binding and activation of the first component of human complement by soluble IgG aggregates, *Immunology,* 45, 705, 1982.
133. **Donaldson, V. H. and Evans, R. R.,** A biochemical abnormality in hereditary angioedema. Absence of serum inhibitor of C1-esterase, *Am. J. Med.,* 35, 37, 1963.
134. **Osler, W.,** Hereditary angioneurotic edema, *Am. J. Med. Sci.,* 95, 362, 1888.
135. **Rosen, F. S., Alper, C. A., Pensky, J., Klemperer, M. R., and Donaldson, V. H.,** Genetically delivered heterogenity of the C1 esterase inhibitor in patients with hereditary angioneurotic edema, *J. Clin. Invest.,* 50, 2143, 1971.
136. **Curd, J. G., Yelvington, M., Ziccardi, R. J., Mathison, D. A., and Griffin, J. H.,** Purification and characterization of two functionally distinct forms of C1 inhibitor from a patient with angioedema, *Clin. Exp. Immunol.,* 45, 261, 1981.
137. **Lachmann, P. J. and Rosen, F. S.,** Genetic defects of complement in man, *Springer Semin. Immunopathol.,* 1, 339, 1978.
138. **Gelfand, J. A., Boss, G. R., Lockard, C., Conley, C. L., Reinhart, R., and Frank, M. M.,** Acquired C1 esterase deficiency and angioedema: a review, *Medicine,* 58, 321, 1979.

139. **Gelfand, J. A., Sherins, R. J., Alling, D. W., and Frank, M. M.,** Treatment of hereditary angioedema with Danazol. Reversal of clinical and biochemical abnormalities, *N. Engl. J. Med.,* 295, 1444, 1976.

140. **Donaldson, V. H., Rosen, F. S., and Bing, D. H.,** Role of the second component of complement (C2) and plasmin in kinin release in hereditary angioneurotic edema (H.A.N.E.) plasma, *Trans. Assoc. Am. Physicians,* 90, 174, 1977.

141. **Curd, J. G., Prograis, L. J., Jr., Cochrane, C. G.,** Detection of active kallikrein in induced blister fluids of hereditary angioedema patients, *J. Exp. Med.,* 152, 742, 1980.

142. **Curd, J. G., Yelvington, M., Burridge, N., Stimler, N. P., Gerard, C., Prograis, L. J., Jr., Cochrane, C. G., and Müller-Eberhard, H. J.,** Generation of bradykinin during incubation of hereditary angioedema plasma, *Mol. Immunol.,* 19, 1365, 1982.

143. **Ruddy, S., Carpenter, C. B., Müller-Eberhard, H. J., and Austen, K. F.,** Mechanisms of inflammation induced by immune reactions, in *Immunopathology, 5th International Symposium,* Miescher, P. A. and Grabar, P., Eds., Grune and Stratton, New York, 1967, 231.

144. **Donaldson, V. H.,** Mechanisms of activation of C1 esterase in hereditary angioneurotic edema plasma in vitro. The role of Hageman Factor, a clot promoting agent, *J. Exp. Med.,* 127, 411, 1968.

145. **Mullertz, S. and Clemmensen, I.,** The primary inhibitor of plasmin in human plasma, *Biochem. J.,* 159, 545, 1976.

146. **Ghebrehiwet, B., Randazzo, B. P., and Kaplan, A. P.,** Studies of complement autoactivatability in HAE: Direct relationship to functional C1-INA and the effect of classical pathway activators, *Clin. Immunol. Immunopathol.,* 32, 101, 1984.

147. **Spath, P. J., Wuthrich, B., and Butler, R.,** Quantification of C1-In functional activities by immuno-diffusion assay in plasma of patients with HAE-evidence of a functionally critical level of C1-In, *Complement,* 1, 147, 1984.

148. **Borsos, T. and Rapp, H.,** Chromatographic separation of C1 and its assay on a molecular basis, *J. Immunol.,* 91, 851, 1963.

149. **Parce, J. W., Kelley, D., and Heinzelmann, K.,** Measurement of antibody dependent binding, proteolysis and turnover of C1s on liposomal antigens localizes the fluidity-dependent step in C1 activation, *Biochim. Biophys. Acta,* 736, 92, 1983.

150. **Ziccardi, R. J.,** Control of Nascent C3b and C4b; a mechanism of feedback inhibition, *J. Immunol.,* 136, 3378, 1986.

151. **Lachmann, P. J.,** A possible homeostatic mechanism in complement fixation: inhibition of the activity of fixed C1 by the fixation of $C1_{3a}$, *Nature,* 210, 140, 1966.

152. **Gabay, Y., Perlmann, J., Perlmann, P., and Sobel, A. T.,** A rosette assay for the determination of C1q receptor bearing cells, *Eur. J. Immunol.,* 9, 797, 1979.

153. **Sobel, A. T. and Bokisch, V. A.,** Receptors for C4b and C1q on human peripheral lymphocytes and lymphoblastoid cells, in *Membrane Receptors of Lymphocytes,* Seligmann, M., Preud'homme, T. L., and Kourilsky, F. M., Eds., North Holland, Amsterdam, 1975, 151.

154. **Tenner, A. J. and Cooper, N. R.,** Analysis of receptor-mediated C1q binding to human peripheral blood mononuclear cells, *J. Immunol.,* 125, 1658, 1980.

155. **Tenner, A. J. and Cooper, N. R.,** Identification of types of cells in human peripheral blood that bind C1q, *J. Immunol.,* 126, 1174, 1981.

156. **Cooper, N. R.,** Activation and regulation of the first complement component, *Fed. Proc.,* 42, 134, 1983.

157. **Ghebrehiwet, B. and Müller-Eberhard, H. J.,** Lysis of C1q-coated chicken erythrocytes by human lymphoblastoid cell lines, *J. Immunol.,* 120, 17, 1978.

158. **Tenner, A. J. and Cooper, N. R.,** Stimulation of a human polymorphonuclear leukocyte oxidative response by the C1q subunit of the first complement component, *J. Immunol.,* 128, 2547, 1982.

159. **Bing, D. H., Almeda, S., Isliker, H., Lahav, J., and Hynes, R. O.,** Fibronectin binds to the C1q component of complement, *Proc. Nat. Acad. Sci. USA,* 79, 4198, 1982.

160. **Menzel, E. J., Smolen, J. S., Liotta, L., and Reid, K. B. M.,** Interaction of fibronectin with C1q and its collagen-like fragment (CLF), *FEBS Lett.,* 129, 188, 1981.

161. **Pearlstein, E., Sorvillo, J., and Gigli, I.,** The interaction of human plasma fibronectin with a subunit of the first component of complement C1q, *J. Immunol.,* 128, 2036, 1982.

162. **Bohnsack, J. R., Tenner, A. J., Laurie, G. W., Kleinman, H. K., Martin, G. R., and Brown, E.,** The C1q subunit of the first component of complement binds to laminin: A mechanism for the deposition and retention of immune complexes in basement membrane, *Proc. Nat. Acad. Sci. USA,* 82, 3824, 1985.

163. **Loos, M.,** The functions of endogenous C1q, a subcomponent of the first component of complement, as a receptor on the membrane of macrophages, *Mol. Immunol.,* 19, 1229, 1982.

164. **Wautier, J. L., Souchon, H., Reid, K. B. M., Peltier, A. P., and Caen, J. P.,** Studies on the mode of reaction of the first component of complement with platelets: interaction between collagen-like portion of C1q and platelets, *Immunochemistry,* 14, 763, 1977.

165. **Ghebrehiwet, B., Silverberg, M., and Kaplan, A. P.,** Activation of the classical pathway of complement by Hageman Factor fragment, *J. Exp. Med.,* 153, 665, 1981.
166. **Boyle, M. D. P. and Young, M.,** Nerve growth factor: Activation of the classical complement pathway by specific substitution for component C1, *Proc. Nat. Acad. Sci. USA,* 79, 2519, 1982.

Chapter 3

# INITIATION AND ACTIVATION OF THE ALTERNATIVE PATHWAY OF COMPLEMENT

**Michael K. Pangburn**

## TABLE OF CONTENTS

# I. INTRODUCTION

The six proteins of the alternative pathway of complement express an intrinsic ability to distinguish self from many non-self organisms. The molecular mechanism of recognition is not yet understood, but it involves only two of the six proteins. The alternative pathway performs a continuous surveillance function that does not require specific antibody or prior exposure to recognize potential pathogens. Discrimination between host and foreign particles occurs because activation of the system is under strict control by regulatory plasma proteins and membrane proteins of the host. Full activation occurs only when the function of these regulators is decreased on the surface of activating particles. Some organisms and nonpathogenic particles which are attacked by the alternative pathway are listed in Table 1.

Activation of the alternative pathway results in covalent attachment of large numbers of C3b molecules to the particle surface. Assembly of the membrane attack complex is initiated by cell-bound alternative pathway enzymes in a manner similar to that of the classical pathway. These events trigger the release of a variety of mediators which induce cellular responses including leukocyte chemotaxis and release of vasoactive amines, hydrolytic enzymes, and arachidonic metabolites. Particle-bound complement proteins also promote adhesion and phagocytosis via cellular receptors.

# II. PROTEINS OF THE ALTERNATIVE PATHWAY

Table 2 lists some of the properties of the six plasma proteins comprising the alternative pathway. The proteins fall into two groups, those that participate in activation and those that regulate the activation process. C3, Factor B, and Factor D are involved in initiation of the pathway and in positive-feedback amplification of cell-bound C3b, which is a unique feature of the alternative pathway.[1-4] Properdin enhances deposition of C3b by stabilizing cell-bound enzymes. Factors H and I function as regulators which limit spontaneous activation and modulate the activation process on cell surfaces. Mixtures of the six isolated proteins have been shown to behave qualitatively and quantitatively like the alternative pathway in serum.[5,6] Furthermore, mixtures of the six proteins were capable of discriminating between known activators of the pathway and host cells. These observations suggest that all of the essential components of the system have been identified and that the recognition ability is intrinsic to the six protein system.

## A. C3

C3 participates in both the classical and alternative pathways and its concentration in plasma is higher than any other complement protein. Its only role in the classical pathway is to form the C5 convertase. In the alternative pathway C3 plays crucial roles in initiation, C3 convertase formation, recognition, C3b amplification and C5 convertase formation. The site through which C3 attaches to particle surfaces[7] has now been defined chemically as an intramolecular thioester bond between a Glu and a Cys residue (Figure 1).[8-11] Proteolytic cleavage of C3 at the C3a-C3b junction generates a metastable species of C3b in which the activated thioester can react with hydroxyl groups on carbohydrates,[12-16] with amino groups,[10,14,17,18] or with water. Reaction with water yields fluid phase C3b which is rapidly inactivated by Factors H and I. Formation of covalent ester or amide bonds links the C3b molecule to surfaces and, in the proper environment, leads to activation of complement.

C3 is a glycoprotein of $M_r$ 185,000 composed of two disulfide linked chains of $M_r$ 110,000 and 75,000.[19-21] Cleavage of the larger chain releases C3a ($M_r = 9,000$), an anaphylatoxin, leaving metastable C3b. The halflife of metastable C3b has been estimated to be only 60 microseconds,[10] during which time the molecule must react with a surface, or its reaction with water (Figure 1) prevents attachment and further participation in complement activation.

## Table 1
## ACTIVATORS OF THE ALTERNATIVE PATHWAY OF HUMAN COMPLEMENT

| Pathogens and particles of microbial origin | Nonpathogens |
|---|---|
| Many strains of Gram-negative bacteria | Pure carbohydrates (Agarose, Inulin) |
| Lipopolysaccharides from Gram-negative bacteria | Rabbit and Guinea pig IgG in complexes |
| Many strains of Gram-positive bacteria | Human IgG, IgA and IgE in complexes |
| Teichoic acid from Gram-positive cell walls | Heterologous erythrocytes (rabbit, mouse, chicken) |
| Fungi and yeast cell walls (zymosan) | Anionic polymers (Dextran sulfate) |
| Some viruses and virus infected cells | Cobra venom factor |
| Some tumor cells (Raji) | Cotton dust, wheat dust and pollen |
| Parasites (trypanosomes) | |

## Table 2
## PROTEINS OF THE ALTERNATIVE PATHWAY

| Symbol | Name | Functions | Mol wt | Serum conc. $\mu$g/m$\ell$ |
|---|---|---|---|---|
| C3 | C3 | Attaches covalently after proteolytic activation generates metastable C3b. C3b fragment is part of C3/C5 convertase. | 185,000 | 1200 |
| B | Factor B | Binds to C3b forming the precursor of the C3/C5 convertase (C3b,Bb). Bb subunit of this complex is a serine protease. | 93,000 | 200 |
| D | Factor D | Serine protease which activates Factor B when B is in complex with C3b. | 24,000 | 1 |
| P | Properdin | Regulator (positive) which enhances activation by binding to and stabilizing the C3/C5 convertase. | 224,000 | 20 |
| H | Factor H | Regulator (negative) which inactivates the C3/C5 convertase by dissociating its subunits. Also a cofactor for Factor I. | 150,000 | 560 |
| I | Factor I | Regulator (negative) which is a serine protease. Inactivates C3b with the aid of Factor H or the C3b receptor (CR1). | 88,000 | 34 |

C3b expresses binding sites for Factors B, H, I, P, C5, and C3b receptors, none of which are present on native C3. A conformational change, which can be detected spectrophotometrically, probably accounts for the appearance of these functions.[22-23] This conformational change can be induced without peptide bond cleavage by any reaction that severs the thioester bond as illustrated in Figure 1. Hydrolysis of the thioester produces $C3(H_2O)$ which is conformationally and functionally C3b-like except that it lacks an attachment site.[11,18,23-25] It is thought that $C3(H_2O)$ formed by spontaneous hydrolysis in plasma initiates the pathway as will be described below.[11,24]

Particle-bound C3b initiates the formation of a bound C3 convertase which like the C4b,2a enzyme of the classical pathway activates C3 and deposits multiple C3b molecules nearby. Each new C3b can repeat this feedback amplification process resulting in rapid deposition of large numbers of C3b molecules. Since C3b is an opsonin, these particles adhere to receptor-bearing cells and are ingested by activated phagocytes.

### B. Factor B

This protein is a serine protease zymogen. It can be activated only when bound in a $Mg^{++}$-dependent complex with C3b. The resulting serine protease is composed of C3b, the larger fragment of Factor B ($M_r$ 60,000) and a single tightly bound magnesium ion.[4,26-28] The C3b,Bb complex is a C3 convertase capable of cleaving C3 to form metastable C3b

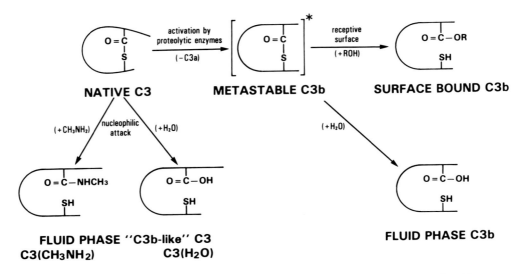

FIGURE 1.   Possible chemical reactions at the thioester site of C3. An intramolecular thioester bond between a glutamic acid side chain and the sulfhydryl group of a cysteine four residues away in C3 becomes the reactive group of the attachment site of metastable C3b. The thioester in native C3 is susceptible to hydrolysis and to attack by nucleophiles. Cleavage of the thioester without proteolytic release of C3a induces a slow conformational change, producing a molecule that is C3b-like in its functions, but which cannot attach to surfaces. (From Pangburn, M. K. and Müller-Eberhard, H. J., *J. Exp. Med.*, 152, 1102, 1980. By copyright permission of The Rockefeller University Press.)

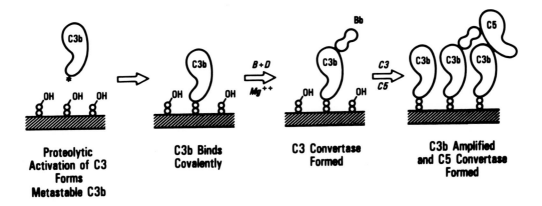

FIGURE 2.   A schematic diagram of the major events in alternative pathway activation. Metastable C3b attaches to surface carbohydrate via an ester bond. C3b binds Factor B which is activated by Factor D forming the surface-bound C3 convertase C3b,Bb. This enzyme activates many C3 molecules depositing numerous C3b nearby. These C3b may in turn form C3 convertases or may bind C5, allowing activation of the C5-9 membranolytic pathway. (From Pangburn, M. K., in *An Introduction to the Complement System*, Ross, G. D., Ed., Academic Press, Orlando, Fla., Chap. 2, 1986. With permission.)

and C3a.[4] The C3b,Bb enzyme in the presence of a second molecule of C3b also cleaves C5[29-30] in a manner exactly analogous to the mechanism of C5 cleavage by C4b,2a in the classical pathway (Figure 2). The catalytic subunits (Bb and C2a) of both enzymes show primary structural homology with typical serine proteases as well as with each other.[31] Their activation mechanism, however, appears to be unique, since the activation peptides are more than 300 residues long and do not contain the characteristic sequence of other serine proteases. C2 and Factor B are genetically linked and are associated with the major histocompatibility locus in man.

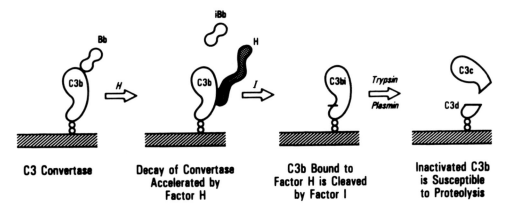

FIGURE 3.   A schematic diagram of the major events in regulation of the alternative pathway. Factor H binds to C3b or to C3b,Bb and rapidly releases Bb. C3b is then irreversibly inactivated by Factor I. (From Pangburn, M. K., in *An Introduction to the Complement System*, Ross, G. D., Ed., Academic Press, Orlando, Fla., Chap. 2, 1986. With permission.)

## C. Factor D

Factor D is a highly specific serine protease[32] that is present in plasma in active form.[4,33-35] Factor D is a trace component of blood and its concentration (1 μg/mℓ is the lowest of all of the complement proteins. It cleaves Factor B only when this protein is bound to C3b or a functionally similar form of C3 such as $C3(H_2O)$.[28,36,37] Upon cleavage by Factor D of an Arg-Lys bond[35,38] in Factor B, the smaller Ba fragment is released leaving the active C3 convertase, C3b,Bb.

## D. Factor P (Properdin)

The existence of an alternative pathway of complement activation, other than the IgG and C1 activated pathway, was recognized through the discovery of properdin in 1954.[39] It has since been shown that, although its presence greatly enhances activation of the pathway, it is not an essential component.[5] Its function is to bind to C3b,Bb and increase the half-life of this complex approximately 10-fold.[40-41] Properdin thus stabilizes both the C3 and C5 convertases of the alternative pathway against intrinsic and regulator-mediated decay (see below).

The structure of properdin has been studied extensively with many differing conclusions. Most of the observations were resolved by the demonstration by electron microscopy that properdin is a heterogeneous polymeric protein with cyclic dimer, trimer, tetramer, and high polymer forms[42] of the basic $M_r$ 56,000 monomer.[43] The properdin monomer appears to be a highly asymmetric flexible molecule 260A long and 30A wide. The unusual amino acid composition of properdin suggested that it might be composed of collagen-like regions, but amino acid sequencing has failed to detect the typical repeated three residue sequences.[44]

## E. Factor H

This protein is the primary regulator of alternative pathway activation. Formerly called β1H, this protein regulates the C3 convertase (C3b,Bb) by inhibiting its formation[45] and by accelerating dissociation of the complex (Figure 3). Factor H binds to C3b and competes with the binding of Factor B thus reducing the efficiency of C3 convertase formation. C3b,Bb has an intrinsic half-life of only 90 sec at 37°C.[46] In the presence of serum concentrations of Factor H the complex dissociates very rapidly (half-life probably less than one sec). Once released, Bb is almost entirely inactive and cannot rebind.[47] C3b may form another C3 convertase[4] unless it remains bound to Factor H and is permanently inactivated by Factor I. Binding of Factor H to C3b also inhibits C5 activation by competing with C5 binding.[48,49]

## F. Factor I

Proteolytic inactivation of both C3b and C4b is mediated by the serine protease Factor I. In both cases a cofactor is required. Either Factor H,[50-51] C4b binding protein,[52] or the C3b receptor (CR1) must be bound to C3b before Factor I can cleave the molecule (Figure 3). Factor I is highly specific and, like Factor D, circulates in plasma as an active protease. Factor I cleaves the alpha-chain of C3b at two sites generating three fragments of $M_r$ 68,000, 43,000, and 3,000.[53-55] The smallest fragment is released, leaving C3bi. C3bi is incapable of participating in complement activation due to the loss of all of the binding sites present on C3b except that for CR1. CR1 promotes an additional cleavage of the 68,000 $M_r$ chain by Factor I generating C3c and C3dg.[56-58] Similar, but not identical, fragments (C3c and C3d) are formed from C3bi by a variety of trypsin-like proteases such as plasmin. Degradation of cell-bound C3b releases the C3c portion ($M_r$ = 150,000) leaving C3d ($M_r$ = 35,000) or C3dg ($M_r$ = 43,000) covalently bound to the cell.

## III. MECHANISMS OF ACTIVATION

Activation of the alternative pathway begins in the fluid phase with the spontaneous and continuous generation of an enzyme that cleaves C3.[24] A small proportion of the resulting metastable C3b attaches to host and foreign particles alike. Discrimination between self and nonself occurs subsequent to this random attachment of C3b and results from rapid inactivation of C3b on host cells.[59] Activation proceeds on pathogenic particles, in effect, by default because the regulatory components of complement are ineffectual or absent on these surfaces. These C3b molecules initiate formation of surface-bound C3 convertases which deposit many more C3b, each of which may repeat the process. This marks the particles for phagocytosis and leads to activation of C5 and cytolysis via the terminal pathway.

### A. Initiation

The current view of the initiation process stems largely from the inability of researchers to identify specific initiators in the alternative pathway which fulfill the roles that IgG and C1 perform in the classical pathway. Once the six proteins just described were rigorously purified and shown to behave as does the alternative pathway in serum,[6] investigations focused on mechanisms intrinsic to this six-protein system.

The proposal most consistent with current evidence suggests that spontaneous hydrolysis of the thioester bond of C3 leads to a gradual conformational change in the molecule.[24] This transition has been studied by inducing thioester cleavage with methylamine.[23] The modified C3 first assumes an intermediate conformation which is characterized by the ability to bind Factor B and form a C3 convertase. This form binds Factor H poorly and is thus not rapidly inactivated allowing the convertase to generate metastable C3b as illustrated in Figure 4. A second conformational transition then leads to the end state $C3(CH_3NH_2)$ or $C3(H_2O)$ which are susceptible to rapid inactivation by Factors H and I. The rate of formation of $C3(H_2O)$ from C3 in plasma has been estimated to be 0.005%/min.[24]

### B. Initial Deposition of C3b

Attachment of C3b via the metastable binding site[7] allows the alternative pathway to focus its biological effects on the surface of the activating particle. Metastable C3b can bind covalently via an ester bond to a wide variety of sugars and polysaccharides allowing it to bind to almost any biological particle. This is important since in the absence of specific antibodies, C3b may be the first host molecule to encounter and initiate a challenge to an invading pathogen.

Deposition of C3b from the fluid phase by the C3 convertase formed from $C3(H_2O)$ is thought to be indiscriminate, i.e., C3b binds to foreign and to autologous cells alike. Evidence

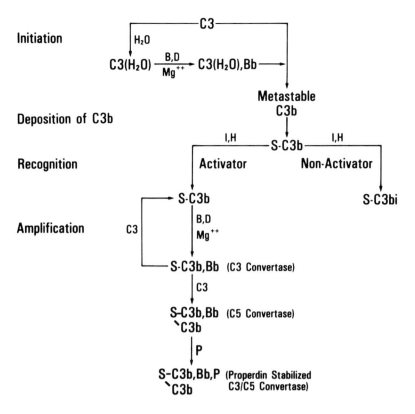

FIGURE 4.    The sequence of reactions in alternative pathway activation. Initiation is a continuous process which begins with spontaneous hydrolysis of the thioester in native C3. C3(H$_2$O) forms a fluid phase C3 convertase and cleaves C3. The resulting metastable C3b attaches randomly on host and nonhost particles. Only on activators of the pathway does C3b escape inactivation by Factors H and I. On these particles C3b is amplified. C5 convertases are formed, and the cytolytic pathway is activated. (From Pangburn, M. K. and Müller-Eberhard, H. J., *Springer Semin. Immunopathol.*, 7, 163, 1984. With permission.)

confirming the randomness of this process has been obtained[2] utilizing the fluorescence activated cell sorter to follow activation on single cells. The pattern observed was consistent with a slow random deposition of the first C3b molecule followed by relatively rapid amplification of bound C3b.

## C. Recognition of Alternative Pathway Activators

Discrimination between host and foreign particles occurs soon after initial deposition of C3b. Its exact mechanism is not at present understood, but two proteins are involved: C3b and Factor H. Fluid phase C3b and C3b bound to host cells are prevented from forming C3 convertases by efficiently binding Factor H. Subsequent cleavage by Factor I inactivates C3b irreversibly. Thus, in the unchallenged host activation of the pathway rarely proceeds beyond formation of fluid phase C3(H$_2$O),Bb and generation by this enzyme of metastable C3b. C3b deposited on activators of the pathway exhibits a three- to ten-fold lower affinity for Factor H.[45,59-61] Because the binding of Factor B and properdin are not affected by the surface to which C3b is bound, formation of cell-bound C3b,Bb occurs. Apparently, a three-fold reduction in Factor H binding permits C3b to be deposited more rapidly than C3b is inactivated on such a surface.

It is not yet clear whether the recognition function of the alternative pathway resides in C3b, Factor H or is expressed jointly by these proteins.[6,45,61-63] Nor is it clear what molecular structures are recognized.[2] Activators include many pure polysaccharides, some immunoglobulins, viruses, fungi, bacteria, tumor cells and parasites (Table 1). The only common feature of these activators is the presence of carbohydrate, but the complexity and variety of carbohydrate structures makes it difficult to envisage the shared molecular determinants which are recognized. One feature shared by most activators is the absence of sialic acid. Sheep erythrocytes, which are extremely weak activators of the human alternative pathway, are converted to efficient activators by removing or modifying surface sialic acid.[45,62] A similar influence of sialic acid on alternative pathway activation has been observed in many systems, reinforcing the original suggestion that a low sialic acid content causes activation.[45,64-69] Mechanistically, sialic acid would function to enhance Factor H binding on nonactivating surfaces. However, low sialic acid concentration is unlikely to be the only deciding feature common to activators, because in several systems activators have been generated by addition of foreign molecules to the cell surfaces without removal of sialic acid. Conversely, treatment of human erythrocytes with neuraminidase or pronase[70] reduces the sialic acid content of the cells to levels similar to or below the levels found on rabbit erythrocytes. Treatment with pronase also inactivates membrane-associated regulatory proteins such as DAF and CR1. Nevertheless, pronase-treated human erythrocytes are not activators of the human alternative pathway at normal pH where rabbit erythrocytes are the most potent activators known.[2,70-72] Incorporation of lipopolysaccharide from E. coli into the membrane of sheep erythrocytes reduces the affinity of Factor H for surface-bound C3b by 60% and causes the cells to become activators of the alternative pathway.[63] Rabbit IgG and Fab′ fragments bound to a variety of particles were shown to activate the alternative pathway.[73-75] Chemical modification of specific residues abolished activation without altering binding. In another study, liposomes did not activate the guinea pig alternative pathway even when a variety of sialo- and asialo-glycolipids were incorporated during their preparation.[76] Upon incorporation of lipids bearing trinitrophenyl groups, the liposomes became efficient activators. Apparently, the absence of sialic acid was not a sufficient condition for activation to occur in this system; however, a modulating role for sialic acid was found. The inclusion of any one of three glycolipids containing sialic acid in the activating liposomes inhibited activation while no inhibition was found with several asialoglycolipids.[69]

## D. Amplification of Cell-Bound C3b

A unique feature of the alternative pathway is its ability to amplify the number of C3b molecules bound to a surface.[4] This process is illustrated in Figure 5. In the absence of regulatory proteins or in environments where their effectiveness is diminished, a spontaneous, C3b-dependent positive feedback process occurs. C3b in the presence of magnesium ions binds Factor B. Once bound, Factor B becomes susceptible to cleavage and activation by Factor D yielding the C3 convertase C3b,Bb. This protease is unstable, exhibiting a half-life under physiological conditions of 90 sec, but it cleaves approximately one C3 per sec,[46] and each of the resulting C3b molecules may repeat the process by forming another C3 convertase with Factor B. Thus, if the system has a C3b doubling time of approximately two sec, then a single C3b could yield $10^9$ C3b in one minute if starting materials were unlimited. Factor H at plasma concentrations accelerates the dissociation of the C3b,Bb complex to an extremely short half-life, preventing amplification unless the complex resides on an activator where regulation is restricted.

Figure 6 illustrates the time course of C3b deposition onto three typical alternative pathway activators.[71] In each case the pattern shows an initial lag phase of variable length, followed by a period of rapid amplification. Finally, a plateau is reached due either to consumption of complement components or to saturation of the surface with C3b.[71] The lag phase cor-

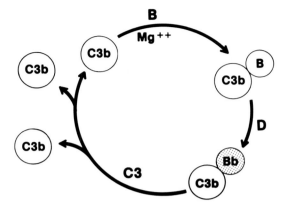

FIGURE 5.   Mechanism of C3b amplification. In the absence of control factors, C3b binds Factor B, which is activated by Factor D to form a C3 convertase (C3b,Bb). This proteolytic enzyme cleaves C3, producing multiple C3b molecules each of which may form C3 convertases and repeat the process. (From Pangburn, M. K., in *An Introduction to the Complement System*, Ross, G. D., Ed., Academic Press, Orlando, Fla., Chap. 2, 1986. With permission.)

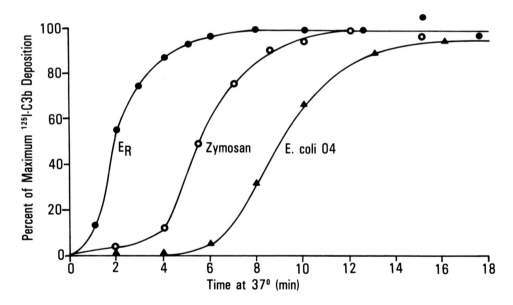

FIGURE 6.   Time course of C3b deposition on alternative pathway activators. Radiolabeled C3 in human serum was used to monitor the time course of attachment of C3b to rabbit erythrocytes ($E_R$), zymosan (yeast cell walls), and E. coli strain 04. Each activator exhibits a lag, a rapid period of amplification, and a plateau phase, which is due to consumption of complement components or saturation of the particle surface. (From Pangburn, M. K., Schreiber, R. D., and Müller-Eberhard, H. J., *J. Immunol.*, 131, 1930, 1983. With permission.)

responds to the time required to deposit the initial C3b molecules on a significant proportion of particles and to amplify these first C3b molecules to detectable levels. Amplification is slower on E. coli 04 than on rabbit erythrocytes, because Factor H function is reduced only 3-fold on this bacteria, while it is reduced approximately 20-fold on $E_r$.[63,71,77]

## E. Activation of C5 and the Terminal Pathway

C5 is activated by the alternative pathway (Figure 4) in a manner exactly analogous to that of the classical pathway. The C3 convertase, C3b,Bb requires a second C3b nearby to bind C5.[29,30,36,49,78,79] This increases the local concentration of C5 and may also modulate C5 for more efficient cleavage. C5 cleavage releases the anaphylatoxin C5a and produces C5b which subsequently binds and activates C6-C9. Because of the large number of bound C3b and the numerous C3 convertases formed from these C3b on activator surfaces, the alternative pathway is an efficient activator of the terminal pathway.

## IV. REGULATION OF ACTIVATION

Five proteins are known to be involved in the regulation of alternative pathway activation: the plasma proteins Factors H, I, and properdin, and the membrane-associated proteins DAF and CR1. All of these regulators are inhibitors of activation except properdin.

### A. Factors H and I

These proteins work in concert to limit the rate of initiation, to prevent fluid phase activation and to prevent amplification of C3b on host cell surfaces. Initiation of the pathway is controlled by inactivation of $C3(H_2O)$ by Factors H and I.[58] Once the full conformational transition occurs in $C3(H_2O)$, it binds Factor H and is inactivated by Factor I.[23] As has been discussed, Factor H binds to fluid phase C3b and to C3b bound to host cells, preventing C3 convertase formation and allowing inactivation by Factor I.

### B. The Role of Properdin

Properdin enhances activation of the alternative pathway. It does this by binding to and stabilizing the C3 convertase making it more resistant to intrinsic and Factor H-mediated decay.[40-41] Native properdin, the form that exists in unactivated serum, does not bind to C3b, nor does it stabilize fluid phase C3b,Bb.[5,30,36,80,81] Interaction with particle-bound C3b,Bb may activate properdin as the result of a conformational rearrangement, but the mechanism of activation and its physiological relevance are still controversial.[81,82] Activated properdin is characterized by the ability to bind to C3b coated particles and to activate complement in serum.

Properdin is not an essential component of the alternative pathway. Activation occurs in its absence, but the activation process is considerably slower.[5,83] For example, in Figure 6 the rate of C3b deposition on rabbit erythroctyes would more closely resemble that on E. coli in the absence of properdin. Participation of properdin is required for effective lysis of measles virus-infected cells.[84] Several families exhibiting homozygous and heterozygous deficiencies of properdin have recently been described.[85,86] The homozygous deficient individuals are characterized by multiple and sometimes fatal meningococcal infections.

### C. Role of Membrane-Associated Regulators

Host cell membranes come under continuous attack from the alternative pathway. Normally the process is benign due to regulation by Factors H and I, but host cells lacking repair mechanisms (erythrocytes and platelets) or cells that come in contact with complement activating particles (erythrocytes, lymphocytes, PMN) may need additional lines of defense. It seems reasonable that those that have been developed reside at the site of attack. Two membrane proteins with complement inhibitory properties have been isolated and characterized and a third has just recently been identified.

The decay accelerating factor (DAF) is clearly the most important membrane-associated regulator of alternative pathway activation. It has been isolated from human erythrocyte membranes,[87] but is present on almost every cell examined.[88,89] DAF is a glycoprotein of 73,000 molecular weight. Its regulatory functions are to accelerate the decay of both the classical and alternative pathway C3 and C5 convertases.[87] Its decay accelerating activity resembles that of Factor H, but DAF does not serve as a cofactor for cleavage of C3b by Factor I,[70] and its binding site on C3 convertases differs from that of Factor H and CR1.[77] All of the decay accelerating activity expressed by intact human erythrocytes is due to DAF.[70] The abnormal erythrocytes of patients with paroxysmal nocturnal hemoglobinuria (PNH) have been shown to lack DAF.[70,90,91] Reinsertion of isolated DAF reduced their sensitivity to lysis by the alternative pathway,[92] and inhibition of DAF on normal human erythrocytes by specific antibody caused the cells to become activators of the pathway.[93] These results strongly suggest that DAF plays a major role in the pathology of PNH.

The C3b receptor (CR1) expresses complement regulatory activities in addition to its receptor function.[94] Since these activities are expressed primarily on adjacent particles, CR1 provides little or no protection from direct attack by complement.[57,70,93] It may protect the cell on which it resides from spillover from activating particles held in close proximity by its receptor function. CR1 acts as a decay accelerating factor[94-96] as a cofactor of Factor I-mediated cleavage of C3b and C4b,[94,96] as a cofactor for cleavage of C3bi yielding C3dg and C3c,[57,58,97] and as an inhibitor of C5 convertase activity by competing with C5 binding to C3b.[98] CR1 on human erythrocytes plays an important role in processing the complement proteins C3b and C4b bound to immune complexes.[57,99]

Erythrocytes have been shown to express a species-specific resistance to lysis by homologous terminal pathway proteins.[100-109] Although the factor responsible has yet to be fully characterized, the sensitivity of PNH erythrocytes to lysis suggest that the more severe form of PNH may be due to a lack of both DAF and the C5-9 inhibitor.

**D. Immunoglobulin Enhancement of Activation**

Activation of the alternative pathway is often enhanced by the presence of specific antibodies.[110-112] In some cases the participation of immunoglobulin has been demonstrated to be essential for effective activation of the pathway. Although measles virus-infected cells activate the alternative pathway in the absence of antibody, significant lysis requires the presence of immune IgG.[113] Similarly, cultured human lymphoid cells, which do not activate complement, activate the alternative pathway when treated with antisera.[114] One mechanism of IgG participation in the alternative pathway may be the diminution of Factor H binding to C3b which is covalently attached to IgG.[115] Another may be the clustering or capping of antigens on the surface of target cells by antibody.

## V. BIOLOGICAL EFFECTS OF ALTERNATIVE PATHWAY ACTIVATION

Both pathways of complement activation are able to activate the cytolytic pathway of complement. Membrane damage by C5-9 is perhaps the major biological effect of complement activation, but complement also stimulates other elements of host defense. Alternative pathway activation generates large quantities of C3a, C5a, C3b, and C3b breakdown products. C3a, an anaphylatoxin, causes vasodilation, resulting in increased blood flow to the area of complement activation. Both C3a and C5a stimulate release of histamine from mast cells, and C5a is chemotactic for human neutrophils. The alternative pathway deposits large numbers of C3b molecules on its targets. Many cells, including neutrophils and mononuclear phagocytes, possess receptors for C3b and its degradation products. These receptors enhance phagocytosis and, in some cases, may mediate phagocytosis of the target without participation of antibodies.

The alternative pathway of complement with the participation of the terminal components and lysozyme expresses potent bactericidal activity toward a wide variety of potentially pathogenic organisms.[1] Individuals genetically lacking C3, properdin, Factor H, or Factor I all suffer from recurrent life-threatening bacterial infections.[116] Bacteria isolated from infected individuals often exhibit a weak or undetectable ability to activate the alternative pathway or an increased resistance to the lytic action of the terminal pathway proteins, or both.

Nucleated cells, viruses, and fungi are also targets of the alternative pathway.[1] Most yeast are strong activators which are rapidly coated with C3b and are ingested by phagocytes. Most molds and other fungi are handled similarly in the uncompromised host. Cultured tumor cells, such as the human lymphoblastoid line Raji, activate and are lysed by the human alternative pathway. Hela cells become activators of the pathway upon infection with measles virus, but efficient lysis requires antiviral antibodies. Vesicular stomatitis virus infected cells have also been shown to activate the pathway. Only a few viruses have been found to activate the alternative pathway directly including sindbis, simian virus-5, and influenza. These examples suggest that the alternative pathway may play a role in the elimination of some tumor and virus-infected cells.

# REFERENCES

1. **Müller-Eberhard, H. J. and Schreiber, R. D.,** Molecular biology and chemistry of the alternative pathway of complement, *Adv. Immunol.,* 29, 1, 1980.
2. **Pangburn, M. K. and Müller-Eberhard, H. J.,** The alternative pathway of complement, *Springer Semin. Immunopathol.,* 7, 163, 1984.
3. **Müller-Eberhard, H. J.,** Complement, *Annu. Rev. Biochem.,* 44, 697, 1975.
4. **Müller-Eberhard, H. J. and Gotze, O.,** C3 proactivator convertase and its mode of action, *J. Exp. Med.,* 135, 1003, 1972.
5. **Schreiber, R. D. and Müller-Eberhard, H. J.,** Assembly of the cytolytic alternative pathway of complement from 11 isolated plasma proteins, *J. Exp. Med.,* 148, 1722, 1978.
6. **Schreiber, R. D., Pangburn, M. K., Lesavre, P., and Müller-Eberhard, H. J.,** Initiation of the alternative pathway of complement: recognition of activators by bound C3b and assembly of the entire pathway from six isolated proteins, *Proc. Nat. Acad. Sci. USA,* 75, 3948, 1978.
7. **Müller-Eberhard, H. J., Dalmasso, A. P., and Calcott, M. A.,** The reaction mechanism of B1c-globulin (C'3) in immune hemolysis, *J. Exp. Med.,* 123, 33, 1966.
8. **Tack, B. F., Harrison, R. A., Janatova, J., Thomas, M. L., and Prahl, J. W.,** Evidence for presence of an internal thiolester bond in third component of human complement, *Proc. Nat. Acad. Sci. USA,* 77, 5764, 1980.
9. **Law, S. K., Lichentenberg, N. A., and Levine, R. P.,** Covalent binding and hemolytic activity of complement proteins, *Proc. Nat. Acad. Sci. USA,* 77, 7194, 1980.
10. **Sim, R. B., Twose, T. M., Paterson, D. S., and Sim, E.,** The covalent-binding reaction of complement component C3, *Biochem. J.,* 193, 115, 1981.
11. **Pangburn, M. K. and Müller-Eberhard, H. J.,** Relation of a putative thioester bond in C3 to activation of the alternative pathway and the binding of C3b to biological targets of complement, *J. Exp. Med.,* 152, 1102, 1980.
12. **Law, S. K. and Levine, R. P.,** Interaction between the third complement protein and cell surface, *Proc. Nat. Acad. Sci. USA,* 74, 2701, 1977.
13. **Law, S. K., Lichtenberg, N. A., and Levine, R. P.,** Evidence for an ester linkage between the labile binding site of C3b and receptive surfaces, *J. Immunol.,* 123, 1388, 1979.
14. **Law, S. K., Minich, T. M., and Levine, R. P.,** Binding reaction between the third human complement protein and small molecules, *Biochemistry,* 20, 7457, 1981.
15. **Mann, J., O'Brien, R., Hostetter, M. K., Alper, C. A., Rosen, F. S., and Babior, B. M.,** The third component of complement: Covalent attachment of a radioactive sugar to the liabile binding site of C3 via the alternative pathway, *J. Immunol.,* 126, 2370, 1981.
16. **Hostetter, M. K., Thomas, M. L., Rosen, F. S., and Tack, B. F.,** Binding of C3b proceeds by a transesterification reaction at the thiolester site, *Nature,* 298, 72, 1982.
17. **Capel, P. J. A., Groeneboer, O., Grosveld, G., and Pondman, K. W.,** The binding of activated C3 to polysaccharides and immunoglobulins, *J. Immunol.,* 121, 2566, 1978.
18. **VonZabern, I., Nolte, R., and Vogt, W.,** Treatment of human complement components C4 and C3 with amines or chaotropic ions, *Scand. J. Immunol.,* 13, 413, 1981.

19. **Bokisch, V. A., Müller-Eberhard, H. J., and Cochrane, C. G.,** Isolation of a fragment (C3a) of the third component of human complement containing anaphylatoxin and chemotactic activity and description of anaphylatoxin inactivator of human serum, *J. Exp. Med.,* 129, 1109, 1969.

20. **Nilsson, U. R., Mandle, R. J., and McConnell-Mapes, J. A.,** Human C3 and C5: subunit structure and modifications by trypsin and C42-C423, *J. Immunol.,* 114, 815, 1975.

21. **Tack, B. F. and Prahl, J. W.,** Third component of human complement: Purification from plasma and physicochemical characterization, *Biochemistry,* 15, 4513, 1976.

22. **Isenman, D. E. and Cooper, N. R.,** The structure and function of the third component of human complement. I. The nature and extent of conformational changes accompanying C3 activation., *Mol. Immunol.,* 18, 331, 1981.

23. **Isenman, D. E., Kells, D. I. C., Cooper, N. R., Müller-Eberhard, H. J., and Pangburn, M. K.,** Nucleophilic modification of human complement protein C3: correlation of conformational changes with acquisition of C3b-like functional properties, *Biochemistry,* 20, 4458, 1981.

24. **Pangburn, M. K., Schreiber, R. D., and Müller-Eberhard, H. J.,** Formation of the initial C3 convertase of the alternative complement pathway. Acquisition of C3b-like activities by spontaneous hydrolysis of the putative thioester in native C3, *J. Exp. Med.,* 154, 856, 1981.

25. **Parkes, C., DiScipio, R. G., Kerr, M. A., and Prohaska, R.,** The separation of functionally distinct forms of the third component of human complement (C3), *Biochem. J.,* 193, 963, 1981.

26. **Medicus, R. G., Götze, O., and Müller-Eberhard, H. J.,** The serine protease nature of the C3 and C5 convertases of the classical and alternative complement pathways, *Scand. J. Immunol.,* 5, 1049, 1976.

27. **Fishelson, Z., Pangburn, M. K., and Müller-Eberhard, H. J.,** C3 convertase of the alternative complement pathway: demonstration of an active, stable C3b,Bb(Ni) complex, *J. Biol. Chem.,* 258, 7411, 1983.

28. **Vogt, W., Dames, W., Schmidt, G., and Dieminger, L.,** Complement activation by the properdin system: Formation of a stoichiometric C3 cleaving complex of properdin Factor B and C3b, *Immunochemistry,* 14, 201, 1977.

29. **Daha, M. R., Fearon, D. T., and Austen, K. F.,** Requirements for formation of alternative pathway C5 convertase, *J. Immunol.,* 117, 630, 1976.

30. **Medicus, R. G., Schreiber, R. D., Götze, O., and Müller-Eberhard, H. J.,** A molecular concept of the properdin pathway, *Proc. Nat. Acad. Sci. USA,* 73, 612, 1976.

31. **Kerr, M. A. and Gagnon, J.,** The purification and properties of the second component of guinea pig complement, *Biochem. J.,* 205, 59, 1982.

32. **Fearon, D. T., Austen, K. F., and Ruddy, S.,** Properdin Factor D: characterization of its active site and isolation of the precursor form, *J. Exp. Med.,* 139, 355, 1974.

33. **Johnson, M. S., Gagnon, J., and Reid, K. B. M.,** Factor D of the alternative pathway of human complement. Purification, alignment and N-terminal amino acid sequences of the major cyanogen bromide fragments, and localization of the serine residue at the active site, *Biochem. J.,* 187, 863, 1980.

34. **Volanakis, J. E., Brown, A. S., Bennett, J. C., and Mole, J. E.,** Partial amino acid sequence of human Factor D: Homology with serine proteases, *Proc. Nat. Acad. Sci. USA,* 77, 1116, 1980.

35. **Lesavre, P. H., Hugli, T. E., Esser, A. F., and Müller-Eberhard, H. J.,** The alternative pathway C3/C5 convertase: Chemical basis of Factor B activation, *J. Immunol.,* 123, 529, 1979.

36. **Medicus, R. G., Götze, O., and Müller-Eberhard, H. J.,** Alternative pathway of complement: Recruitment of precursor properdin by the labile C3/C5 convertase and the potentiation of the pathway, *J. Exp. Med.,* 144, 1076, 1976.

37. **Lesavre, P. and Müller-Eberhard, H. J.,** Mechanism of action of Factor D of the alternative complement pathway, *J. Exp. Med.,* 148, 1498, 1978.

38. **Christie, D. L. and Gagnon, J.,** Isolation, characterization and N-terminal sequence of the cyanogen bromide fragments of Factor B. Localization of a free thiol group and a sequence defining the site cleaved by Factor D, *Biochem. J.,* 201, 555, 1982.

39. **Pillemer, L., Blum, L., Lepow, I. H., Ross, O. A., Todd, E. W., and Wardlaw, A. C.,** The properdin system and immunity. I. Demonstration and isolation of a new serum protein, properdin, and its role in immune phenomena, *Science,* 120, 279, 1954.

40. **Fearon, D. T. and Austen, K. F.,** Properdin: Binding to C3b and stabilization of the C3b-dependent C3 convertase, *J. Exp. Med.,* 142, 856, 1975.

41. **Schreiber, R. D., Medicus, R. G., Götze, O., and Müller-Eberhard, H. J.,** Properdin and nephritic factor-dependent C3 convertases: Requirement of native C3 for enzyme formation and the function of bound C3b as properdin receptor, *J. Exp. Med.,* 142, 760, 1975.

42. **Smith, C. A., Pangburn, M. K., Vogel, C. W., and Müller-Eberhard, H. J.,** Molecular architecture of human properdin, a positive regulator of the alternative pathway of complement, *J. Biol. Chem.,* 259, 4582, 1984.

43. **Minta, J. O. and Lepow, I. H.,** Studies on the subunit structure of human properdin, *Immunochemistry,* 11, 361, 1974.

44. **Reid, K. B. M. and Gagnon, J.,** Amino acid sequence studies of human properdin-N-terminal sequence analysis and alignment of the fragments produced by limited proteolysis with trypsin and the peptides produced by cyanogen bromide treatment, *Molec. Immunol.,* 18, 949, 1981.

45. **Pangburn, M. K. and Müller-Eberhard, H. J.,** Complement C3 convertase: cell surface restriction of βIH control and generation of restriction on neuraminidase treated cells, *Proc. Nat. Acad. Sci. USA,* 75, 2416, 1978.

46. **Pangburn, M. K. and Müller-Eberhard, H. J.,** The C3 convertase of the alternative pathway of human complement: enzymatic properties of the bimolecular protease, *Biochem. J.,* 235, 723, 1986.

47. **Fishelson, Z. and Müller-Eberhard, H. J.,** Residual hemolytic and proteolytic activity expressed by Bb after decay-dissociation of C3b,Bb, *J. Immunol.,* 132, 1425, 1984.

48. **Fischer, E. and Kazatchkine, M. D.,** Surface-dependent modulation by H of C5 cleavage by the cell-bound alternative pathway C5 convertase of human complement, *J. Immunol.,* 130, 2821, 1983.

49. **Isenman, D. E., Podack, E. R., and Cooper, N. R.,** The interaction of C5 with C3b in free solution: A sufficient condition for cleavage by fluid phase C3/C5 convertase, *J. Immunol.,* 124, 326, 1980.

50. **Pangburn, M. K., Schreiber, R. D., and Müller-Eberhard, H. J.,** Human complement C3b inactivator: Isolation, characterization, and demonstration of an absolute requirement for the serum protein β1H for cleavage of C3b and C4b in solution, *J. Exp. Med.,* 146, 257, 1977.

51. **Crossley, L. G. and Porter, R. R.,** Purification of the human complement control protein C3b inactivator, *Biochem. J.,* 191, 173, 1980.

52. **Fujita, T. and Nussenzweig, V.,** The role of C4-binding protein and β1H in proteolysis of C4b and C3b, *J. Exp. Med.,* 150, 267, 1979.

53. **Davis, A. E., Harrison, R. A., and Lachmann, P. J.,** Physiologic inactivation of fluid phase C3b: isolation and structural analysis of C3c, C3dg (alpha-2D) and C3g, *J. Immunol.,* 132, 1960, 1984.

54. **Harrison, R. A. and Lachmann, P. J.,** The physiological breakdown of the third component of human complement, *Mol. Immunol.,* 17, 9, 1980.

55. **Sim, E., Wood, A. B., Hsiung, L., and Sim, R. B.,** Patterns of degradation of human complement fragment, C3b, *FEBS Lett.,* 132, 55, 1981.

56. **Medicus, R. G. and Arnaout, M. A.,** Release of C3c from Bound C3bi by C3b inactivator, *Mol. Immunol.,* 19, 1386, 1982.

57. **Medof, M. E., Iida, K., Mold, C., and Nussenzweig, V.,** Unique role of the complement receptor CR1 in the degradation of C3b associated with immune complexes, *J. Exp. Med.,* 156, 1739, 1982.

58. **Ross, G. D., Lambris, J. D., Cain, J. A., and Newman, S. L.,** Generation of three different fragments of bound C3 with purified factor I or serum. I. Requirements for factor H vs. CR1 cofactor activity, *J. Immunol.,* 129, 2051, 1982.

59. **Fearon, D. T. and Austen, K. F.,** Activation of the alternative complement pathway due to resistance of zymosan-bound amplification convertase to endogenous regulatory mechanisms, *Proc. Nat. Acad. Sci. USA,* 74, 1683, 1977.

60. **Fearon, D. T. and Austen, K. F.,** Activation of the alternative complement pathway with rabbit erythrocytes by circumvention of the regulatory action of endogenous control proteins, *J. Exp. Med.,* 146, 22, 1977.

61. **Horstmann, R. D., Pangburn, M. K., and Müller-Eberhard, H. J.,** Species specificity of recognition by the alternative pathway of complement, *J. Immunol.,* 134, 1101, 1985.

62. **Fearon, D. T.,** Regulation by membrane sialic acid of βIH-dependent decay-dissociation of amplification C3 convertase of the alternative complement pathway, *Proc. Nat. Acad. Sci. USA,* 75, 1971, 1978.

63. **Pangburn, M. K., Morrison, D. C., Schreiber, R. D., and Müller-Eberhard, H. J.,** Activation of the alternative complement pathway: recognition of surface structures on activators by bound C3b, *J. Immunol.,* 124, 977, 1980.

64. **Kazatchkine, M. D., Fearon, D. T., and Austen, K. F.,** Human alternative complement pathway: membrane-associated sialic acid regulates the competition between B and βIH for cell-bound C3b, *J. Immunol.,* 122, 75, 1979.

65. **Nydegger, U. E., Fearon, D. T., and Austen, K. F.,** Autosomal locus regulates inverse relationship between sialic acid content and capacity of mouse erythrocytes to activate human alternative complement pathway, *Proc. Nat. Acad. Sci. USA,* 75, 6078, 1978.

66. **Kazatchkine, M. D., Fearon, D. T., Silbert, J. E., and Austen, K. F.,** Surface-associated heparin inhibits zymosan-induced activation of the human alternative pathway by augmenting the regulatory action of the control proteins on particle-bound C3b, *J. Exp. Med.,* 150, 1202, 1979.

67. **Edwards, M. S., Kasper, D. L., Jennings, H. F., Baker, C. J., and Nicholson-Weller, A.,** Capsular sialic acid prevents activation of the alternative complement pathway by type III, group B streptococci, *J. Immunol.,* 128, 1278, 1982.

68. **Okada, H., Tasuda, T., Tsumita, T., and Okada, H.,** Membrane sialoglycolipids regulate the activation of the alternative complement pathway by liposomes containing trinitrophenyl-aminocaproxyldipalmitoylphosphatydylethanolamine, *Immunology,* 48, 129, 1983.

69. **Okada, N., Yasuda, T., and Okada, H.,** Restriction of alternative complement pathway activation by sialosylglycolipids, *Nature,* 299, 261, 1982.

70. **Pangburn, M. K., Schreiber, R. D., and Müller-Eberhard, H. J.,** Deficiency of an erythrocyte membrane protein with complement regulatory activity in paroxysmal nocturnal hemoglobinuria, *Proc. Nat. Acad. Sci. USA,* 80, 5430, 1983.

71. **Pangburn, M. K., Schreiber, R. D., and Müller-Eberhard, H. J.,** C3b deposition during activation of the alternative complement pathway and the effect of deposition of the activating surface, *J. Immunol.,* 131, 1930, 1983.

72. **Pangburn, M. K., Schreiber, R. D., and Müller-Eberhard, H. J.,** Characterization of the complement regulatory functions of the decay accelerating factor and the C3b receptor on normal human erythrocytes, in preparation.

73. **Ernst, A.,** Separate pathways of C activation by measles virus cytotoxic antibodies: Subclass analysis and capacity of Fab molecules to activate C via the alternative pathway, *J. Immunol.,* 121, 1206, 1978.

74. **Sission, J. G. P., Cooper, N. R., and Oldstone, M. B. A.,** Alternative complement pathway-mediated lysis of measles virus infected cells: Induction by IgG antibody bound to individual viral glycoproteins and comparative efficacy of F(ab')2 and Fab' fragments, *J. Immunol.,* 123, 2144, 1979.

75. **Albar, J. P., Juarez, C., Vivanco-Martinez, F., Bragado, R., and Ortiz, F.,** Structural requirements of rabbit IgG F(ab')2 fragment for activation of the complement system through the alternative pathway. I. Disulfide bonds, *Mol. Immunol.,* 18, 925, 1981.

76. **Okada, N., Yasuda, T., Tsumita, T., and Okada, H.,** Activation of the alternative complement pathway of guinea pig by liposomes incorporated with trinitrophenylated phosphatidyl thanolamine, *Immunology,* 45, 115, 1982.

77. **Pangburn, M. K.,** Differences between the binding sites of the complement regulatory proteins DAF, CR1 and Factor H on C3 convertases, *J. Immunol.,* 136, 2216, 1986.

78. **DiScipio, R. G.,** The binding of human complement proteins C5, factor B, βIH and properdin to complement fragment C3b on zymosan, *Biochem. J.,* 199, 485, 1981.

79. **Vogt, W., Schmidt, G., von Buttlar, B., and Dieminger, L.,** A new function of the activated third component of complement: Binding to C5, an essential step for C5 activation, *Immunology,* 34, 29, 1978.

80. **Götze, O., Medicus, R. G., and Müller-Eberhard, H. J.,** Alternative pathway of complement: non-enzymatic, reversible transition of precursor to active properdin, *J. Immunol.,* 118, 525, 1977.

81. **Medicus, R. G., Esser, A. F., Fernandez, H. N., and Müller-Eberhard, H. J.,** Native and activated properdin: interconvertibility and identity of amino- and carboxy-terminal sequences, *J. Immunol.,* 124, 602, 1980.

82. **Farries, T. C., Finch, J. T., Lachmann, P. J., and Harrison, R. A.,** 'Activated' properdin is an artefact of isolation, *Biochem. J.,* 243, 507, 1987.

83. **Schreiber, R. D., Morrison, D. C., Podack, E. R., and Müller-Eberhard, H. J.,** Bactericidal activity of the alternative complement pathway generated from eleven isolated plasma proteins, *J. Exp. Med.,* 149, 870, 1979.

84. **Sissons, J. G. P., Schreiber, R. D., Perrin, L. H., Cooper, N. R., Müller-Eberhard, H. J., and Oldstone, M. B. A.,** Lysis of measles virus-infected cells by the purified cytolytic alternative complement pathway and antibody, *J. Exp. Med.,* 150, 445, 1979.

85. **Sjoholm, A. G., Braconier, J., and Soderstrom, C.,** Properdin deficiency in a family with fulminant meningococcal infections, *Clin. Exp. Immunol.,* 50, 291, 1982.

86. **Sjoholm, A. G., Braconier, J., and Soderstrom, C.,** Properdin deficiency in a family with fulminant meningococcal infections, *Clin. Exp. Immunol.,* 50, 291, 1982.

87. **Densen, P., Weiler, J., and Griffiss, J. M.,** Genetic, immunologic, and functional studies of a family with properdin deficiency and fatal meningococcal disease, *Clin. Res.,* 33, 400a, 1985.

88. **Nicholson-Weller, A., March, J. P., Rosen, C. E., Spicer, D. B., and Austen, K. F.,** Surface membrane expression by human leukocytes and platelets of decay-accelerating factor, a regulatory protein of the complement system, *Blood,* 65, 1237, 1985.

89. **Nicholson-Weller, A., Spicer, D. B., and Austen, K. F.,** Deficiency of the complement regulatory protein, ''decay-accelerating factor'', on membranes of granulocytes, monocytes and platelets in paroxysmal nocturnal hemoglobinuria, *N. Engl. J. Med.,* 312, 1091, 1985.

90. **Pangburn, M. K., Schreiber, R. D., Trombold, J. S., and Müller-Eberhard, H. J.,** Paroxysmal nocturnal hemoglobinuria: Deficiency in Factor H-like functions of the abnormal erythrocytes, *J. Exp. Med.,* 157, 1971, 1983.

91. **Nicholson-Weller, A., March, J. P., Rosenfeld, S. I., and Austen, K. F.,** Affected erythrocytes of patients with paroxysmal nocturnal hemoglobinuria are deficient in the complement regulatory protein, decay-accelerating factor, *Proc. Nat. Acad. Sci. USA,* 80, 5066, 1983.

92. **Medof, M. E., Kinoshita, T., Silber, R., and Nussenzweig, V.,** Amelioration of lytic abnormalities of paroxysmal nocturnal hemoglobinuria with decay-accelerating factor, *Proc. Nat. Acad. Sci. USA,* 82, 2980, 1985.

93. **Horstman, R. D., Pangburn, M. K., and Müller-Eberhard, H. J.,** Species specificity of recognition by the alternative pathway of complement, *J. Immunol.,* 134, 1101, 1985.

94. **Fearon, D. T.,** Regulation of the amplification C3 convertase of human complement by an inhibitory protein isolated from human erythrocyte membrane, *Proc. Nat. Acad. Sci. USA,* 76, 5867, 1979.

95. **Fearon, D. T.,** Identification of the membrane glycoprotein that is the C3b receptor of the human erythrocyte, polymorphonuclear leukocyte, B lymphocyte, and monocyte, *J. Exp. Med.,* 152, 20, 1980.

96. **Iida, K. and Nussenzweig, V.,** Functional properties of membrane-associated complement receptor CR1, *J. Immunol.,* 130, 1876, 1983.

97. **Medicus, R. G. and Arnaout, M. A.,** Surface restricted control of C3b INA-dependent C3c release from bound C3bi molecules, *Fed. Proc.,* 41, 848 (abstr.), 1982.

98. **Fishelson, Z., Schreiber, R. D., Pangburn, M. K., and Müller-Eberhard, H. J.,** Complement regulatory functions of the C3b receptor: Regulation of C5 convertase activity, in preparation.

99. **Nelson, R. A.,** The immune adherence phenomenon: a hypothetical role of erythrocytes in defense against bacteria and viruses, *Proc. R. Soc. Exp. Biol. Med.,* 49, 55, 1956.

100. **Hansch, G. M., Hammer, C. H., Vanguri, P., and Shin, M. L.,** Homologous species restriction in lysis of erythrocytes by terminal complement proteins, *Proc. Nat. Acad. Sci. USA,* 78, 5118, 1981.

101. **Hu, V. W. and Shin, M. L.,** Species-restricted target cell lysis by human complement: complement-lysed erythrocytes from heterologous and homologous species differ in their ratio of bound to inserted C9, *J. Immunol.,* 133, 2133, 1984.

102. **Yamamoto, K.,** Lytic activity of C5-9 complexes for erythrocytes from species other than sheep: C9 rather than C8 dependent variation in lytic activity, *J. Immunol.,* 119, 1482, 1977.

103. **Zalman, L. S., Wood, L. M., and Müller-Eberhard, H. J.,** Isolation of a human erythrocyte membrane protein capable of inhibiting expression of homologous complement transmembrane channels, *Proc. Natl. Acad. Sci. U.S.A.,* 83, 6975, 1986.

104. **Shin, M., Hansch, G., Hu, V., and Nicholson-Weller, A.,** Membrane factors responsible for homologous species restriction of complement-mediated lysis: DAF operates at the C3/C5 convertase, while a second pronase sensitive factor(s) operates at C8 and C9 reaction, *J. Immunol.,* 136, 1776, 1986.

105. **Okada, H., Okada, N., Yamaguchi, S., Kai, C., and Hoshino, H.,** Resistance to homologous complement of adult T cell leukemia cells, *Complement,* 2, 58, 1985.

106. **Schonermark, S., Rauterberg, E. W., Roelcke, D., Loke, S., and Hansch, G. M.,** A C8-binding protein on the surface of human erythrocytes: the inhibitor of lysis in a homologous system, *Immunobiology, Workshop 12, Complement,* 103, 1985.

107. **Schonermard, S., Rauterberg, E. W., Shin, M. L., Löke, S., Roelcke, D., and Hänsch, G. M.,** Homologous species restriction in lysis of human erythrocytes: a membrane-derived protein with C8-binding capacity functions as an inhibitor, *J. Immunol.,* 136, 1772, 1986.

108. **Jenkins, D. E. and Leddy, J. P.,** Enhanced reactive lysis of paroxysmal nocturnal hemoglobinuria erythrocytes by C5b-9 does not involve increased C7 binding or cell-bound C3b, *J. Immunol.,* 134, 506, 1985.

109. **Houle, J. J. and Hoffmann, E. M.,** Evidence for restriction of the ability of complement to lyse homologous erythrocytes, *J. Immunol.,* 133, 1444, 1984.

110. **Nelson, B. and Ruddy, S.,** Enhancing role of IgG in lysis of rabbit erythrocytes by the alternative pathway of human complement, *J. Immunol.,* 122, 1994, 1979.

111. **Schenkein, H. A. and Ruddy, S.,** The role of immunoglobulins in alternative complement pathway activation by zymosan. 1.Human IgG with specificity for zymosan enhances alternative pathway activation by zymosan, *J. Immunol.,* 126, 7, 1981.

112. **Winkelstein, J. A. and Shin, H. S.,** The role of immunoglobulin in the interaction of pneumococci and the properdin pathway: evidence for its specificity and lack of requirement for the Fc portion of the molecule, *J. Immunol.,* 112, 1635, 1974.

113. **Sissons, J. G. P., Oldstone, M. B. A., and Schreiber, R. D.,** Antibody-independent activation of the alternative complement pathway by measles virus-infected cells, *Proc. Nat. Acad. Sci. USA,* 77, 559, 1980.

114. **Theofilopoulos, A. N. and Perrin, L. H.,** Binding of components of the properdin system to cultured human lymphoblastoid cells and B lymphocytes, *J. Exp. Med.,* 143, 271, 1976.

115. **Fries, L. F., Gaither, T. A., Hammer, C. H., and Frank, M. M.,** C3b covalently bound to IgG demonstrates a reduced rate of inactivation by Factors H and I, *J. Exp. Med.,* 160, 1640, 1984.

116. **Alper, C. A. and Rosen, F. S.,** Inherited deficiencies of complement proteins in man, *Springer Semin. Immunopathol.,* 7, 251, 1984.

117. **Pangburn, M. K.,** The alternative pathway, in *An Introduction to the Complement System,* Ross, G. D., Ed., Academic Press, Orlando, Florida. Chap. 2, 1986.

Chapter 4

# DECAY ACCELERATING FACTOR AND THE DEFECT OF PAROXYSMAL NOCTURNAL HEMOGLOBINURIA

**M. Edward Medof**

## TABLE OF CONTENTS

# I. INTRODUCTION

Upon activation of the complement cascade by a target of immune attack, C4b and C3b fragments associate covalently with molecules on the target's surface (reviewed in References 1 and 2). Once bound, the C4b and C3b polypeptides serve as anchors for the assembly of the C3 convertases, C4b2a and C3bBb. Amplification of C3 activation by these central enzymes of the cascade allows progression of the complement sequence and permits the formation of ligands which facilitate interaction of the target with host inflammatory cells (reviewed in Reference 3). The deposition of C4b and C3b on target surfaces is thus a key step in target processing and disposal.

C4b and C3b polypeptides bind to target constituents in a nonspecific manner. Hydroxyester and amide bonds form (see Chapter 10) when activated thioester groups within the α' chains of nascent C4b and C3b encounter nucleophilic hydroxyl or amino groups contained in surface molecules. Generation of nascent fragments via the classical pathway is localized to the site of antibody binding. However, prior to initial C3b uptake, the alternative pathway-mediated process is unfocused, and nascent C3b formation, in principle, can be initiated wherever appropriate acceptor groups are accessible. Moreover, during complement activation mediated by either pathway, nascent C4b and C3b fragments may condense with nucleophiles on surfaces of nearby host cells as well as on the surface of the target. Strict discrimination between appropriate and inappropriate sites of complement activation, therefore, must occur *following C4b and C3b deposition* to avoid host cell damage.

Despite intimate and prolonged contact with serum complement proteins, host blood cells continuously circumvent autologous complement attack. Efficient control processes providing for this circumvention must therefore be present within host cell membranes to ensure that cell damage does not occur directly via spontaneous (alternative pathway) activation or in the event of recognition by autoantibody, or as a consequence of bystander effects arising from their proximity to targets engaged by complement.

The molecular mechanisms underlying the ability of host cells to recognize autologous C4b and C3b deposition as inappropriate, and to control the function of the deposited fragments so as to avoid consequent cell injury have been subjects of extensive investigations. Important insights into general mechanisms of regulation of bound C3b function have come from studies of factors responsible for differences in alternative pathway activation by different types of substrates.[1,2] These analyses have employed heterologous erythrocytes and other foreign particles, e.g., bacteria or zymosan, and data derived from them have accounted for many of the variables which regulate efficiency of complement activation on such substrates. C3b function on foreign particles is governed primarily by susceptibility of the deposited C3b polypeptides to the action of serum factor H (see Chapter 10). When the foreign particles are activators of the cascade [e.g., rabbit erythrocytes (E$^r$), zymosan, or E. coli], the binding affinity of Factor H for the deposited C3b is low and the C3 convertase, C3bBb, can be assembled. The removal or addition of certain constituents from particle surfaces prior to C3b deposition alters the affinity of factor H binding and the resultant efficiency of C3bBb formation. For example, prior desialization of nonactivating sheep or mouse erythrocytes (E$^{sh}$ or E$^{mo}$) both diminishes the affinity of factor H binding to the deposited C3b and converts the cells into activators.[4,5] Conversely, coupling of heparin glycosaminoglycan to zymosan facilitates factor H binding to C3b deposited on the zymosan and diminishes the activating efficiency of the particles.[6]

Information gained from studies of complement activation on foreign particles, however, has not been sufficient to account for experimental observations made in studies of complement activation on host cells. The finding that the presence of sialic acid in cell membranes is associated with low affinity factor H binding to cell-bound C3b, and the fact that human erythrocytes (E$^{hu}$) are rich in sialic acid while human complement activating E$^r$ are not, suggested that the higher sialic acid content of $E^{hu}$ could explain the greater resistance of human cells to lysis in autologous serum. Desialization of $E^{hu}$, however, neither reduces the affinity of factor H binding nor enhances the susceptibility of $E^{hu}$ to lysis in autologous serum,[5] indicating that other factors must be involved.

## II. HISTORICAL

The possibility that a distinct entity inhibitory to complement activation might reside in the membranes of host cells was first suggested by Hoffman in 1969.[7,8] He demonstrated that lysis of antibody-sensitized sheep erythrocyte intermediates ($E^{sh}A$) in guinea pig serum could be markedly inhibited by addition of 1% deoxycholate or 20% butanol extracts of $E^{hu}$ stroma to the intermediates. Inhibitory activity in the extracts was localized in the aqueous phase and could be recovered in a narrow band following preparative electrophoresis. Butanol extraction at high ionic strength yielded an $E^{hu}$ fraction (designated I-H) that appeared to bind to the $E^{sh}$, interfering with lysis at all steps of the cascade and that gave a single arc upon immunoelectrophoresis (IEP) with rabbit anti-$E^{hu}$ stromal antiserum. Extraction at low ionic strength yielded an $E^{hu}$ fraction (designated I-L) that selectively inhibited $E^{sh}AC142$, $E^{sh}AC1423$, and $E^{sh}AC14235$ and that with the same antiserum gave two arcs on IEP, one of which appeared to correspond to the arc observed with the high ionic strength product. Although Hoffman incorrectly speculated that the inhibitory activity resembled C3, he suggested it might serve as a control device to reduce hemolysis of cells inadvertently sensitized by antibody in vivo. In subsequent studies,[9] he showed that a parallel activity able to inhibit lysis of $E^{sh}$ by guinea pig complement could be detected in extracts of $E^r$ and of guinea pig erythrocytes ($E^{gp}$) but not those of five other species. Because the low ionic strength activity (I-L) resembled a serum factor described by Opferkuch, Loos and Borsos[10] which accelerated decay of $E^{sh}AC142$ and which was termed decay accelerating factor (DAF), Hoffman adopted the same nomenclature and designated his activity cellular DAF.

Further work on cellular DAF awaited characterization of the serum regulatory proteins [factor H, C4 binding protein (C4bp), and the C3b/C4b inactivator (factor I)] and elucidation of their roles in regulation of the cascade in the fluid phase, and in initiation of alternative pathway activation on foreign substrates (see above). The inability of the actions of the serum regulators to account for the capacity of desialated $E^{hu}$ to circumvent lysis by human complement redirected attention back to cell membranes. The search for $E^{hu}$ surface constituents that could inhibit alternative pathway activation led to the isolation by Fearon[11] of a 205 kDa glycoprotein (gp205) that could dissociate properdin (P)-stabilized C3bBb and the subsequent identification[12] of gp205 as the $E^{hu}$ C3b/C4b receptor (CR1). The unanticipated detection and purification of CR1 by its ability to inhibit C3 convertase function raised the possibility that this CR1 activity is responsible for host cell protection. It is known that CR1 is expressed in high levels on leukocytes that come into close contact with complement activators, making this hypothesis attractive. The demonstration that CR1 also possesses C4bp-like activity[13,14] and can inhibit formation of classical pathway C3 and C5 convertases, as well as C3bBbP, showed that the molecule is a general complement inhibitor, lending further support to the notion that it could be protective. Human cell types lacking CR1, however, resist lysis even following desialization,[15] arguing that this CR1 activity is not essential and implying the existence of other mechanisms.

The finding that factor H and C4bp-like activities reside in CR1 established the existence of specific membrane-associated factors which can regulate complement activation. In an effort to ascertain the relationship between CR1 and the inhibitory factor(s) termed cellular DAF by Hoffman, Nicholson-Weller, Burge, and Austen extracted $E^{gp}$ (Reference 16) and $E^{hu}$ (Reference 17) stroma with 20% aqueous butanol according to his procedures and purified the active component(s). Sequential chromatographies on DEAE-Sephacel, Hydroxyapatite,

Phenyl-Sepharose, and Trypan Blue-Sepharose revealed that, in the case of the $E^{hu}$ extract, the decay accelerating activity migrates on SDS-PAGE with an apparent $M_r$ of ~70K and that it is distinct from CR1. Hemolytic studies using $E^{sh}$ intermediates bearing classical and alternative pathway C3 convertases suggested that, in contrast to CR1 which is more active in decaying C3bBbP, DAF is more effective in decaying C4b2a. The addition of rabbit antibody raised against each factor neutralized the respective inhibitory activity demonstrating that DAF and CR1 are immunochemically as well as structurally distinct.

## III. DIFFERENTIAL ROLES OF DAF AND CR1 IN REGULATION OF C3b AND C4b

In the isolated state, both cellular DAF and CR1 could be shown to accelerate decay-dissociation of C3bBb and C4b2a. Moreover, in contrast to initial findings with $E^{sh}$ intermediates, DAF and CR1 were shown by Pangburn[18] to have comparable activities in dissociating Bb from zymosan particles bearing C3bBb. The identification of two entities, with similar factor H- and C4bp-like activites in $E^{hu}$ membranes was puzzling and raised questions concerning their respective physiological functions and the reason for the apparent redundancy in their functional properties.

In studies employing $Ni^{++}$-stabilized C3bBb complexes [C3bBb($Ni^{++}$)] assembled on intact $E^{hu}$, Pangburn et al.[18] observed that the decay rate of the enzyme on the $E^{hu}$ surface was 5-fold faster than that on the $E^{sh}$ surface or in the fluid phase. Pretreatment of the $E^{hu}$ with trypsin (1 mg/m$\ell$ at 37°C for 30 min) prior to C3b deposition and convertase formation, inactivated immune adherence activity of the red cells, but had no effect on the shortened half-life of the cell-bound enzyme. Since immune adherence is a CR1-dependent function, this finding suggested that the accelerated enzyme decay rate of $E^{hu}$ was not mediated by CR1. In contrast to the effects of trypsin however, pretreatment of the $E^{hu}$ with pronase (5 mg/m$\ell$ at 37°C for 30 min) not only abolished immune adherence but also abrogated the cell-associated enhancement of convertase decay rate. To more precisely evaluate the role of CR1 and that of DAF in the accelerated decay of C3 convertase complexes assembled on $E^{hu}$ membranes, Pangburn et al. examined the effects of treating $E^{hu}$ bearing C3bBb($Ni^{++}$) with rabbit anti-CR1 or anti-DAF antibodies. Incubation of the $E^{hu}$ intermediates with anti-DAF antibodies increased the half-time of the cell-bound convertase to that of the unregulated fluid-phase enzyme. In contrast, incubation of the cells with anti-CR1 antibodies had no effect on convertase decay rate but completely blocked cleavage of C3b in the presence of serum factor I. The lack of effect of anti-CR1 antibodies on C3bBb decay rate was surprising in view of the marked accelerating effect of isolated CR1 on decay of the enzyme[11,19] and raised the possibility that CR1 might not express this function *in situ*. The association of DAF with convertase decay acceleration and of CR1 with C3b cofactor activity appeared to provide an explanation for the requirement of both factors in cells. Interpretation of the results in this experimental system was complicated, however, by the possibility that the effects of the two regulatory proteins on C3 convertase activity could be mediated by DAF and CR1 molecules within the same or on neighboring $E^{hu}$.

In the initial investigations of DAF function employing $E^{sh}AC142$, it had been assumed that membrane DAF acted similarly to C4bp which inactivates C3 convertase sites by competitively displacing C2a from C4b.[13,14] In experiments designed to directly examine the mechanism of the DAF-mediated reaction,[20] aliquots of highly purified DAF were added to samples of $E^{sh}AC14$, prior to, as well as after the addition of C2, and the effects of the added DAF on the resulting C3 convertase activity on the two cell types compared. Unexpectedly, DAF treatment inhibited the assembly of C3 convertase activity on $E^{sh}AC14$ as markedly as it reduced the activity of preassembled C4b2a complexes on $E^{sh}AC142$. The curve of convertase inhibition as a function of DAF dose was identical for the two intermediates. Extensive washing of the DAF-treated $E^{sh}AC14$ prior to C2 addition did not diminish the DAF inhibitory effect. To establish whether the inhibition of convertase assembly on the $E^{sh}AC14$ was due to association of the added DAF with cell-bound C4b fragments, the effects of DAF treatment on $E^{sh}A$ (prior to addition of C1 and C4) as well as on unsensitized $E^{sh}$ were investigated. Comparable impairment in the efficiency of subsequent C4b2a assembly was observed in all cases. The findings, taken together, suggested that DAF was interacting with the $E^{sh}$ membrane and that in the conventional C4b2a decay assay, it was incorporating into the cells before exerting its inhibitory effect. To test this hypothesis and to quantitate the efficiency of the inhibitory effect, experiments were performed using $^{125}I$-labeled DAF. These studies showed that DAF protein was in fact associating with the $E^{sh}$ membrane and that as few as 50 to 70 incorporated DAF molecules had a striking effect in inhibiting subsequent assembly of C4b2a. NP40 extraction of the $E^{sh}$ stroma and analysis of the extract by SDS-PAGE/radioautography revealed the presence of the 70 kDalton $^{125}I$-DAF band.

To investigate the characteristics of the incorporation process, an impure radiolabeled DAF preparation was added to $E^{sh}$ intermediates and extracts of cells analyzed for incorporated radiolabel. $^{125}I$-DAF was taken up but the contaminants remained in the incubation medium, indicating that the process was selective. The incorporated $^{125}I$-DAF could not be removed by washing the cells with high salt (1M NaCl). The incorporation process required 37°C for 20 to 30 min for an optimal inhibitory effect. The rate of $^{125}I$-DAF uptake into pronase- or trypsin-pretreated $E^{sh}$ was the same as into untreated $E^{sh}$, suggesting that protein membrane receptors were not involved. The DAF incorporation was blocked, however, by the addition of serum lipoproteins (HDL or LDL) or of serum albumin to the reaction mixture. Of importance, the inhibitory effect of these proteins could be observed only before and not after addition of the isolated DAF to the $E^{sh}$. Collectively the data were consistent with direct interaction of a hydrophobic domain of the DAF molecule with the $E^{sh}$ lipid bilayer. The temperature dependence of the process suggested that it required membrane motility, and the inability of lipoproteins or albumin to interfere with DAF function after cell uptake implied that the domain of DAF which was interacting with these proteins was inserting into the lipid membrane. The capacity of a small number of incorporated DAF molecules to inhibit C4b2a complexes subsequently assembled randomly on the DAF-bearing cells indicated that, once inserted, the incorporated DAF molecules must be mobile within the plane of the cell membrane in order to interact with C4b2a formed elsewhere on the surface of the cells.

The ability to insert DAF into $E^{sh}$ membranes before or after addition of individual complement components permitted analysis of the precise effect of DAF on each step of the complement cascade (independently of CR1). Treatment of $E^{sh}A$ with highly purified DAF markedly inhibited lysis of the cells in guinea pig or human complement.[20] The inhibitory effect was completely blocked by monospecific anti-DAF antibody, and treatment of the cells with purified glycophorin A had no effect. Determination of the specificity of DAF in this inhibition was important to establish, in view of reports by Okada et al.[21,22] that erythrocytes could be protected from lysis with heterologous complement by pretreatment of the red cells with partially purified glycophorin preparations homologous to the source of complement used. The presence of incorporated DAF in $E^{sh}A$ had no effect on the efficiency of uptake of C1 or of C4. The incorporated DAF molecules, however, completely blocked the uptake of C2. On DAF-treated $E^{sh}AC14_{lim}$ cells, the DAF inhibitory effect could not be overcome by augmenting C2 concentration, regardless of the concentration used. These findings appeared to explain earlier observations by Brown et al.[23] that following antibody sensitization, $E^{hu}$ accumulate C1 and C4, but do not consume C2. The effect of DAF sensitization on alternative pathway activation was similar. The presence of incorporated DAF in $E^{sh}AC43$ completely blocked the uptake of factor B, and the block could not be reversed by augmenting factor B concentration. The DAF inhibitory effect was similar in the presence of P. The presence of DAF in $E^{sh}AC143$ cells also completely prevented the formation of C5 convertase sites. Taken together, the inhibitory action of DAF in preventing uptake of C2 by bound C4b and of factor B by bound C3b appeared to partially explain Hoffman's original observations[8] regarding the selective inactivation by I-L or $E^{sh}AC142$, $E^{sh}AC1423$, and $E^{sh}AC14235$. The finding that following membrane incorporation, exogenous DAF abolished the hemolytic activity of C4b and C3b sites on $E^{sh}AC14$ and $E^{sh}AC43$ suggested that endogenous cell-associated DAF molecules could function to preclude the assembly of amplification convertases as well as to accelerate decay of convertases after formation. Initial prevention of convertase assembly provided a mechanism to avoid C2 and factor B consumption, as well as C3 activation.

The efficiency with which incorporated DAF molecules inhibited the activities of subsequently deposited C4b or C3b fragments suggested that DAF functions *intrinsically* in cells, i.e., acts upon C4b and C3b molecules deposited on the same membrane. To investigate this issue and to determine if membrane-associated DAF can also function *extrinsically*, i.e., inhibit C4b and C3b fragments deposited on adjacent cells or other substrates, three types of experiments were performed. In the first, DAF-treated $E^{sh}AC142$ were suspended into progressively larger volumes of buffer and rate of decay of C4b2a activity compared. As would be predicted for an intrinsic mode of DAF action, no reductions in decay rate with cell dilution were observed. In the second set of studies, DAF-treated $E^{sh}A$ were mixed with an equal number of untreated $E^{sh}AC142$, and the effect of the DAF-containing cells on the decay rate of C4b2a on the untreated intermediates was assessed. Even though control studies showed that the presence of DAF in the DAF-treated $E^{sh}A$ markedly inhibited formation of C4b2a on these cells, C4b2a decay rate on the untreated $E^{sh}AC142$ in the presence of the DAF-containing $E^{sh}A$ was identical to that in the absence of the DAF-containing cells. In the third set of studies, intact $E^{hu}$ were used as a source of membrane DAF. The $E^{hu}$ were added in increasing numbers to $E^{sh}AC142$, and the effect of the added cells on C4b2a decay rate on the $E^{sh}$ intermediates was measured. The $E^{hu}$ inhibited C4b2a enzymatic activity on the $E^{sh}$ intermediates in a dose-dependent fashion but the inhibitory activity was unaffected by anti-DAF monoclonal antibodies, whereas it was completely reversed by anti-CR1 monoclonals, indicating that the extrinsic inhibitory effect was mediated by CR1. The results thus indicated that DAF functions only within the membranes of the same cells which bear C3 convertases, i.e., it is strictly an intrinsic inhibitor (Figure 1). CR1, in contrast, can interact with convertases on neighboring cells. The assignment of intrinsic convertase inhibitory activity to DAF and extrinsic activity to CR1 appeared to further clarify the respective roles of the two factors. To ascertain the overall influence of membrane DAF activity on complement activation on cell surfaces, increasing amounts of DAF were incorporated into $E^r$, and the effect on lysis of the activators in $Mg^{++}$-EGTA human serum examined. The amount of human complement required for lysis of the $E^r$ increased as a function of the DAF dose added to the cells.

The ability of membrane-associated DAF to prevent deposited C4b and C3b fragments from not only serving as sites for the assembly of C4b2a and C3bBb but also from consuming available C2 or factor B in the reaction mixture suggested that DAF molecules might exert their inhibitory activity by interacting with C3b and C4b polypeptides in the membrane and interfering with their ability to take up C2 and factor B zymogens. Incubation of DAF-treated $E^{sh}AC14$ with anti-DAF antibodies restored initial C4b hemolytic activity to the intermediates, indicating that the inhibition of C4b by DAF does not irreversibly alter C4b structure.[20] In accordance with this interpretation, SDS-PAGE/autoradiographic analysis of DAF-treated $[^{125}I]$C4-labeled $E^{sh}AC14_{lim}$ and $[^{125}I]$C3-labeled $E^{sh}AC43_{lim}$ (on which hemolytic activity in each case was completely blocked) revealed only intact C4b and C3b peptides.

The mechanism of DAF action was further investigated in two studies employing different

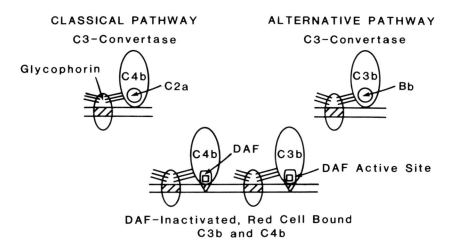

FIGURE 1. Inhibition of C4b and C3b fragments by DAF when C4b or C3b is bound to host cells. C4b or C3b that is bound to a target surface is accessible to C2 or factor B, respectively, and the C3 convertases, C4b2a and C3bBb, are able to assemble. C4b or C3b that is bound to a host cell (e.g., a red cell usually via glycophorin) is blocked by the association of DAF, and the convertases thus cannot assemble.

experimental approaches. In one, Kinoshita et al.[24] added increasing amounts of purified [125]I-labeled DAF to E^shAC14 and E^shAC43_lim[3] prepared with increasing amounts of C4 and C3, respectively. After incubation of the DAF-treated intermediates with cross-linking agents and extraction of the cell membranes with NP40, DAF in the extracts was immunoprecipitated with anti-DAF antibodies and the immunoprecipitates analyzed on SDS-PAGE gels for DAF conjugates with C4 and C3 peptides. These analyses revealed high $M_r$ C4 and C3 specific bands which increased in intensity with C4b and C3b dose, directly demonstrating association of DAF molecules with C4b and C3b fragments within cell membranes. In the other study, Pangburn[25] added increasing concentrations of soluble C3b, Bb, C3bBb, C3bB, C4b, or C4b2a to a fixed concentration of purified DAF and examined the respective abilities of the various proteins or complexes to inhibit DAF-mediated dissociation of [125]I]Bb-labeled C3bBb preassembled on zymosan particles. Inhibition of DAF-mediated decay acceleration was greater with C3bBb, C3bB, and C4b2a than with C3b or C4b alone, whereas in parallel analyses of CR1- and factor H-mediated decay acceleration, inhibition by the biomolecular complexes and by uncomplexed C3b and C4b fragments were comparable. These observations suggested that DAF may recognize conformational determinants in C3 convertases. Although such recognition could provide an explanation for the ability of a small number of membrane-associated DAF molecules to inhibit the function of a large number of deposited C4b or C3b fragments, the relationship of the findings to those obtained in the more physiologic experimental system of Kinoshita et al.[24] and the mechanisms by which C2 and factor B consumption are prevented remain to be further clarified.

## IV. DEFICIENCY OF DAF IN PAROXYSMAL NOCTURNAL HEMOGLOBINURIA (PNH)

PNH is an acquired hemolytic disorder in which blood cells are abnormally sensitive to the lytic action of autologous complement. The disease is thought to result from the clonal expansion of blood cell progenitors altered by somatic mutation (reviewed in Reference 26). Affected blood elements accumulate increased numbers of C3b fragments on their surfaces in vivo and take up excessive amounts of C3b in vitro following sensitization with antibody.

The findings that DAF and CR1 possess factor H-like activities raised the possibility that an abnormality in one or both of these factors might account for the exaggerated C3b uptake and heightened complement sensitivity of affected cells in this condition.

Comparative analyses by Pangburn et al.[18] of the decay rate of preassembled C3 convertase complexes on PNH and normal $E^{hu}$ [using the assays described above employing $C3bBb(Ni^{++})$] revealed that the half-time of the cell-bound enzyme on PNH $E^{hu}$ was 3.5-fold greater than that on normal $E^{hu}$, an extent of stabilization that approached the prolonged half-time of the (presumably) unregulated enzyme on $E^{sh}$. The investigations additionally found that assembly of the enzyme on PNH $E^{hu}$ was 3-fold more efficient than on normal $E^{hu}$. In accordance with these findings, following nephritic factor-stabilized deposition of fluorescein isothio-cyanate (FITC)-labeled C3b on unseparated PNH $E^{hu}$, fluorescence activitated cell sorter (FACS) analyses showed that affected $E^{hu}$ took up 8-fold more C3b than unaffected $E^{hu}$ (Reference 27). In addition to the diminution in C3 convertase decay rate that was observed on the PNH $E^{hu}$, analyses of bound C3b structure on the PNH $E^{hu}$ following incubation with factor I (in the absence of added factor H) revealed reduced conversion to iC3b. In one patient a 100-fold higher concentration of factor I was required to obtain a rate of C3b cleavage on the affected $E^{hu}$ equivalent to that on normal $E^{hu}$. Treatment (prior to C3b deposition) of the PNH $E^{hu}$ with trypsin (under conditions which abolished CR1 immune-adherence activity of normal $E^{hu}$) had no further damping effect on the diminished rate of C3b cleavage on the PNH $E^{hu}$, suggesting that no CR1 cofactor activity was present in the membranes of the affected PNH $E^{hu}$. In support of this suggestion, the PNH $E^{hu}$ took up lesser amounts of CR1 ligand (C3b dimer) than did normal $E^{hu}$. The results of the several studies indicated that affected PNH $E^{hu}$ were markedly deficient in membrane associated factor H-like activities compared to normal $E^{hu}$. The defects, in the PNH $E^{hu}$, of factor I cofactor activity and of C3b dimer uptake, in addition to the defect of convertase decay acceleration, raised the possibility that abnormalities in both CR1 and DAF were involved in the complement sensitivity of affected PNH cells.

Using assays employing anti-DAF antibodies, Nicholson-Weller et al.[28] and Pangburn et al.,[18] in simultaneous investigations, examined endogenous DAF protein in PNH $E^{hu}$. Nicholson-Weller et al.[28] surface labeled $E^{hu}$ from normal individuals and three PNH patients with $^{125}I$, added anti-DAF antibodies to NP40 extracts of the stroma, and analyzed the immunoprecipitated DAF by SDS-PAGE/radioautography. Two of the patients studied had >90% type III $E^{hu}$ [15 to 25-fold more sensitive to complement than normal $E^{hu}$ as assessed by the complement lysis sensitivity (CLS) assay of Rosse and Dacie[29]], and one had >90% type II $E^{hu}$ (3 to 5 fold more sensitive). Anti-DAF precipitates of normal $E^{hu}$ stroma exhibited $^{125}I$-labeled 70 kDalton DAF while those from the PNH patients with type III $E^{hu}$ exhibited no DAF, and that from the patient with type II $E^{hu}$ exhibited markedly reduced amounts of labeled DAF. In contrast, anti-CR1 precipitates of stroma from all the PNH patients exhibited $^{125}I$-labeled CR1 which, in one of the patients with type III cells, was present in normal levels. In another set of experiments, the normal and PNH $E^{hu}$ were incubated with a limited concentration of anti-DAF antibodies and residual antibody titer in the supernatants assayed. While $3.3 \times 10^7$ normal $E^{hu}$ adsorbed 30% of the antibody, $2 \times 10^8$ PNH type II $E^{hu}$ were required to adsorb the same amount of antibody, and $2 \times 10^8$ type III PNH $E^{hu}$ adsorbed no antibody. Pangburn et al.[18] $^{125}I$-surface labeled unfractionated $E^{hu}$ from a PNH patient (T. J.) with 44% affected $E^{hu}$, separated the complement-sensitive and -insensitive $E^{hu}$ subpopulations by acid lysis, and examined DAF in NP40 extracts of the stroma of the two $E^{hu}$ populations by immunoprecipitation followed by SDS-PAGE/radioautography. In addition to a nonspecifically precipitated 90 kDalton band thought to correspond to $E^{hu}$ Band 3 protein, the complement-insensitive $E^{hu}$ population showed a DAF band (73 kDalton in their system) similar to that in normal $E^{hu}$, while the complement-sensitive cells showed only the 90 kDalton band and no DAF band. CR1 was detected in the abnormal cells by an enzyme-linked immunoassay, but the number of CR1 per affected PNH $E^{hu}$ was 40% of that of a pool of five normal $E^{hu}$. The results of the two studies thus indicated that affected PNH $E^{hu}$ are DAF-deficient and suggested that this molecular defect could underlie the abnormal complement sensitivity of the affected cells. The differing results in the two studies concerning CR1, however, left the role of CR1 deficiency in the abnormality of PNH unanswered. Additionally, the finding in the first study of an apparent partial reduction in DAF in type II $E^{hu}$ raised the question of whether the more profound DAF deficiency observed in the type III $E^{hu}$ might account for the markedly greater complement sensitivity of PNH type III cells than of type II cells in the CLS assay.

The abilities to selectively block DAF function in normal $E^{hu}$ with anti-DAF antibodies and to restore DAF activity to DAF-deficient PNH $E^{hu}$ with isolated DAF [20] permitted direct analysis of the role of DAF deficiency in the heightened sensitivity of PNH cells to complement. A characteristic abnormality found in PNH is susceptibility of affected $E^{hu}$ to lysis in (pH 6.5) acidified serum. The acid lysis susceptibility as measured in a hemolytic assay termed the Ham test[30] is a major criterion in the laboratory diagnosis of the disorder.[26] In studies by Pangburn et al.[18] pretreatment of normal $E^{hu}$ with pronase rendered the normal cells susceptible to acid lysis, while pretreatment of the normal $E^{hu}$ with trypsin, which abrogates CR1 function, had no effect in this assay. To determine if induction of acid lysis sensitivity of normal $E^{hu}$ by pronase was in fact mediated via an effect on membrane DAF and to establish if acid lysis susceptibility of affected PNH $E^{hu}$ is a consequence of DAF deficiency, the effects of anti-DAF treatment of normal $E^{hu}$ and DAF treatment PNH $E^{hu}$ on acid lysis sensitivity as measured by the Ham test were investigated. Exposure of normal $E^{hu}$ to monospecific anti-DAF antibodies rendered the normal cells PNH-like in acid lysis sensitivity.[31,32] Conversely, reconstitution of affected PNH $E^{hu}$ with exogenous DAF reduced the characteristic acid lysis sensitivity of the PNH $E^{hu}$.[32] The ameliorating effect of the DAF treatment of the PNH $E^{hu}$, however, was incomplete. Uptake of $\sim$ 600 DAF molecules per $E^{hu}$, as determined by immunoradiometric assay of NP40 extracts of the treated cells, decreased the complement sensitivity in 30% acidified serum by only $\sim$ 65%. Although the amount of incorporated DAF corresponded to only 20% of the endogenous DAF level (see below) in normal $E^{hu}$ and the failure to achieve complete correction could therefore have resulted from insufficient DAF incorporation, this finding raised the possibility that, in the membrane of the PNH $E^{hu}$, another primary or secondary defect might be present which could preclude complete reversal of the abnormality by DAF. Of relevance, Shin et al.[33] reported that acidification of complement not only increases the affinity of C3bBb interaction but also augments the formation and cell binding of C5b6.

To investigate the consequence of DAF deficiency of PNH $E^{hu}$ on the early steps of complement activation on the cells under physiological conditions, the comparative efficiencies of assembly of classical pathway C3 convertase on affected PNH $E^{hu}$ and normal $E^{hu}$ were quantitated, and the influence of DAF reconstitution on C3 convertase assembly on the PNH $E^{hu}$ evaluated.[32] For this purpose, preliminary titrations were performed with anti-DAF-treated normal $E^{hu}$ to establish the number of deposited C4b and concentration of C2 required for lysis of the cells upon addition of (guinea pig) C3-9 in the absence of DAF activity. Whereas no lysis of buffer- or anti-CR1-treated normal $E^{hu}$AC1 was induced following deposition of $16 \times 10^3$ C4b per cell, 15% lysis of anti-DAF-treated $E^{hu}$AC1 occurred following deposition of only $1 \times 10^3$ C4b per cell and complete lysis was induced by $6 \times 10^3$ deposited C4b per cell. Similarly, while control normal $E^{hu}$AC14 bearing $23 \times 10^3$ C4b per cell showed no lysis following treatment with 1:10 C2, anti-DAF treated-$E^{hu}$AC14 bearing $19 \times 10^3$ C4b per cell gave 50% lysis upon addition of 1:160 C2 and >95% lysis following addition of 1:40 C2. When the latter titration was repeated with PNH $E^{hu}$AC14 bearing $19 \times 10^3$ C4b per cell, the curve of percent lysis as a function of added C2 concentration paralleled that of the anti-DAF treated normal $E^{hu}$AC14. Reconstitution of the PNH $E^{hu}$AC14 at 30°C for 1 hr with purified DAF (140 ng/m$\ell$) reduced the assembly of C4b2a on the affected cells to near normal levels irrespective of the added C2 concentration. These findings provided further evidence that restriction of autologous C4b2a formation and subsequent C3b deposition on normal E$^{hu}$ is mediated by DAF, and demonstrated directly that DAF deficiency in affected PNH E$^{hu}$ is causally related to the exaggerated C3b uptake which characterizes the abnormal cells.

## V. DISTRIBUTION OF DAF IN BLOOD CELLS OF NORMAL INDIVIDUALS AND PATIENTS WITH PNH

The demonstration of the crucial role of DAF in protecting E$^{hu}$ from complement-mediated damage raised the questions of whether the membrane molecule might serve the same function in other blood elements in intimate contact with serum complement proteins. This question was investigated in two simultaneous studies, one employing assays based on monoclonal anti-DAF antibodies and the other, assays based on polyclonal antibodies.

In the first set of studies carried out by Kinoshita et al.,[34] three murine clones (IA10, IIH6, and VIIIA7) producing anti-DAF antibodies were identified by selective reactivity with 70 kDalton DAF on Western blots of impure glycophorin-containing E$^{hu}$ DAF preparations. Upon addition to DAF-treated E$^{sh}$AC14, the pooled antibodies reversed DAF-mediated inhibition of C4b sites on the intermediates. The antibodies did not interfere with each other in binding to DAF immobilized on plates, indicating that each was directed against a different DAF epitope. The three monoclonals were used to examine various blood cell types for DAF, employing a number of different methods. Immunoprecipitation of NP40 extracts of PMN, blood monocytes, and tonsillar B- and T-lymphocytes with IA10-bearing protein-A sepharose, yielded a DAF band in each case, indicating that each of the cell types contained DAF. The DAF band was recognized on Western blots by $^{125}$I-labeled IIH6 and VIIIA7, as well as by IA10, demonstrating that the DAF from all cell types shared at least three epitopes with E$^{hu}$ DAF. The apparent M$_r$ of the DAF recovered from each cell type varied however; DAF from PMN and platelets was ~ 5 kDalton larger than E$^{hu}$ DAF, while DAF from monocytes and lymphocytes was of intermediate size. Quantitations of DAF concentrations in the NP40 extracts of the various cell types with a two-site radioimmunometric assay, employing IA10 as capturing reagent and $^{125}$I-labeled IIH6 as revealing reagent, showed that PMN and monocytes contained the largest amounts of DAF, 85 and $68 \times 10^3$ molecules per cell, respectively, while B-lymphocytes contained $54 \times 10^3$, T-lymphocytes $9 \times 10^3$, E$^{hu}$ $3.3 \times 10^3$, and platelets $2.1 \times 10^3$ DAF molecules per cell. Analysis of the surface expression of DAF on each of the cell types by flow cytometry revealed that, within each cell type, DAF levels varied widely in individual cells. The levels were normally distributed in PMN and monocytes, while in lymphocytes some cells overlapped with the negative control, and in E$^{hu}$ the distribution was skewed with some cells having relatively high levels. It was noted that the relative fluorescence intensity of PMN following anti-DAF staining was lower than expected from the DAF content of the PMN as determined by radioimmunometric assay, suggesting the possibility that some of the PMN DAF was intracellular. The presence of an intracellular DAF pool in resting PMN was verified in subsequent studies by Berger et al[35] which showed that, upon activation of the cells with N-formyl-methionyl-leucyl-phenylalanine (f-MLP) or C5a, intracellular DAF contained in PMN translocates to the PMN surface in a process mediated by changes in intracellular [Ca$^{++}$].

In the second set of studies carried out by Nicholson-Weller et al.,[36] rabbit anti-DAF IgG raised against E$^{hu}$ DAF was purified on Protein A Sepharose and used without removal of contaminating anti-glycophorin A, since glycophorin is expressed only by E$^{hu}$. F(ab')$_2$ fragments of the anti-DAF IgG were employed to examine blood cells for DAF by flow cytometry and in direct binding assays, and intact anti-DAF IgG used to analyze NP40 extracts of $^{125}$I-surface-labeled cells by immunoprecipitation. FACS analyses of buffy coat cells yielded results essentially similar to those above. All cell populations showed a unimodal distribution of DAF on their surfaces with the highest fluorescence intensity in the case of monocytes and with a nonuniform distribution of DAF in the case of $E^{hu}$ and lymphocytes. Although difficulty was encountered in distinguishing specific anti-DAF fluorescence on platelets, Scatchard analyses of the binding of $^{125}$I-anti-DAF to platelets indicated 2240 molecules of anti-DAF F(ab')$_2$ bound at saturation, yielding a value for DAF comparable to that obtained by Kinoshita et al..[34] Examination of the molecular forms of DAF on the different cell types following addition of anti-DAF IgG to NP40 extracts of $^{125}$I-surface-labeled cells and analysis of the immunoprecipitates on SDS-PAGE/radioautography revealed that each cell type expressed a single DAF species. Consistent with the results above, in a gel system in which the apparent $M_r$ of $E^{hu}$ DAF was 75K, PMN DAF migrated with an apparent $M_r$ of 83K while monocyte and lymphocyte DAF migrated with an $M_r$ of 78 to 79K, and platelet DAF 75 to 80K.

Application by Nicholson-Weller et al.[37] of the FACS and immunoprecipitation methodology to analyses of buffy coat cells from PNH patients revealed that affected PMN, monocytes, and platelets, as well as $E^{hu}$ are DAF-deficient in this disorder. In contrast to cells from normal subjects, which exhibited a unimodal distribution of anti-DAF fluorescent intensity, PMN and blood monocytes of four PNH patients exhibited two distinct populations of anti-DAF F(ab')$_2$ fluorescence, one overlapping with the nonimmune control. The percentage of DAF-negative PMN and monocytes from the four patients correlated with the severity of PNH and was as high as 99% in one patient with 50% type III $E^{hu}$. SDS-PAGE/autoradiographic analysis of anti-DAF immunoprecipitates of NP40 extracts of $^{125}$I-surface-labeled PMN from this patient revealed no DAF antigen. FACS analyses of platelets from three of the patients did not resolve DAF-negative and -positive platelet populations but showed reduced mean fluorescence. As found with PMN, however, immunoprecipitation of extracts of platelets from one of the patients revealed no DAF protein under conditions in which DAF was recovered from normal platelets. Analyses of lymphocytes from the four patients yielded equivocal results. The average mean fluorescence of the patients' lymphocytes was 241 as compared to 285 for (patient) control cells and 329 for normal cells; and the proportions of DAF-negative cells were 42% as compared to 31% and 23%, respectively. The finding that DAF deficiency in PNH involves PMN, monocytes, and platelets, as well as $E^{hu}$, argued that the cell alteration leading to this defect arises in a stem cell. The inability to demonstrate involvement of lymphocytes suggested that the defect might originate at the level of pluripotent rather than more primitive totipotent stem cells.

Analyses by Kinoshita et al[34] of buffy coat cells of PNH patients using methodology based on monoclonal anti-DAF antibodies demonstrated that affected subpopulations of platelets could be distinguished and that in some PNH patients lymphocytes were normal, while in others, lymphocytes were abnormal. In one patient (SB) with 60% type III $E^{hu}$ and with (complement-insensitive) type I $E^{hu}$ which showed DAF levels comparable to normal $E^{hu}$, 77% of PMN, 80% of monocytes, and 78% of platelets segregated on FACS in DAF-deficient peaks which overlapped with the negative controls. The lymphocytes from this patient appeared normal with respect to anti-DAF staining. In two other patients (GC and VR) with 40% and 30% affected type III $E^{hu}$, respectively, PMN, monocytes and platelets were entirely DAF-deficient by FACS. The absence of DAF in platelets of one of the patients was confirmed by two-site immunoradiometric assay. In these two patients, DAF levels on lymphocytes were undetectable or very low. It was noted that, while affected $E^{hu}$ of these two patients and of the former patient were both totally DAF-deficient, in contrast to type I $E^{hu}$ of the former patient (SB) which showed normal DAF levels, the type I $E^{hu}$ of the latter two patients showed markedly reduced DAF levels compared to $E^{hu}$ of normal controls.

These observations by Kinoshita[34] concerning these three patients provided further evidence that PNH cells arise from the clonal expansion of abnormal bone marrow progenitors. The finding that lymphocytes were uninvolved in one patient but were profoundly DAF-deficient in two others suggested that the defect giving rise to DAF deficiency can occur in totipotent cells as well as more committed pluripotent cells. The findings of the two studies that leukocytes and platelets as well as $E^{hu}$ are affected by the defect underlying PNH may help to explain longstanding clinical observations that the hemolysis that occurs in PNH is frequently associated with venous thromboses and/or leukocyte abnormalities[24] and may account for previous experimental findings that the in vitro uptake of C3b by PNH platelets and PMN is greater than normal.[38,39]

## VI. NATURE OF THE PNH DEFECT

A number of different functional abnormalities of the membranes of PNH $E^{hu}$ have been described.[26] Affected $E^{hu}$ are not only abnormal with respect to their inability to restrict autologous C3b uptake, but are also characteristically deficient in membrane acetylcholinesterase (AChE) activity. Moreover, while type II $E^{hu}$ (found in some PNH patients) are 5-fold more sensitive to complement than normal $E^{hu}$, type III $E^{hu}$ (present in the majority of PNH patients) are 25-fold more sensitive. The type III $E^{hu}$ are markedly more susceptible than normal $E^{hu}$ to bystander lysis by fluid phase terminal pathway complexes (i.e., C5b-9). There is experimental evidence indicating that the resistance of normal $E^{hu}$ to this passive lysis results from a natural capacity of normal $E^{hu}$ membranes to restrict insertion and/or polymerization of autologous C9[40,41] and that the vulnerability of PNH type III $E^{hu}$ is due to a defect in membrane restriction at this level[42,43] as well as at the level of C3. The detection of DAF deficiency in affected PNH cells raised the question of whether the DAF defect was somehow involved in the AChE abnormality and whether it played a role in the heightened sensitivity of type III PNH $E^{hu}$ to bystander lysis as well as in the exaggerated uptake of C3b.

Examination of the relationship between the DAF defect and the AChE abnormality of affected PNH $E^{hu}$ was facilitated by the development by Fambrough and Rosenberry[44] of murine monoclonal antibodies directed against $E^{hu}$ AChE. Using these antibodies, Chow and Rosse[45] showed that the defect in AChE enzyme activity in PNH $E^{hu}$ resided in the complement-sensitive $E^{hu}$ subpopulation and that the complement-sensitive cells contained no anti-AChE precipitable protein. In collaborative studies[46] undertaken to establish whether AChE deficiency coincided in the same cells as DAF deficiency, the cell distribution of the two defects among complement-sensitive and -insensitive PNH $E^{hu}$ were correlated by purifying AChE-negative $E^{hu}$ and analyzing them for DAF expression. The AChE-negative $E^{hu}$ subpopulations of the PNH patients were isolated by addition of AChE antibody to unfractionated PNH $E^{hu}$, passage of the antibody-treated $E^{hu}$ through protein-A columns, and collection of the nonadherent cells. Isolation of the AChE-negative $E^{hu}$ subpopulations from eight PNH patients by this method and analysis of the purified cells for DAF by two-site radioimmunometric assay employing anti-DAF monoclonals revealed complete absence of DAF protein in the nonadherent cells in all cases.

Examination of the nonadherent cells by flow cytometry using anti-AChE and anti-DAF monoclonals verified that the isolated cells were totally AChE-deficient and confirmed that the AChE and DAF defects completely overlap in the same cells. These investigations additionally showed that type II and type III $E^{hu}$ are both totally AChE- and DAF-deficient. Moreover, the defects in these two proteins in the PNH $E^{hu}$ differ from the CR1 abnormality in the cells in that the DAF and AChE deficits segregated precisely with the complement-sensitive cell population while the CR1 deficit was equally distributed between complement-sensitive and -insensitive $E^{hu}$ populations. Interestingly, in patients with type III $E^{hu}$, partial deficiencies of AChE and DAF were additionally present in the complement-insensitive (type I) $E^{hu}$ subpopulations.

$E^{hu}$ AChE is (a dimer) composed of 75 kDalton subunits. Because of the similarity in size to 70 kDalton $E^{hu}$ DAF, the possibility existed that the dual abnormality in affected PNH cells might represent a single defect in the same protein. To clarify this issue, functional and structural studies employing the anti-DAF and anti-AChE antibodies were carried out. Pretreatment of normal $E^{hu}AC14$ with high concentrations of pooled anti-AChE antibodies did not diminish the natural resistance of the cells to assembly of autologous C4b2a under conditions in which 10-fold lower concentrations of pooled anti-DAF monoclonals completely overcame this DAF-mediated resistance. Conversely, pretreatment of normal $E^{hu}$ with sufficient amounts of anti-DAF antibodies to render them PNH-like in acid lysis had no effect on their membrane AChE enzyme activity under conditions in which 10-fold lower concentrations of pooled AChE antibodies completely abrogated enzyme function. Finally, addition of the anti-DAF and anti-AChE monoclonals to NP40 extracts of $^{125}I$-surface labeled $E^{hu}$ stroma precipitated two discrete proteins that differed slightly in apparent $M_r$ (Figure 2). Parallel studies with neuraminidase-pretreated $E^{hu}$ revealed that the enzyme markedly reduced the apparent $M_r$ of DAF but had no effect on that of AChE. The results thus indicated that AChE and DAF are distinct entities with independently mediated activities and that the concomitant defects of the two factors in PNH $E^{hu}$ constitute separate abnormalities.

The heightened sensitivity of lytic terminal pathway complexes which distinguishes type III PNH $E^{hu}$ from type II $E^{hu}$ is demonstrable in vitro by markedly greater sensitivity[47] of type III $E^{hu}$ in the CLS assay of Rosse and Dacie and susceptibility of type III $E^{hu}$ to lysis in zymosan- or cobra venom factor (CoVF)-treated serum.[42,43] By means of binding and photolabeling studies, Hu and Nicholson-Weller[48] showed that the enhanced susceptibility of type III cells toward lysis is correlated with C9 binding 5 to 6-fold greater than to normal $E^{hu}$ and with the absence of a characteristic lag time that is observed with normal $E^{hu}$ between C9 uptake and cell lysis. The intrinsic membrane defect responsible for this abnormality was not characterized.

To determine whether the diminished resistance to membrane attack constitutes a third defect of PNH type III $E^{hu}$, the capacity of normal $E^{hu}$ to restrict lysis by human C5-9 and the effects of anti-DAF and anti-AChE antibodies on this restriction were evaluated.[46] Although treatment of normal $E^{hu}AC1423$ bearing $10^4$ C3b per cell with pooled monoclonal or polyclonal anti-DAF antibodies rendered the intermediates readily susceptible to immediate lysis upon addition of (small amounts of) human C2 and guinea pig C5-9, the same treatment did not render the C3b bearing cells susceptible to lysis in human C5-9 irrespective of the amount of C2 added. The simultaneous treatment of the cells with anti-AChE antibodies in addition to the anti-DAF antibodies did not overcome the resistance of the $E^{hu}AC1423$ to lysis in human C5-9, indicating that it is mediated by another entity. In contrast, without any antibody pretreatment, (type III) PNH $E^{hu}AC1423$ bearing only $2 \times 10^3$ C3b per cell lysed as readily in human C5-9 as in guinea pig C5-9, indicating that a defect in this resistance is present in the type III cells.

To investigate the relationship between the activity responsible for this terminal pathway resistance and DAF, the effects of anti-DAF treatment of normal $E^{hu}$ and of DAF reconstitution of PNH $E^{hu}$ on the hemolytic sensitivities of the respective cells in the CLS and CoVF assays were evaluated.[46] Treatment of normal $E^{hu}AC14$ with sufficient polyclonal or pooled monoclonal anti-DAF antibody to overcome the natural resistance of the normal $E^{hu}$ to C4b2a assembly and C3b uptake increased their sensitivity in CLS only (~ 5-fold) to the level of type II $E^{hu}$. Augmenting the concentration of anti-DAF antibodies 3 to 5-fold further had no additional effect. Conversely while restoration of DAF activity to type II PNH $E^{hu}$ reduced their sensitivity in CLS to near normal levels, incorporation of sufficient DAF (585 DAF

# Immunoprecipitation of DAF and AChE

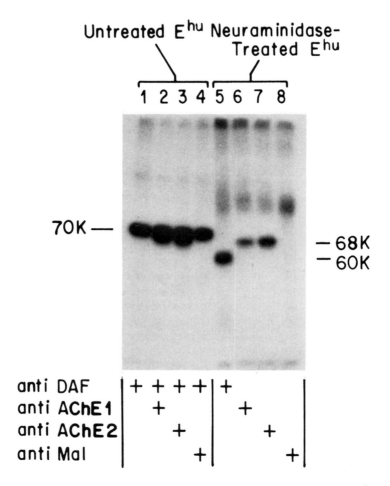

| anti DAF | + + + + | + | |
| anti AChE1 | + | + | |
| anti AChE2 | + | + | |
| anti Mal | + | + | |

FIGURE 2.   Comparison between DAF and $E^{hu}$ AChE. $E^{hu}$, untreated or pretreated with neuraminidase, were surface labeled with $^{125}I$ and, following hypotonic lysis, the membranes extracted with NP40. Extracts of untreated $E^{hu}$ were incubated with either pooled monoclonal anti-DAF antibodies (lane 1), anti-DAF and anti-AChE monoclonal AEI together (lane 2), anti-DAF and anti-AChE monoclonal AEII together (lane 3), or anti-DAF and pooled nonrelevant anti-malarial monoclonals (lane 4). Extracts of neuraminidase-treated cells were incubated with either pooled anti-DAF monoclonals (lane 5), anti-AChE AEI alone (lane 6), anti-AChE AEII alone (lane 7), or pooled anti-malaria monoclonals (lane 8). After addition of protein A-agarose, the immunoprecipitated proteins were extracted with SDS, subjected to SDS-PAGE on 7.5% gels, and radioautographs prepared. The anti-DAF and anti-AChE monoclonals precipitated different proteins and, unlike DAF, membrane AChE did not decrease in size following pretreatment of the $E^{hu}$ with neuraminidase.

molecules/$E^{hu}$) into PNH type III $E^{hu}$ to restore the ability of the PNH cells to completely restrict uptake of C3b had only a minimal effect on the (15 to 25-fold) greater sensitivity of the type III $E^{hu}$ in CLS. Similar results were obtained in the CoVF-serum assay. Whereas no lysis of normal $E^{hu}$ occurred following incubation of the cells in 1:8 CoVF serum, complete lysis of type III PNH $E^{hu}$ occurred in 1:64 CoVF serum.[46] Prior treatment of the normal cells with polyclonal anti-DAF antibodies did not abrogate their inherent resistance to passive lysis, and reconstitution of the PNH cells with DAF did not diminish their increased sensitivity to lysis in this assay. The results thus argued that the defect in terminal pathway restriction in PNH type III E[hu] is distinct from the defect in DAF. The coincidence in the same cells of this defect, together with the DAF and AChE defects, indicates that type III E[hu] must be deficient in at least three factors.

Membrane factors which can inhibit C9 polymerization, and thereby limit the activity of the membrane attack complex have been reported in extracts of E[hu] stroma by Podack (personal communication) and by Zalman and Müller-Eberhard.[49] The activity detected by Podack elutes from DEAE-Sephacel at higher ionic strength than DAF and migrates as an 80 kDalton molecule on SDS-PAGE, while that described by Zalman and Müller-Eberhard has an apparent $M_r$ of 38K. Another terminal pathway inhibitory factor with the ability to bind to C8 and block its interaction with C9 has been isolated from extracts of E[hu] stroma by Schonermark et al.[50] The relationship, however, of this factor to the above inhibitors of C9 polymerization has not yet been investigated.

PNH occurs frequently in association with bone marrow failure.[26] Current evidence indicates that the disease arises as a result of a somatic mutation in a stem cell that favors proliferation and is expressed during marrow regeneration. The detection of DAF deficiency in affected PNH cells suggested that this mutation might involve the DAF structural gene. Such a mutation leading to nonfunction or deletion of the DAF gene appeared to provide a simple mechanism which could account for both disease etiology and pathogenesis. Since the presence of multiple protein deficits in PNH E[hu] cannot be explained by this mechanism, the detection of this situation in PNH argued that the PNH defect is more complex.

As discussed above, only $\sim$ 3000 DAF molecules are present per normal E[hu]. Because of this relatively low DAF level and because red cells have a long lifetime in the circulation and do not synthesize new protein, the presence of small amounts of DAF antigen on PNH E[hu] would be difficult to detect. In the course of the analyses by Kinoshita et al.[34] of PNH leukocytes discussed above, it was observed that although DAF expression by affected cells was severely impaired (>95%), in many cases, low levels of anti-DAF fluorescence above that of nonrelevant control antibody were detectable on PNH leukocytes. In an independent set of studies using fluorescence-labeled polyclonal anti-DAF antibody, Moore et al.[51] found that affected bone marrow progenitor cells from PNH patients are initially DAF-positive but become DAF-negative when placed in tissue culture. Although the mechanism of this phenomenon is unclear, their findings indicated that the PNH defect could be predetermined in altered progenitors and expressed during proliferation. Analyses by Berger et al.[35] of PMN from PNH patients following stimulation with f-MLP showed that affected cells not only lack surface DAF but are also devoid of intracellular DAF. The demonstration in the same studies that the affected cells contained apparently intact intracellular pools of CR1 and of iC3b receptors (CR3) and could upregulate these proteins in a normal fashion, argued that DAF deficiency occurs at the time of synthesis or packaging of DAF for intracellular storage and cannot be explained by loss of DAF from the cell membrane. These lines of evidence raised the possibility that the membrane alterations that occur in PNH could represent an abnormality in regulation or in a posttranslational event, resulting in the formation of abnormal proteins.

The realization that multiple membrane proteins are deficient in PNH suggested the possibility that the deficient proteins might share a common structural element that is missing or defective in PNH. AChE deficiency was the first chemical abnormality reported in PNH E[hu].[52] Of relevance to data that will be discussed below, multiple forms of both cellular and extracellular AChE molecules exist (reviewed in Reference 53). Structural analyses of the catalytic subunit of E[hu] AChE by Rosenberry and co-workers[54-56] showed that it is an amphipathic molecule. Like DAF,[20] in the isolated state, it aggregates into detergent micelles.[52] The purified E[hu] AChE subunit can be converted into a soluble AChE form $\sim$ 2 kDalton smaller in apparent size on gels than the intact enzyme, by digestion with papain which cleaves a dipeptide (His-Gly) attached to a glycolipid structure at the C-terminus of the molecule.[54] The C-terminal glycolipid structure is composed of phospholipid linked to an oligosaccharide containing ethanolamine and nonacetylated glucosamine.[55,56] Similar glycolipid structures have been found at the C-termini of Thy-1 antigen of murine lymphocytes[57,58] and of "membrane form" variant surface glycoproteins (mfVSGs) of Trypanosome and Leishmania parasites.[59-62] There is evidence from studies of mfVSG biosynthesis[63-65] that the non-amino acid structure is added to mfVSG molecules during a posttranslational modification that occurs immediately after formation of VSG polypeptide.

## VII. VARIANTS OF DAF ON EPITHELIAL CELL SURFACES AND IN BODY FLUIDS

In the course of investigations of DAF expression by blood cells, plasma and urine samples obtained from some of the cell donors were assayed for DAF along with cell extracts in the two-site radioimmunometric assay employing anti-DAF monoclonals.[66] Unexpectedly, substantial amounts of DAF antigen were consistently detectable in plasma, and relatively large amounts measurable in urine. The antigen concentration in "spot" urine specimens from some donors exceeded 500 ng/m$\ell$, >15% of the total cell-associated DAF concentration in whole blood ($\sim$ 3 $\mu$g/m$\ell$). The fact that positivity in the assay depended on reactivity with two monoclonal anti-DAF antibodies directed against different epitopes of the E$^{hu}$ DAF molecule argued that the results were not artifactual and suggested that the antigens detected might contain a significant portion of the E$^{hu}$ DAF structure.

To characterize the nature of the DAF reactivity, plasma and urine specimens from the donors were fractionated, concentrates of the plasma and urine antigens prepared, and the concentrates compared to E$^{hu}$ membrane DAF on Western blots. The plasma antigen bound to DEAE-Sephacel in 0.01 M PO$_4$, pH 8.0, and eluted between 2 and 5 mS. The urine antigen was excluded on Sephadex G25 and, following lyophilization and redissolution, was retained upon dialysis. When examined next to E$^{hu}$ membrane DAF (70 kDalton) on radioautographs (Figure 3) of the Western blots (developed with $^{125}$I-labeled anti-DAF monoclonal IIH6), the plasma antigen migrated with higher apparent M$_r$ ($\sim$ 100 kDalton) and the urine antigen with slightly lower apparent Mr ($\sim$ 67 kDalton).

To further investigate the structural properties of the extracellular DAF species and to allow functional studies, the more abundant DAF variant, urine DAF, was isolated by affinity chromatography. Anti-DAF Sepharose beads were prepared using low affinity monoclonal anti-DAF antibody IA10 and antigen was eluted with pH 11.5 triethylamine buffer.[67] Approximately 100 $\mu$g of urine DAF was recovered from about 500 m$\ell$ of urine. Western blot analysis of the affinity purified product (following development with several antibodies) showed a single band at $\sim$ 67 kDalton. To determine whether the urine DAF molecule possesses functional activity and, if so, how its function compares with that of purified E$^{hu}$ membrane DAF, hemolytic studies with sheep cell intermediates were performed. Like E$^{hu}$ membrane DAF, the urine DAF variant accelerated C4b2a decay on EAC142$_{lim}$ cells, but, on a molar basis, its activity was 20-fold less than that of purified E$^{hu}$ DAF. The lesser efficiency of urine DAF in decay acceleration was comparable to that of the serum C4b2a inhibitor, C4bp. When the functional comparison of the two DAF species was repeated using EAC14 cells in an assay designed to require DAF incorporation for an effect, the activity of E$^{hu}$ DAF was identical to that measured in the assay with EAC142$_{lim}$, whereas no activity of urine DAF was observed.[66] These results suggested that urine DAF lacks the ability to membrane incorporate. This was verified in studies with the $^{125}$I-labeled purified urine DAF molecule. One possible explanation is that urine DAF retains its ligand binding site but (in analogy to E$^{hu}$ AChE) is devoid of a domain that mediates its anchorage in the

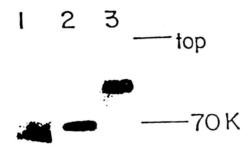

FIGURE 3.   Western blot analysis of plasma and urine DAF molecules. Affinity purified preparations of urine (lane 1), E$^{hu}$ membrane (lane 2) and plasma (lane 3) DAF were subjected to SDS-PAGE on 7.5% gels. After electrophoresis, the separated proteins were transferred to nitrocellulose, the blots incubated with $^{125}$I-labeled monoclonal anti-DAF antibody (IIH6) and, after washing, radioautographs prepared. The plasma DAF species migrated with an apparent M$_r$ of ~100K, and the urine DAF species with an apparent M$_r$ of ~67K.

lipid bilayer, and that the loss of this domain accounts for the slightly increased mobility of the urine molecule on SDS/PAGE.

Levels of plasma DAF, and amounts of urine DAF produced per 24 hr, were quantitated in healthy individuals. Plasma levels varied from 25 to 50 ng/m$\ell$; 24-hr urinary amounts ranged from 200 to as high as 500 μg. Surprisingly, the urine values represent 0.5 to as much as 3.3% of the total intravascular blood cell DAF. Importantly, similarly high values were also documented in urine specimens from PNH patients (unpublished results). Since some of the patients had very little DAF detectable on their blood cells, this result suggested that the urine DAF either must arise locally, i.e., from a non-blood cell site, or might represent an abnormal form of the molecule. In studies employing cultured umbilical endothelium, Asch et al.[68] showed that endothelial cells synthesize high levels of DAF ($>10^5$ molecules DAF/cell). The expression of DAF by vascular endothelium, which, like blood cells, are in intimate and prolonged contact with serum complement proteins, is consistent with the postulated role of the blood cell molecule in protecting blood cells against complement-mediated damage. The possibility existed that endothelial cells could be the source of urine DAF but in this circumstance transport of ~ 70 kDalton DAF molecules across the glomerulus would be required.

Using pooled anti-DAF monoclonal antibodies, immunohistochemical analyses of various tissues were undertaken to investigate the distribution of DAF in cells surrounding the urinary tract and elsewhere outside the vascular space. In a set of studies directed at determining the origin of the urine DAF, investigations of renal cortex and urinary tract were performed. Under conditions in which anti-CR1 monoclonals stained podocytes in the same section and in which anti-DAF monoclonals showed reactivity with lymphocytes in tonsil sections, no localized anti-DAF staining of CR1-positive glomerular cells was observed. In contrast, marked anti-DAF staining of tubular epithelium was noted adjacent to glomeruli in cortex and throughout renal medulla. Similarly strong staining of epithelium was observed in ureter and bladder.[66]

To test the possibility that DAF could also be present in other body fluids and secretions, samples of saliva, tears, cerebrospinal fluid (CSF) and (osteoarthritic) joint fluid were assayed

# Cornea

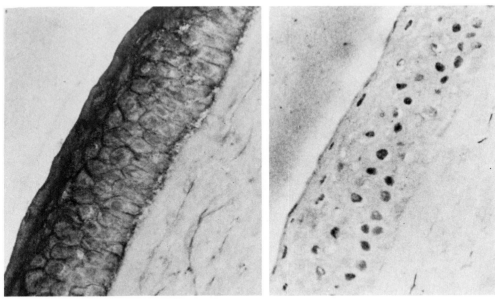

anti -DAF                    anti - CR I

FIGURE 4A.   Various tissues were examined immunohistologically for DAF using monoclonal anti-DAF antibodies and the peroxidase method. Optimal conditions for fixation and staining were established in preliminary experiments with lymph nodes containing B lymphocytes which express large amounts of DAF and pooled anti-CR1 monoclonals were used as control. Anti-DAF and anti-CR1-stained sections of *cornea* are shown. Marked anti-DAF staining of corneal epithelium is apparent. The staining is localized to the epithelial cell membrane and increases in intensity in upper epithelial cell layers. (From Medof, M. E., Walter, E. I., Rutgers, J. L., Knowles, D. M., and Nussenzweig, V., *J. Exp. Med.*, 165, 848, 1987. With permission of The Rockefeller University Press.)

for DAF in the two-site assay. The results, shown in Table 2, revealed $>100$, 200, 35, and 100 ng/m$\ell$ of DAF antigen, respectively. Immunoprecipitation of the antigens in saliva and tears with anti-DAF monoclonals and analysis of the immunoprecipitated proteins on Western blots showed that soluble DAF molecules in these fluids are larger ($\sim 100$ kDalton) than urine DAF.[64] In view of the anti-DAF staining of urothelium, sections of cornea, conjunctiva, oral mucosa, and synovium were examined. Strong anti-DAF staining of epithelial cells in all sites including cornea (Figure 4, panel A), glandular cells in conjunctiva (panel B) and oral mucosa was observed. Marked anti-DAF staining was similarly seen of mucosa and exocrine glandular cells throughout the GI tract, of pleura and pericardium, and of vaginal epithelium and uterine endometrium.

To confirm that epithelial cells synthesize DAF, primary cultures of foreskin epithelium were obtained and, after growth on coverslips, were fixed and examined immunohistochemically for anti-DAF reactivity. Strong and specific anti-DAF staining similar to that observed with the tissue sections was noted (Figure 4, panel C). Another portion of the foreskin cells were extracted with NP40 and the extract assayed for DAF by two-site radioimmunoassay. An amount of DAF ($2 \times 10^5$ mol/cell) $>$ 3-fold higher[66] than that present in the same number of blood PMN[32] was measured. When DAF antigen in the extract was examined next to E$^{hu}$ membrane DAF on Western blots, it was slightly larger in apparent size ($\sim 72$ vs. $\sim 70$ kDalton).

# Conjunctiva

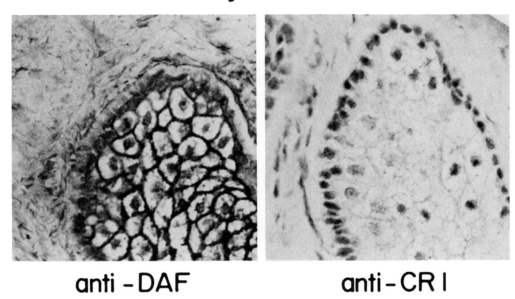

anti - DAF          anti - CR I

FIGURE 4B. Tissues were fixed and stained as in Figure 4A. Sections of tarsal conjunctiva are shown. Prominent anti-DAF-staining of glandular tissues is apparent. (From Medof, M. E., Walter, E. I., Rutgers, J. L., Knowles, D. M., and Nussenzweig, V., *J. Exp. Med.*, 165, 848, 1987. With permission of The Rockefeller University Press.)

The concurrent findings of soluble DAF antigen in fluids contained in extracellular spaces and of large amounts of membrane DAF on the surfaces of adjacent epithelial cells and glandular cells lining the extracellular compartments suggested that the extracellular DAF variants arise from the epithelial cells. The function of DAF in these locations remains unclear. The observation however that urine DAF has C4bp (or factor H)-like activity shows that it could inhibit fluid-phase activation of the cascade and thus could have a protective role similar to that of blood cell DAF. Alternatively, the extracellular DAF variants could serve some other noncomplement-related function.

## VIII. STEPS IN DAF BIOSYNTHESIS

In view of the possibility (see above) that a defect in posttranslational processing could underlie the deficient expression of membrane proteins in affected PNH cells and the observation that both membrane and soluble DAF forms are produced by epithelial cells, it was of interest to analyze the sequence of the steps which take place in DAF biosynthesis.

To identify an optimal model to study DAF biosynthesis, different human cell lines were collected. Following expansion in culture, the lines were examined for DAF expression by two-site radioimmunometric DAF assay (Table 1) and by flow cytometry. Among lymphoid lines, expression by Raji cells was highest ($4 \times 10^4$ molecules/cell). Little if any DAF was found in Daudi cells or in the CLL line 119. The levels in EB + cells were in general higher than in EB − cells. Baseline DAF expression by the HL-60 myeloid line was $\sim 10^4$ molecules/cell and increased during 12-0-tetradecanoylphorbol-13-acetate (TPA)-induced differentiation along the macrophage pathway (Table 2). Some of these as well as other cell lines were examined by FACS for both DAF and AChE using monoclonal anti-DAF and anti-AChE

# Foreskin epithelium     Hela cells

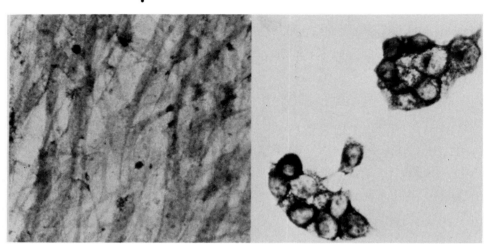

## anti-DAF                    anti-DAF

FIGURE 4C.   Human foreskin epithelium and the HeLa cell line were cultured and then stained as done with tissues (Figure 4ab). Immunohistological analyses of the cultured cells showed strong anti-DAF staining. Immunoradiometric assays of the HeLa cell extracts revealed $> 2 \times 10^5$ DAF molecules per cell. Western blot analyses demonstrated that the epithelial cell DAF is slightly larger in size (72 vs. 70 kDalton) than $E^{hu}$ DAF. (From Medof, M. E., Walter, E. I., Rutgers, J. L., Knowles, D. M., and Nussenzweig, V., *J. Exp. Med.*, 165, 848, 1987. With permission of The Rockefeller University Press.)

## Table 1
## DAF AND CR1 EXPRESSION BY MYELOID
## AND LYMPHOID CELL LINES

| Cell line | DAF (mol/cell $\times$ 10³) | CR1 (mol/cell $\times$ 10³) |
|---|---|---|
| Myeloid lines | | |
| HL60 | 12 | 0.7 |
| Lymphoid lines | | |
| EB(−) | | |
| ST486 | 0.7 | 0 |
| JD38 | 14 | 0 |
| CA46 | 10 | 0 |
| MC116 | 10 | 0 |
| EB(+) | | |
| Raji | 40 | 0 |
| Daudi | 0.7 | 0 |
| P3HR1 | 34 | 0 |
| PA682 | 22 | 0 |
| EBV2 | 5.2 | 0 |
| CLL 119 | 0 | 0 |
| RBC control | 2.3 | 0.7 |

**Table 2**
**DAF AND CR1 EXPRESSION DURING**
**DIFFERENTIATION OF HL60 CELLS**

| | DAF (mol/cell × 10³) time (hr) | | | CR1 (mol/cell × 10³) time (hr) | | |
|---|---|---|---|---|---|---|
| | **0** | **48** | **72** | **0** | **48** | **72** |
| Control | 12 | | 14 | 0.7 | 1 | |
| TPA[a] | | 50 | 45 | | 7 | 9 |

> [a]  12-0-tetradecanoylphorbol-13-acetate.

antibodies. These analyses revealed that the erythroleukemia line, K562, and the epithelial line, HeLa, express both proteins. Measurements with the two-site radioimmunometric DAF assay showed that undifferentiated K562 cells express about $2 \times 10^4$ molecules of DAF per cell, and the expression of both DAF and AChE by K562 cells increases when the cells are treated with sodium butyrate.[69,70] The HeLa cells which are of epithelial origin, express 2 to $3 \times 10^5$ DAF mol/cell, in accordance with the findings of large amounts of DAF in epithelial cells in multiple sites in immunohistochemical analyses and of similarly large amounts of membrane DAF in cultured foreskin epithelium in in vitro studies (see above). Surface-labeling of the HeLa cells with $^{125}$I and examination of the HeLa-cell associated DAF molecule by SDS-PAGE/radioautography showed that it is comparable in apparent size (~72 kDalton) to foreskin epithelial DAF.

Two independent investigations of DAF biosynthesis were conducted, one employing HeLa cells, and the other, by Lublin et al.,[71] employing differentiated HL-60 cells. In the studies by Lublin et al. the oligosaccharide content of DAF was first investigated by analyzing the effect of endoglycosidase digestions on SDS-PAGE mobility of $E^{hu}$ DAF. Endoglycosidase-F treatment, which cleaves complex N-linked glycans, lowered the apparent $M_r$ (74K in their system) of $E^{hu}$ DAF by only 3K while sequential neuraminidase and endo-α-N-acetylgalactosaminidase treatment, which removes O-linked oligosaccharides, reduced its apparent $M_r$ to 48K. Neuraminidase treatment alone accounted for 18 kDalton of this shift. The effects of the N-linked and O-linked glycan-specific treatments on SDS-PAGE mobility were additive. These findings suggested that $E^{hu}$ DAF contains a relatively large number of oligosarchides in O-glycosidic linkage to serine or threonine residues. The 3 kDalton size reduction observed with endoglycosidase-F is consistent with the presence of a single complex N-linked oligosaccharide unit in the molecule.

To investigate the nature of intracellular DAF precursors, 1,25-dihydroxy vitamin-$D_3$ differentiated HL-60 cells were labeled with [$^{35}$S]-Met and extracts of the cells analyzed by anti-DAF immunoprecipitation followed by SDS-PAGE/fluorography.[71] These studies revealed two intracellular DAF species of ~43 and 46 kDalton. Pulse chase analyses showed that both were DAF precursors and that the 46 kDalton molecule was an intermediate product which arose from the 43 kDalton precursor during the first 10 min of labeling. Digestions with endoglycosidase-H (which cleaves high-mannose N-linked glycans) and repeat studies performed in the presence of tunicamycin yielded intermediates, ~3 kDalton smaller in apparent size (in accordance with the effects of endoglysosidase-F on mature DAF), indicative of a single N-linked glycan in the molecule. Biosynthetic studies with K562 erythroleukemia cells revealed DAF precursors the same size as those in HL-60 cells, suggesting that the differences in apparent size between mature DAF molecules on $E^{hu}$ and blood monocytes are due to differences in O-linked glycosylation.

In the other set of investigations of DAF biosynthesis employing HeLa cells,[72] labeling experiments were performed with [$^{35}$S]-Cys. Similar to the results obtained by Lublin et al.,

# Pulse Chase Analysis of
# DAF Biosynthesis in HeLa Cells

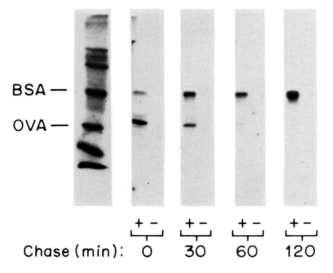

FIGURE 5A.    Pulse-chase study of DAF biosynthesis in HeLa cells. After 1 hr incubation with Cys-free RPMI and 15 min pulse with [$^{35}$S]-Cys, the cells were chased for the time periods shown. The monolayers were extracted with SDS and labeled DAF proteins isolated by immunoprecipitation and analyzed by SDS-PAGE/fluorography. The lanes designated ( − ) show the results of control studies with nonrelevant monoclonal antibodies. (From Medof, M. E., Walter, E. I., Roberts, W. L., Haas, R., and Rosenberry, T. L., *Biochemistry*, 25, 6740, 1986. Copyright 1986 American Chemical Society. With permission.)

pulse chase studies demonstrated a 48-kDalton intracellular DAF precursor which chased into mature DAF with a half time of ~30 min (Figure 5, panel A). Th 48-kDalton DAF precursor labeled with [$^3$H]-mannose (panel B) in accordance with the presence in this molecule of N-linked glycans. Treatment of the precursor with endoglycosidase-H lowered its apparent $M_r$ by ~4K, and a pro-DAF species of identical size was observed when biosynthetic studies were performed in the presence of tunicamycin (10 μg/mℓ). The mature DAF molecule (Figure 5, panel B) but not the 48-kDalton DAF precursor labeled with [$^3$H]-N-acetylgalactosamine, a precursor of O-linked sugars, and the mature DAF protein was reduced only ~4K in apparent $M_r$ following treatment with endoglycosidase-F, again indicating that most of the sugars in mature DAF are O-linked.

Analysis of culture supernatants of HeLa cell monolayers by two-site DAF radioimmunoassay revealed that these cells release DAF antigen, in contrast to DAF-positive K562 cells in suspension which do not (Figure 6). Isolation of the fluid-phase DAF species by immunoprecipitation with pooled anti-DAF monoclonals and analysis of the immunoprecipitated proteins by Western blotting revealed a 67 kDalton DAF form which resembled urine DAF in gel mobility. Studies with cultured foreskin epithelium yielded results similar to those obtained with HeLa cells. As observed in the isolation of mfVSGs,[59-61] rapid extraction of the cells with 2% SDS was required to prevent degradation of endogenous HeLa membrane DAF into the smaller (67 kDalton) DAF form. In view of the possible relationship of these in vitro fluid phase DAF species to in vivo soluble DAF forms, the HeLa and cultured epithelial cell systems could provide good models to investigate the structural differences between membrane and soluble DAF forms and the mechanism of formation of the latter.

HeLa cell RNA was isolated, messenger RNA (mRNA) purified, and the mRNA translated

# Ethanolamine Incorporation into DAF

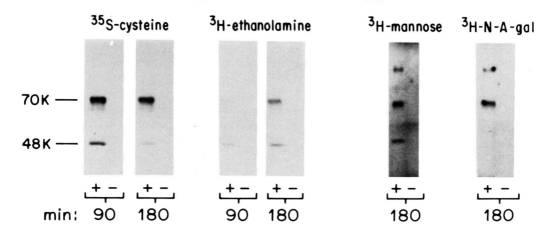

FIGURE 5B. [³H]-mannose, [³H]-N-acetylgalactosamine, and [³H]-ethanolamine incorporation into DAF. After continuous labeling for the times shown, the cells were extracted and label incorporation analyzed. The results of control studies are designated ( − ) as in Figure 5A, above. [³H]-mannose incorporated into 48 kDalton DAF precursor and 72 kDalton mature DAF, whereas [³H]-N-acetylgalactosamine incorporated only into mature 72 kDalton DAF. The appearance of [³H]-ethanolamine paralleled those of[³⁵S]-Cys and [³H]-mannose. (From Medof, M. E., Walter, E. I., Roberts, W. L., Haas, R., and Rosenberry, T. L., *Biochemistry,* 25, 6740, 1986. Copyright 1986 American Chemical Society. With permission.)

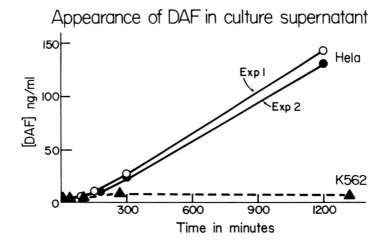

FIGURE 6. HeLa cells were cultured, and during log phase growth, the culture supernatant was assayed at different times for DAF antigen by radiometric assay. While no DAF antigen was detectable in the supernatant of K562 erythroleukemia cells, progressively increasing levels of DAF antigen were measurable in the HeLa cell supernatants. (From Medof, M. E., Walter, E. I., Rutgers, J. L., Knowles, D. M., and Nussenzweig, V., *J. Exp. Med.,* 165, 848, 1987. With permission of The Rockefeller University Press.)

in the presence of wheat germ and [³⁵S]-Met. The in vitro-translated DAF product was immunoprecipitated with anti-DAF monoclonals and compared on SDS-PAGE gels to pro-DAF detected in tunicamycin-treated cells in the HeLa cell biosynthetic studies. The mRNA translation product migrated with an apparent $M_r$ ~6K larger than the nonglycosylated DAF precursor (generated in tunicamycin-treated cells) consistent with the presence of one or more signal sequences (unpublished data). This finding is relevant to features of posttranslational processing of DAF that will be discussed in the section below.

## IX. MECHANISM OF DAF ANCHORAGE IN CELL MEMBRANES

To provide quantities of protein sufficient for structural analyses, large scale purifications of $E^{hu}$ DAF were undertaken by affinity chromatography. A single step procedure similar to that described (see above) for purification of urine DAF was developed. In a typical isolation, 3 mg of DAF was recovered from 12 units of packed $E^{hu}$. The product was homogenous on silver stains of SDS-PAGE gels, free of contaminating glycophorin on Western blots, and after radioiodinating with Iodogen, gave only characteristic DAF bands[20] on radioautographs of SDS-PAGE gels. Because of the structural analogies between membrane and soluble forms of $E^{hu}$ DAF and AChE and the common deficits of the two factors in PNH, the purified DAF protein was employed in a set of experiments designed to analyze $E^{hu}$ DAF for a C-terminal anchoring structure analogous to that found in $E^{hu}$ AChE[54-56] and similarly described in mfVSGs of Typanosomes[59-61] and Leishmania,[62] and in Thy-1 antigen[57,58] of murine thymocytes.

The glycolipid anchoring structure of trypanosome mfVSGs was shown to contain 1,2-dimyristylphosphatidylinositol linked through an oligosaccharide[60,61] to ethanolamine that is in amide linkage with the C-terminal amino acid of VSG polypeptide.[59] One characteristic of this glycolipid structure[61] and of the less well-characterized but similar C-terminal glycolipid anchoring structure in Thy-1 antigen,[58] is susceptibility to cleavage by phosphatidylinositol (PI) specific phospholipase C (PLC) purified from *S. aureus*. PI-PLC cleaves within PI releasing inositol-monophosphate from diacylglycerol. As one approach to determine whether DAF might be anchored by an interaction involving PI, the susceptibility of endogenous membrane DAF in intact $E^{hu}$ to exogenous PI-PLC cleavage was investigated.[73] Upon incubation of $E^{hu}$ at 37°C for 60 min with the enzyme, ~15% of the membrane DAF was released as determined by assaying the supernatant and cells for DAF antigen by two-site radiometric DAF assay. In contrast, <1% of membrane DAF was released by 10-fold higher concentrations of phosphatidylcholine-specific PLC from *B. cereus*, phospholipase A2, or trypsin, the last of which totally cleaved $E^{hu}$-associated CR1. Isolation of the PI-PLC released DAF species by specific immunoprecipitation and comparison of the derivative to native $E^{hu}$ DAF by SDS-PAGE/radioautography (after repeating the digestion using $^{125}$I surface-labeled $E^{hu}$) revealed that it was smaller in apparent $M_r$ by ~3K. Analysis of the purified derivative revealed that this 67 kDalton product differed from $E^{hu}$ membrane DAF in that it did not adsorb to Phenyl-Sepharose. To assess whether it retained the ability to membrane incorporate, it was added to $E^{sh}AC14$ and its effect on C4b hemolytic sites evaluated. In marked contrast to $E^{hu}$ membrane DAF, no inhibition of hemolytic activity was observed. The PI-PLC derivative closely resembled urine DAF,[66] however, in that it accelerated decay of preassembled C4b2a on $E^{sh}AC142$ intermediates with comparable efficiency. The addition of pooled monoclonal anti-DAF antibodies completely reversed the inhibition, confirming that the activity resided in the released DAF form. In independent studies carried out simultaneously by Davitz et al.[74] a similar result was observed. Approximately 12% of endogenous DAF was released from $E^{hu}$ by PI-PLC, and the cleavage was associated with loss of the ability of the DAF molecule to membrane incorporate. Interestingly, a larger proportion of membrane DAF (as much as 50%) was released from PMN and blood lymphocytes as assessed in flow cytometric analyses employing anti-DAF monoclonals.

Reductive methylation converts primary amine-containing constituents of proteins into their mono- and di-methylated derivatives, which can be identified following protein hydrolysis by coelution with radiomethylated standards in an amino-acid analyzer.[75] Purified

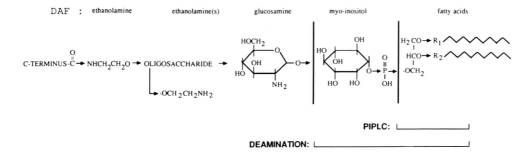

FIGURE 7. Schematic representation of the structure of the membrane DAF anchor based on studies of the $E^{hu}$ DAF, $E^{hu}$ AChE, and the mfVSG anchors. The glycolipid anchoring structure is held in the membrane by alkyl groups (designated $R_1$ and $R_2$) which are inserted into the lipid bilayer. In mfVSGs, these are fatty acid (myristate) components of PI. The PI is linked to an oligosaccharide via a glycosidic bond between inositol and nonacetylated glucosamine. In mfVSGs and in $E^{hu}$ AChE, the oligosaccharide is linked to the respective polypeptides via an amide bond between an ethanolamine and the C-terminal amino acid. PI-PLC and deamination cleavage sites are shown. (Prepared in conjunction with Drs. W. Roberts and T. L. Rosenberry.)

$E^{hu}$ DAF was radiomethylated with $^3$HCHO and NaCNBH$_3$ and the product subjected to automated amino acid analysis.[73] In addition to 18 moles of $\epsilon$-radiomethylated Lys per $E^{hu}$ DAF polypeptide and one mole of $\alpha$-radiomethylated Asp indicative of N-terminal Asx, this analysis revealed labeled ethanolamine and glucosamine as present in the $E^{hu}$ AChE anchor.[55] Moreover, the amounts of these two sugars detected were comparable to those of the corresponding components in $E^{hu}$ AChE. Radiomethylated $E^{hu}$ DAF was digested with papain and the product isolated by gel-exclusion chromatography. SDS-PAGE analysis revealed that it consisted of two large fragments that appeared 9 and 15 kDalton smaller in size on gels than intact $E^{hu}$ membrane DAF. Amino acid analysis of these fragments demonstrated that Asp and Lys were quantitatively retained while labeled ethanolamine and glucosamine had been completely removed. The presence of labeled N-terminal Asp and complete retention of all labeled Lys indicated that, as in the case of $E^{hu}$ AChE,[55] ethanolamine and glucosamine were localized in the small released C-terminal fragments. A schematic representation of the $E^{hu}$ DAF is shown in Figure 7.

To relate the nonacetylated glucosamine detected in $E^{hu}$ DAF directly to the DAF anchor and to further investigate the relationship of the DAF membrane anchor to that of $E^{hu}$ AChE, the two proteins were subjected to nitrous acid deamination. This procedure cleaves at nonacetylated glucosamine[76] and was used to demonstrate that glucosamine in the mfVSG anchor is immediately adjacent to PI in glycosidic linkage with inositol.[61] To aid the interpretation of results, the two proteins were first labeled with the probe 3-(trifluoromethyl)-3-(m-[$^{125}$I] iodophenyl) diazirine ([$^{125}$I]-TID) which binds covalently to lipids[77] and was shown to have specificity for the phospholipid moiety of the $E^{hu}$ AChE anchor.[78] When the $^{125}$I-TID labeled $E^{hu}$ DAF and AChE molecules were cleaved at nonacetylated glucosamine by nitrous acid deamination, the label was quantitatively released from both proteins in a parallel fashion. Loss of the label from DAF correlated with loss of the ability of DAF to associate with detergent micelles or liposomes. Previous studies of $E^{hu}$ AChE showed that the ethanolamine with free amino group that is detected by radiomethylation is contained within the oligosaccharide moiety of the glycolipid and that another ethanolamine is in amide linkage to AChE C-terminal Gly.[55] Radiomethylation of the deaminated DAF and AChE products demonstrated that they retained ethanolamine but not glucosamine, establishing that the nonacetylated glucosamine in the $E^{hu}$ DAF and AChE anchors,[73] like that in the mfVSG anchor,[61] is C-terminal to the internal oligosaccharide moiety.[55] Analysis of the released $^{125}$I-TID labeled DAF and AChE anchor fragments by extraction with chloroform:methanol:water and examination of the organic phase on silica thin layer chromatography (chloroform:methanol:water 65:25:4) demonstrated that they were identical. Except for a minor component, however, they did not correspond to PI or to [125]I-TID labeled PI standards (unpublished observations), suggesting differences between the phospholipid components in E[hu] DAF and AChE and those in mfVSGs.

The cDNA which encodes for VSGs predicts that VSGs should contain a C-terminal hydrophobic extension[79] which is not found in mature VSGs and thus appears to be removed prior to incorporation of the C-terminal glycolipid. It has been suggested[63-65] that this C-terminal extension might serve as a stop sequence which functions to appropriately position the VSG mRNA translation product in the endoplasmic reticulum, and that it might then be removed and the C-terminal glycolipid anchor substituted *en bloc* in a two-dimensional reaction. A similar body of data has led to the same suggestion for Thy-1 antigen.[80]

To further verify that ethanolamine is present in E[hu] DAF and to develop a system to investigate the mechanism of its incorporation, biosynthetic experiments in HeLa cells were performed with [³H]-ethanolamine.[73] Both mature membrane DAF and the 48 kDalton HeLa DAF precursor labeled with this probe (Figure 5, panel B) confirming the presence of this component in DAF and demonstrating that it is incorporated prior to the addition of O-linked sugars to pro-DAF in the Golgi. These biosynthetic analyses thus provide evidence that the anchor structure in E[hu] DAF is incorporated at an early step in DAF biosynthesis, similar to findings with mfVSGs.[63-65]

## X. DIRECTIONS FOR FUTURE STUDY

The experiments summarized in this review indicate that some DAF antigen can be detected in affected PNH cells, suggesting that the PNH defect is not due to nonfunction or deletion of the DAF structural gene. Moreover, the defect is not limited to DAF; expression of AChE and other membrane molecules, i.e., a putative (80 kDalton) terminal complement pathway inhibitor, are also deficient. The evidence that the structural gene can function and the presence of abnormalities of multiple membrane components raise the possibility that a regulatory or posttranslational abnormality exists in affected cells.

Structural studies of DAF have shown that, like AChE on E[hu],[54-56] it is an amphipathic protein which is linked to the E[hu] membrane at its C-terminus by a glycolipid containing both ethanolamine and glucosamine with unblocked primary amino groups. Experimental studies completed so far of similar anchoring structures present at the C-terminal ends of trypanosome mfVSGs[59-61] and preliminary analyses of the structure present in DAF[73] indicate that this non-amino-acid anchor is added to the DAF molecule in a posttranslational process. The glycolipid anchoring structure may be preassembled in cells and attached *en bloc* to glycolipid anchored proteins immediately after translation.[59-61,73] The possibility exists that a defect, or defects, in the incorporation of this structure into the DAF molecule is involved in the abnormal DAF expression that occurs in PNH. In support of this idea, studies by Low et al.[81] have shown that another protein deficient in PNH cells,[82] alkaline phosphatase, can be released by PI-PLC and thus may be anchored by a similar structure. Elucidation of the site of the abnormality in PNH cells could yield information about the mechanism of the PNH defect. The investigation of this problem could additionally provide an experimental system which would permit studies of a general biological process that is involved in the expression of several membrane proteins.

Cloning of the genes for Thy-1 antigen[80] and for trypanosome VSGs[79] has shown that the cDNAs encoding these proteins predict hydrophobic C-terminal extensions (like those that serve as conventional anchors) that are not present in mature Thy-1[57] or mfVSG proteins.[60,61] This finding, in conjunction with biosynthetic data[63-65] indicate that these C-terminal extensions are replaced by the corresponding C-terminal glycolipid anchors immediately following their release from ribosomes. Analysis of DAF cDNA will establish whether a similar C-terminal extension is predicted and will facilitate the investigation of intracellular events which take place in the assembly and attachment of the anchor structure into the DAF molecule. In addition, the availability of a DAF cDNA probe would permit Southern blot analyses to determine the number of genes homologous to DAF in the normal genome and ascertain whether any abnormalities are present in the vicinity of the DAF gene of PNH patients, as well as Northern blot analyses to assess the comparative levels of DAF message in the normal and affected cells and to determine if any aberrant DAF mRNA transcripts are synthesized. The results of such studies could formally establish whether the PNH defect involves abnormal DAF gene expression, elaboration of abnormal DAF message, or is at the translational or posttranslational level.

The similarity in structure and function between cellular and extracellular DAF variants raises questions concerning the mechanism of formation of the extracellular DAF species. It is possible that the soluble DAF forms arise from different genes than membrane DAF molecules, are products of a secretory pathway, or alternatively are derived from membrane DAF molecules. Of relevance, an endogenous membrane associated PI-PLC activity is present in trypanosomes[83] which can convert mfVSGs to soluble VSGs, suggesting a mechanism by which a cell might regulate the distribution of the two forms. Further biosynthetic studies and structural analyses of the extracellular DAF species (e.g., for components of the anchor proximal to the site of PI-PLC cleavage) could provide insights concerning their formation. The expression of DAF by epithelial cells and the presence of DAF variants in numerous bodily fluids indicate that DAF is a widespread protein not restricted to the hematological system and raise the possibility that the molecule could be important in these sites, possibly also in inhibiting complement or in serving some as yet undefined alternative function.

# REFERENCES

1. **Müller-Eberhard, H. J. and Schreiber, R. D.,** Molecular biology and chemistry of the alternative pathway of complement, *Advances in Immunology* Vol. 29, Academic Press, 1980, 1.
2. **Tack B. F.,** The β-cys-γ-glu thiolester bond in human C3, C4, and $\alpha_2$-macroglobulin, *Springer Semin. Immunopathol.,* 6, 259, 1983.
3. **Ross, G. D. and Medof, M. E.,** Membrane complement receptors specific for bound fragments of C3, *Adv. Immunol.,* 37, 217, 1985.
4. **Fearon, D. T.** Regulation by membrane sialic acid of β1H-dependent decay-dissociation of the amplification C3 convertase of the alternative complement pathway, *Proc. Nat. Acad. Sci. USA,* 75, 1971, 1978.
5. **Pangburn, M. K. and Müller-Eberhard, H. J.,** Complement C3 convertase: cell surface restriction of β1H control and generation of restriction on neuraminidase-treated cells, *Proc. Nat. Acad. Sci. USA.* 75, 2416, 1978.
6. **Kazatchine, M. D., Fearon, D. T., Silbert J. E., and Austen, K. F.,** Surface-associated heparin inhibits zymosan-induced activation of the human alternative complement pathway by augmenting the regulatory action of the control proteins on particle-bound C3b, *J. Exp. Med.,* 150, 1202, 1979.
7. **Hoffman, E. M.,** Inhibition of complement by a substance isolated from human erythrocytes. I. Extraction from human erythrocyte stromata, *Immunochemistry,* 6, 391, 1969.
8. **Hoffman, E. M.,** Inhibition of complement by a substance isolated from human erythrocytes. II. Studies on the site and mechanism of action, *Immunochemistry,* 6, 405, 1969.
9. **Hoffman, E. M. and Etlinger, H. M.,** Extraction of complement inhibitory factors from the erythrocytes of non-human species, *J. Immunol.,* 111, 946, 1973.
10. **Opferkuch, W., Loos, M., and Borsos, T.,** Decay of SAC42: Evidence for three acccelerating factors in serum, *Fed. Proc.,* 31, 740, 1972.
11. **Fearon, D. T.,** Regulation of the amplification C3 convertase of human complement by an inhibitory protein isolated from human erythrocyte membrane, *Proc. Nat. Acad. Sci. USA,* 76, 5867, 1979.
12. **Fearon, D. T.,** Identification of the membrane glycoprotein that is the C3b receptor of the human erythrocyte, polymorphonuclear leukocyte, B lymphocyte and monocyte, *J. Exp. Med.,* 152, 20, 1980.

13. **Gigli, I., Fujita, T., and Nussenzweig, V.**, Modulation of the classical pathway C3 convertase by plasma proteins C4 binding protein and C3b inactivator, *Proc. Nat. Acad. Sci. USA*, 76, 6596, 1979.
14. **Fujita, T. and Nussenzweig, V.**, The role of C4-binding protein and β1H in proteolysis of C4b and C3b, *J. Exp. Med.*, 150, 267, 1979.
15. **Okada, H., Tanaka, H., and Okada, N.**, Prevention of complement activation on the homologous cell membrane of nucleated cells as well as erythrocytes, *Eur. J. Immunol.*, 13, 340, 1983.
16. **Nicholson-Weller, A., Burge, J., and Austen, K. F.**, Purification from guinea pig erythrocyte stroma of a decay-accelerating factor for the classical C3 convertase, C4b, 2a, *J. Immunol.*, 127, 2035, 1981.
17. **Nicholson-Weller, A., Burge, J., Fearon, D. T., Weller, P. F., and Austen, K. F.**, Isolation of a human erythrocyte membrane glycoprotein with decay accelerating activity for C3 convertases of the complement system, *J. Immunol.*, 129, 184, 1982.
18. **Pangburn, M. K., Schreiber, R. D., and Müller-Eberhard, H. J.**, Deficiency of an erythrocyte membrane protein with complement regulatory activity in paroxysmal nocturnal hemoglobinuria, *Proc. Nat. Acad. Sci. USA*, 80, 5430, 1983.
19. **Iida, K. and Nussenzweig, V.**, Complement receptor is an inhibitor of the complement cascade, *J. Exp. Med.*, 153, 1138, 1980.
20. **Medof, M. E., Kinoshita, T., and Nussenzweig, V.**, Inhibition of complement activation on the surface of cells after incorporation of decay-accelerating factor (DAF) into their membranes, *J. Exp. Med.*, 160, 1558, 1984.
21. **Okada, H., Yasuda, T., Tsumita, T., Shinomiya, H., Utsumi, S., and Okada, H.**, Regulation by glycophorin of complement activation via the alternative pathway, *Biochem. Biophys. Res. Commun.*, 108, 770, 1982.
22. **Okada, H., and Tanaka, H.**, Species-specific inhibition by glycophorin fraction of complement activation via the alternative pathway, *Mol. Immunol.*, 20, 1233, 1983.
23. **Brown, E. J., Ramsey, J., Hammer, C. H., and Frank, M. M.**, Surface modulation of classical pathway activation: C2 and C3 convertase formation and regulation on sheep, guinea pig, and human erythrocytes, *J. Immunol.*, 131, 403, 1983.
24. **Kinoshita, T., Medof, M. E., Hong, K., and Nussenzweig, V.**, Inactivation of red cell-bound C4b and C3b by endogenous association with complement receptor CR1, *Fed. Proc.*, 45, 247 (Abstr.)., 1986.
25. **Pangburn, M. K.**, Differences between the binding sites of the complement regulatory proteins DAF, CR1, and Factor H on C3 convertases, *J. Immunol.*, 136, 2216, 1986.
26. **Rosse, W. F. and Parker, C. J.**, Paroxysmal nocturnal haemoglobinuria, *Clin. Haematol.*, 14, 105, 1984.
27. **Pangburn, M. K., Schreiber, R. D., Trombold, J. S., and Müller-Eberhard, H. J.**, Paroxysmal nocturnal hemoglobinuria; deficiency in factor H-like functions of the abnormal erythrocytes, *J. Exp. Med.*, 157, 1971, 1983.
28. **Nicholson-Weller, A., March, J. P. Rosenfeld, S. I., and Austen, K. F.**, Affected erythrocytes of patients with paroxysmal nocturnal hemoglobinuria are deficient in the complement regulatory protein, decay accelerating factor, *Proc. Nat. Acad. Sci. USA*, 80, 5066, 1983.
29. **Rosse, W. F. and Dacie, J. V.**, Immune lysis of normal human and paroxysmal nocturnal hemoglobinuria (PNH) red blood cells. I. The sensitivity of PNH red cells to lysis by complement and specific antibody, *J. Clin. Invest.*, 45, 736, 1966.
30. **Ham, T. H.**, Chronic hemolytic anemia with paroxysmal nocturnal hemoglobinuria, *N. Eng. J. Med.*, 217, 915, 1937.
31. **Pangburn, M. K. and Müller-Eberhard, H. J.**, Regulation of complement by membrane-associated proteins: defect in paroxysmal nocturnal hemoglobinuria, *Fed. Proc. Fed. Am. Soc. Exp. Biol.*, 43, 1765 (Abstr.), 1984.
32. **Medof, M. E., Kinoshita, T., Silber, R., and Nussenzweig, V.**, Amelioration of the lytic abnormalities of paroxysmal nocturnal hemoglobinuria with decay-accelerating factor, *Proc. Nat. Acad. Sci. USA*, 82, 2980, 1985.
33. **Hammer, C. H., Hänsch, G., Gresham, H. D., and Shin, M. L.**, Activation of the fifth and sixth components of the human complement system: C6-dependent cleavage of C5 in acid and the formation of a bimolecular lytic complex, C5b, $6^{a1}$, *J. Immunol.*, 131, 892, 1983
34. **Kinoshita, T., Medof, M. E., Silber, R., and Nussenzweig, V.**, Distribution of decay accelerating factor in the peripheral blood of normal individuals and patients with paroxysmal nocturnal hemoglobinuria, *J. Exp. Med.*, 162, 75, 1985.
35. **Berger, M. and Medof, M. E.**, Increased expression of complement decay accelerating factor during activation of human neutrophils, *J. Clin. Invest.*, 79, 214, 1987.
36. **Nicholson-Weller, A., March, J. P., Rosen, C. E., Spicer, D. B., and Austen, K. F.**, Surface membrane expression by human blood leukocytes and platelets of decay accelerating factor, a regulatory protein of the complement system, *Blood*, 65, 1237, 1985.

37. **Nicholson-Weller, A., Spicer, D. B., and Austen, K. F.,** Deficiency of the complement regulatory protein "decay accelerating factor" on membranes of granulocytes, monocytes, and platelets in paroxysmal nocturnal hemoglobinura, *N. Engl. J. Med.,* 312, 1091, 1985.

38. **Dixon, R. H. and Rosse, W. F.,** Mechanism of complement-mediated activation of human blood platelets in vitro, *J. Clin. Invest.,* 59, 360, 1977.

39. **Stern, M. and Rosse, W. F.,** Two populations of granulocytes in paroxysmal nocturnal hemoglobinuria, *Blood,* 53, 928, 1979.

40. **Hansch, G. M., Hammer, C. H., Vanguri, P., and Shin, M. L.,** Homologous species restriction in lysis of erythrocytes by terminal complement proteins, *Proc. Nat. Acad. Sci. USA,* 78, 5118, 1981.

41. **Hu, V. W. and Shin, M. L.,** Species-restricted target cell lysis by human complement: complement-lysed erythrocytes from heterologous and homologous species differ in their ratio of bound to inserted C9, *J. Immunol.,* 133, 2133, 1984.

42. **Pachman, C. H., Rosenfeld, S. I., Jenkins. D. E., Jr., Thiem, P. A., and Leddy, J. P.,** Complement lysis of human erythrocytes; differing susceptibility of two types of paroxysmal nocturnal hemoglobinuria cells to C5b-9, *J. Clin. Invest.,* 64, 428, 1979.

43. **Rosenfeld, S. I., Jenkins, D. E., and Leddy, J. P.,** Enhanced reactive lysis of paroxysmal nocturnal hemoglobinuria erythrocytes by C5b-9 does not involve increased C7 binding or cell-bound C3b, *J. Immunol.,* 134, 506, 1985.

44. **Fambrough, D. M., Engel, A. G., and Rosenberry, T. L.,** Acetylcholinesterase of human erythrocytes and neuromuscular junctions: homologies revealed by monoclonal antibodies, *Proc. Nat. Acad. Sci. USA,* 79, 1078, 1982.

45. **Chow, F. L., Hall, S. E., Rosse, W. F., and Telen, M. J.,** Separation of the acetylcholinesterase-deficient red cells in paroxysmal nocturnal hemoglobinuria erythrocytes, *Blood,* 67, 893, 1986.

46. **Medof, M. E., Nussenzweig, V., Kinoshita, T., Gottlieb, A., Hall, S., Silber, R., and Rosse, W. F.,** Nature of the PNH defect, *Complement* 5, 53 (Abstr.), 1985.

47. **Rosse, W. F.,** Variations in the red cells in paroxysmal nocturnal haemoglobinuria, *Brit. J. Haematol.,* 24, 327, 1973.

48. **Hu, V. W. and Nicholson-Weller, A.,** Enhanced complement-mediated lysis of type III paroxysmal nocturnal hemoglobinuria erythrocytes involves increased C9 binding and polymerization, *Proc. Nat. Acad. Sci. USA,* 82, 5520, 1985.

49. **Zalman, L. S. and Müller-Eberhard, H. J.,** Anti-C9 reactive protein in the granules of large granular human lymphocytes, *Complement,* 2, 90 (Abstr.), 1985.

50. **Schonermark, S., Rauterberg, E. W., Roelcke, D., Lobe, S., and Hansch, G. M.,** A C8-binding protein on the surface of human erythrocytes is the inhibitor of lysis in a homologous system, *Immunobiology,* 68, 103 (Abstr.), 1984.

51. **Moore, J. C., Frank, M. M., and Müller-Eberhard, H. J.,** Decay accelerating factor is present on PNH progenitor cells but is lost during in vitro erythropoiesis, *J. Exp. Med.,* 162, 1182, 1985.

52. **Auditore, J. V., Hartman, R. C., Flexner, J. M., and Balchum, O. J.,** The erythrocyte acetylcholinesterase enzyme in paroxysmal nocturnal hemoglobinuria, *Arch. Pathol.,* 69, 534, 1960.

53. **Brimijoin, J.,** Molecular forms of acetylcholinesterase in brain, nerve and muscle: nature, localization and dynamics, *Prog. Neurobiol.,* 21, 291, 1983.

54. **Kim, B. H. and Rosenberry, T. L.,** A small hydrophobic domain that localizes human erythrocyte acetylcholinesterase in liposomal membranes is cleaved by papain digestion, *Biochemistry,* 24, 3586, 1985.

55. **Haas, R., Brandt, P. T., Knight, J., and Rosenberry, T. L.,** Identification of amine components in the glycolipid membrane binding domain of the C-terminus of human erythrocyte acetylcholinesterase, *Biochemistry,* 25, 3098, 1986.

56. **Roberts, W. L. and Rosenberry, T. L.,** Identification of covalently attached fatty acid hydrophobic membrane-binding domain of human erythrocyte acetylcholinesterase, *Biochem. Biophys. Res. Comm.,* 133, 621, 1985.

57. **Tse, A. G.-D., Barclay, A. N., Watts, A., and Williams, A. F.,** A glycophospholipid tail at the carboxyl terminus of the Thy-1 glycoprotein of neurons and thymocytes, *Science,* 230, 1003, 1985.

58. **Low, M. G. and Kincade, P. W.,** Phosphatidylinositol is the membrane-anchoring domain of the Thy-1 glycoprotein, *Nature,* 318, 62, 1985.

59. **Holder, A. A.,** Carbohydrate is linked through ethanolamine to the C-terminal amino acid of *Trypanosoma brucei* variant surface glycoprotein, *Biochem. J.,* 209, 261, 1983.

60. **Ferguson, M.A.J., Haldar, K., and Cross, G.A.M.,** *Trypanosomal brucei* variant surface glycoprotein has a sn-1,2-dimyristyl glycerol membrane anchor at its COOH terminus, *J. Biol. Chem.,* 260, 4963, 1985.

61. **Ferguson, M.A.J., Low, M. G., and Cross, G.A.M.,** Glycosyl-sn-1,2-dimyristylphosphatidylinositol is covalently linked to *Trypanosoma brucei* variant surface glycoprotein, *J. Biol. Chem.,* 260, 14547, 1985.

62. **Bordier, C., Etges, R. J., Ward, J., Turner, M. J., and Cardoso de Almeida, M. L.** *Leishmania* and *Trypanosoma* surface glycoproteins have a common glycophospholipid membrane anchor, *Proc. Nat. Acad. Sci. USA,* 83, 5988, 1986.

63. **Rifkin, M. R. and Fairlamb, A. H.,** Ethanolamine and its incorporation into the variant surface glycoprotein of bloodstream forms of *Trypanosoma brucei, Molec. Biochem. Parasitol.,* 15, 245, 1985.

64. **Ferguson, M.A.J., Duszenko, M., Lamont, G. S., Overath, P., and Cross, G.A.M.,** Biosynthesis of *Trypanosoma brucei* variant surface glycoprotein, *J. Biol. Chem.,* 261, 356, 1986.

65. **Bangs, J. D., Hereld, D., Krakow, J. L., Hart, G. W., and Englund, P. T.,** Rapid processing of the carboxyl terminus of a trypanosome variant surface glycoprotein, *Proc. Nat. Acad. Sci. USA,* 82, 3207, 1985.

66. **Medof, M. E., Walter, E. I., Rutgers, J. L., Knowles, D. M., and Nussenzweig, V.,** Identification of the complement decay accelerating factor (DAF) on epithelium and glandular cells and in body fluids, *J. Exp. Med.,* 165, 848, 1987.

67. **Spinella, D. G., Shah, D. D., Hale, P. D., and Levine, R. P.,** Monoclonal antibodies to human C4. I. The purification of hemolytically active C4 from small volumes of normal serum, *Complement,* 1, 184, 1984.

68. **Asch, A., Kinoshita, T., and Nussenzweig, V.,** Decay-accelerating factor is present on cultured human umbilical vein endothelial cells, *J. Exp. Med.,* 162, 221, 1985.

69. **Andersson, L. C. and Gahmberg, C. G.,** A human leukemia cell line inducible to erythroid differentiation, in *In Vivo and In Vitro Erythropoiesis: The Friend System,* Rossi, G. E., Ed., Elsevier/North Holland Biomedical Press, 1980, 457.

70. **Guerrasio, A., Vainchenker, W., Breton-Gorius, J., Testa, U., Rosa, R., Thomopoulos, P., Titeux, M., Guichard, J., and Beuzard, Y.,** Embryonic and fetal hemoglobin synthesis in K562 cell line, *Blood Cells,* 7, 165, 1981.

71. **Lublin, D. M., Kresek-Staples, J., Pangburn, M. K., and Atkinson, J. P.,** Biosynthesis and glycosylation of the human complement regulatory protein decay-accelerating factor, *J. Immunol.,* 137, 1629, 1986.

72. **Medof, M. E., Mann, W. H., and Rosenfeld, M.,** Biosynthesis of human decay accelerating factor, in preparation.

73. **Medof, M. E., Walter, E. I., Roberts, W.L., Haas, R., and Rosenberry, T. L.,** Decay accelerating factor of complement is anchored to cells by a C-terminal glycolipid, *Biochemistry* 25, 6740, 1986.

74. **Davitz, M., Low, M., and Nussenzweig, V.,** Release of decay-accelerating factor (DAF) from the cell membrane by phosphatidylinositol-specific phospholipase C (PIPLC), *J. Exp. Med.,* 163, 1150, 1986.

75. **Haas, R. and Rosenberry, T. L.,** Quantitative identification of N-terminal amino acids in proteins by radiolabeled reductive methylation and amino acid analysis: application to human erythrocyte acetylcholinesterase, *Analyt. Biochem.,* 148, 154, 1985.

76. **Shively, J. E. and Conrad, H. E.,** Formation of anhydrous sugars in the chemical depolymerization of heparin, *Biochemistry,* 15, 3932, 1976.

77. **Brunner, J. and Semenza, G.,** Selective labeling of the hydrophobic core of membranes with 3-(Trifluoromethyl)-3-(m-[$^{123}$I]iodophenyl)diazirine, a carbene-generating reagent, *Biochemistry,* 20, 7174, 1981.

78. **Roberts, W. L. and Rosenberry, T. L.,** Selective radiolabeling and isolation of the hydrophobic membrane-binding domain of human erythrocyte acetylcholinesterase, *Biochemistry,* 25, 3091, 1986.

79. **Turner, M. J.,** The biochemistry of the surface antigens of the African trypanosomes, *Br. Med. Bull.,* 41, 137, 1985.

80. **Seki, T., Moriuchi, T., Chang, H. C., Denome, R., and Silver, J.,** Structural organization of the rat thy-1 gene, *Nature,* 313, 485, 1985.

81. **Low, M. G. and Zilversmit, D. B.,** Role of phosphatidylinositol in attachment of alkaline phosphatase to membranes, *Biochemistry,* 19, 3913, 1980.

82. **Lewis, S. M. and Dacie, J. V.,** Neutrophil (leukocyte) alkaline phosphatase in paroxysmal nocturnal haemoglobinuria, *Brit. J. Haematol.,* 11, 549, 1965.

83. **Bülow R. and Overath, P. O.,** Purification and characterization of the membrane-form variant surface glycoprotein hydrolates of *Trypanosoma brucea, J. Biol. Chem.,* 261, 11918, 1986.

*Section I.B: Recognition — Killer Lymphocytes*

Chapter 5

# T CELL SPECIFICITY AND THE T CELL RECEPTOR α, β and γ CHAINS

**David H. Raulet**

## TABLE OF CONTENTS

# I. INTRODUCTION

Since the mid 1970s it has been known that helper and cytotoxic T cells recognize foreign antigenic determinants "in the context" of normal self-cell surface components, the major histocompatibility complex (MHC) encoded proteins.[1-5] In the 10 years following the discovery of these basic phenomena, a vast number of studies of T cell specificity were performed which led to a rather thorough understanding of T cell recognition at the phenominological level. However, since the T cell antigen receptor molecule was not identified until the early 1980s, analysis of the molecular basis of T cell specificity was not possible until recently. In the first part of this review, I will summarize some of the recent studies of the T cell receptor α and β chain proteins, and the genes that encode them. These studies represent the initial effort at developing an understanding of the molecular basis of MHC-restricted T cell recognition. In anticipation of the conclusions of this review, I note that the current status of the studies does not allow solid conclusions to be drawn as to the structural basis of T cell specificity for MHC and antigens. Nonetheless, several models have been ruled out and the basis has been laid for the eventual solution to this problem.

The second part of this chapter is devoted to a description of the murine T cell γ gene family. the γ gene was first isolated in attempts to clone the α subunit of the T cell antigen receptor,[6] and remains a gene family of unknown function. As will be described, the γ genes have striking similarities to the α and β T cell receptor genes, including unambiguous homology of the predicted γ chain protein to immunoglobulins, and clear structural similarities of the genes and proteins to those of the α and β subunits. Of particular significance is that like the α and β genes, the γ genes undergo somatic gene rearrangements and are expressed specifically in cells of the T lineage. The most striking clue to the function of the γ gene is that unlike the α and β genes, the γ genes are generally expressed most actively in the least mature developing thymocytes, strongly suggesting a specific function for the genes in the events of early T cell development. Hence, some current models of γ gene function suggest a role for the γ chain in selection of T cells with specificity for self-MHC proteins, a process known to occur in T cell development. Following a detailed description of the genes and their behavior, I will summarize some speculative models as to how the γ chain may be involved in selection of the T cell specificity repertoire.

# II. T CELL SPECIFICITY AND THE T CELL RECEPTOR

## A. T Cell Specificity

It is important to emphasize from the outset that as of the present, T cell receptor interactions have never been measured in conventional molecular binding assays in which Scatchard curves can be generated and affinities measured. The problem has been that the receptor and (at least) one of the ligands, the MHC proteins, are intrinsic membrane proteins. In lieu of such binding data, T cell receptor interactions are measured indirectly by assays of the triggering of T cell functions such as cytolysis of targets (CTL) or lymphokine production (helper T cells). Hence, while in the following discussion I will refer to the reactivity or lack of reactivity of T cells with various ligands, it must be kept in mind that the threshold affinities for triggering T cell functions are not known and therefore lack of a reaction in a functional assay does not necessarily imply a negligible receptor affinity for a given ligand.

## 1. MHC Restriction

The remarkable property of recognition by T cells is that they not only distinguish closely related antigenic determinants, but they also discriminate allelic forms of the highly polymorphic MHC-encoded proteins expressed by the cells which present the antigens.[1-5] Thus, no reaction is apparent unless both the MHC protein and the antigen are of the correct type.

The early studies further suggested indirectly that the affinity of T cell receptors for antigen or MHC protein alone is considerably lower than for the combination of the two. In addition, many early studies, particularly those of genetically determined low responsiveness to antigens (the immune response or Ir genes), led to the concept that MHC proteins and antigens must physically interact in some way for T cell recognition to occur.[8,9]

The detailed evidence, too lengthy to review here, suggests that the T cell receptor recognizes a molecular complex of MHC proteins and antigen (or a fragment of the antigen), and reacts poorly to either the MHC protein or antigen in the absence of the other. From the point of view of the T cell, the debate centered on whether there are two types of T cell receptors on a given T cell, one specific for antigen, the other for allelic determinants on MHC proteins, or a single receptor that in some way recognizes the molecular complex of antigen and MHC proteins. As summarized below, the current evidence argues that there is a single two chain T cell receptor molecule which is responsible for both antigen and MHC specificity. However, the present data do not allow a definitive resolution as to whether the T cell receptor has two more or less independent contact sites (for MHC protein and antigen), or alternatively a single contact site which is created by the unique interaction of a given antigen/MHC protein pair. Although this basic issue may be definitively resolved only by future X-ray diffraction studies of the appropriate complexes, the emerging analyses from many laboratories concerning the primary structures of T cell receptors with given specificities, some of which are summarized in this review, should lay the basis for a firm prediction to be made.

## 2. T Cell Fine Specificity

Although most H-2 restricted T cell clones appear to have strict specificity for a given MHC protein, exceptional clones have been noted which cross-react at the level of MHC restriction. The detailed properties of such clones strongly argue that the MHC proteins and the antigen do not behave independently from the point of view of the T cell receptor. For example, rare T cell clones exist which can react with an antigen, X, in the context of an MHC protein, H-2$^a$, and also cross-react with an antigen, Y, in the context of H-2$^b$. Such clones, however, do not react with the antigen X in the context of H-2$^b$ or antigen Y in the context of H-2$^a$.[10-12] These and other studies argue that the T cell receptor can recognize determinant(s) created by idiosyncratic interactions of given MHC protein-antigen pairs. There are other examples in which a T cell clone reacts with the same antigen in the context of two quite different MHC proteins. However, the cross-reactivity of such T cell with related forms of the antigen (fine specificity) is often different when presented by the different MHC proteins, again arguing for an MHC-antigen interaction.[11,12] As discussed below, such clones are useful in analyzing the contribution of T cell receptor segments to specificity. MHC restricted T cells often cross-react on a foreign MHC molecule in the absence of antigen.[13-15] Again such cross-reactive T cells will be useful in analyzing the contribution of α and β gene segments to specificity, and hopefully shed light on why such reactions are common or uncommon in the first place.

One sort of T cell crossreaction is notable because it has *not* been documented. Most CTL are restricted by the MHC Class I proteins (K, D, and L in the mouse),[7] whereas most helper T cells are restricted by the MHC Class II proteins (IA and IE in the mouse).[2,16,17] In the cross-reactions discussed in the previous paragraphs, T cells restricted by (or specific for, in the case of alloreactive cells) Class I or Class II proteins crossreact on a different Class I or Class II protein, respectively (i.e., an allelic variant or a product of a different locus of the same class). However no convincing case of a Class I restricted T cell cross-reacting on a Class II protein, or vice-versa, has been reported. The possible role of the accessory molecules Lyt-2 and L3T4 in encouraging Class I[18] or Class II[19] specific reactions, respectively, may be partly responsible for this, but may not be the complete explanation since Class I specific, Lyt-2[18] clones[18] and Class II specific L3T4[20] clones[20] have been described. Thus, comparisons of the components of Class I vs. Class II specific T cell receptors have been of particular interest.

*3. Thymus Education*

Germane to the studies of the molecular basis of T cell specificity are the studies of the ontogenic acquisition of T cell specificity within the thymus. Many studies have shown that T cells prefer to react with antigens in the context of those MHC proteins they encounter within the thymus during their differentiation, which may, by experimental manipulation, be different from their own.[17,21,22] Thus T cell receptors appear to be "fitted" ontogenetically to the MHC proteins of the host. The "fitting" process, called thymus education, is presumed to involve a positive selection process acting on those developing thymocytes which express the appropriate T cell receptors. The biology of thymus education presents several conundrums. In particular, it is a mystery as to how T cell receptors restricted by self-MHC proteins can be selected if, in fact, such receptors have no or negligible affinity for self-MHC proteins in the absence of antigen. Hence, there is currently considerable interest in analysis of the molecular and cellular mechanisms whereby self-restricted T cells are selected during ontogeny. The molecular basis of restricted recognition by mature T cells is obviously pertinent to these studies.

## B. The T Cell Receptor

*1. The α and β Chains*

The strategy which eventually succeeded in the isolation of the T cell receptor depended upon production of monoclonal antibodies which distinguish one T cell clone from another, and, hence, react with determinants created by the variability of the antigen receptor.[23-25] Such clonotypic antibodies react with the now-familiar molecular complex composed of the clonally variable, disulfide-linked α and β glycoproteins (each approximately 40 to 45 kDaltons apparent molecular weight, Figure 1) and the noncovalently associated, clonally invariable T3 accessory molecules. Parallel subtractive cDNA cloning studies yielded the genes encoding the β and α chains shortly thereafter.[26-30] In addition, this approach yielded a third similar gene, originally presumed to encode the α chain, which is called γ.[6] All three gene families undergo T cell specific gene rearrangements, are transcribed specifically in T cells, and encode proteins with distinct homology to the immunoglobulin (Ig) heavy (H) and light (L) chains. All three gene families have distinct variable (V), joining (J) and constant (C) gene segments [the β family but perhaps not the α and γ families include diversity (D) segments as well]. Productive rearrangement of a V segment to a J segment produces the functional transcription unit. The properties of the murine α and β gene families (Figure 2) are summarized below. The γ family will be discussed in the second half of this review.

*2. The β Genes*

The β gene family includes two neighboring C gene segments, C1 and C2, which differ in predicted amino acid sequence by only four residues. Each C gene has an associated cluster of six functional J segments. At least two Dβ segments have been isolated.[31,32]

Approximately 20 V gene segments are in the Vβ family.[33] Most of the Vβ genes are quite distinct from each other (ca. 16 to 50% amino acid homology compared to the immunoglobulins, which show greater than 45% homology) although two three-membered cross-hybridizing Vβ gene subfamilies have been described.

With the exception of somatic hypermutation, which appears not to occur in the α, β, or γ genes, the mechanisms for generating diversity in the β genes appears similar to the H-chain Ig genes.[33] Thus, combinatorial diversity and junctional diversity have been well

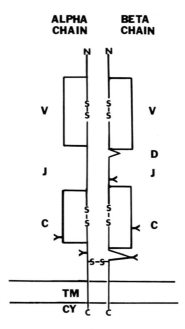

FIGURE 1.   Schematic structure of the α/β heterodimeric T cell receptor, drawn approximately to scale. Putative intra- and inter-chain disulfide linkages are indicated as are potential sites on the constant region for N-linked glycosylation (Y). Glycosylation sites on the variable regions are not indicated, as they are different on different V genes.

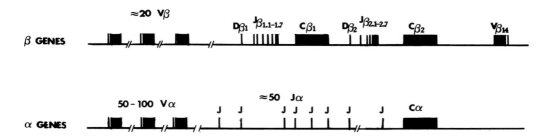

FIGURE 2.   Genomic organization of α and β gene segments. Intron-exon structures of the constant regions are *not* indicated. The Jα segments span at least 60 kb of DNA, whereas the Jβ segments are closely linked in two groups. The Vβ14 segment is located 3′ to the Cβ gene segments, and rearranges to Jβ segments by inversion.[33]

documented in studies of Vβ gene rearrangements. At least two additional mechanisms for increasing diversity are operative in the β genes, compared with the H chain genes. Unlike the H chain genes, β gene rearrangements sometimes do not include a D segment. In addition, D segments in β gene rearrangements can be functionally rearranged in all three translational reading frames, unlike the H chain D segments, which are only read in one reading frame. In addition, the greater divergence in the germline Vβ sequences compared to the IG-V genes can be considered a source of greater diversity. However, there are many more VH (100 to 1000) and Vκ (Ca. 100) genes than Vβ genes.

### 3. The α Genes

The α family[33-36] includes a single C gene, perhaps 50 J segments and ca. 50 to 100 V genes. The Vα genes are generally organized in cross-hybridizing subfamilies of 3 to 10 members. Like the Vβ genes, the predicted amino acid homologies between Vα subfamilies is lower (16 to 50%) than between Ig-V gene subfamilies (>45% homology). The unusually large number of Jα segments may be an important source of diversity in the α gene family. As of the present, no Dα segments have been isolated, and there may be none. Sequence analyses suggest that junctional diversity resulting from small deletions and possible additions of nucleotides at the Vα-Jα junction is also a source of α gene variability.[33-36]

### 4. The α/β Heterodimer

A critical question in assessing T cell specificity is whether the α/β heterodimer is responsible for both antigen and MHC recognition. A variety of functional studies suggest this is the case. A now classic study[37] showed that MHC and antigen recognition are not accomplished by two completely independent receptors. Thus, the cell-fusion product of two T cell hybridomas with distinct antigen and MHC restriction specificities did not result in a cell with a "mixed" specificity (i.e., the antigen specificity of one parent plus the MHC restriction specificity of the other). Another important experiment demonstrated that an anti-idiotypic antibody, which reacts with the α/β heterodimer of a particular T cell hybridoma with defined MHC and antigen fine specificity, predicts both antigen and MHC fine specificity of freshly isolated T cell hybridomas.[38] Recently, it was demonstrated that transfection of both the α and β genes from a T cell clone of defined specificity into an unrelated T cell hybrid conferred upon the recipient the antigen and MHC specificity of the donor cell.[39] This result strongly suggests that the α and β genes are the only clonally variable genes which confer antigen and MHC specificity, although additional confirming experiments with other antigen-reactive T cells will be necessary for a solid conclusion to be drawn.

## C. T Cell Receptor Gene Usage and Specificity

### 1. Constant Regions and Specificity

A clear conclusion of all the studies to date is that CTL and helper T cells use the same Cα and Cβ genes. Although there are two Cβ genes, they are extremely similar to each other, and appear to be used interchangably in T cells with specificity for Class I and Class II MHC proteins.[33] Although the C gene would not be expected to influence the specificity of a receptor, it was possible that different T cells (e.g., those specific for Class I vs. Class II MHC) might use entirely different T cell receptor gene families; this is apparently not the case.

### 2. V, D, and J Gene Usage and Specificity for Class I and Class II MHC

Several studies indicate that particular T cell clones specific for Class I and clones specific for Class II may use the same germline Vβ gene segment. For example, a CTL clone specific for allo-H2-D$^b$ (Class I) uses the Vβ6 gene segment which is also used by a helper clone specific for a chicken red blood cell antigen plus IA$^b$ (Class II).[40] Similarly, members of the three-membered Vβ8 subfamily are used by many Class II-restricted helper T cells,[41,42] as well as by the CTL clone 2C, allo-specific for L$^d$ (Class I) (the 2C clone, originally thought to use the Vβ7 segment, actually uses a Vβ8 gene[43]). Furthermore, monoclonal antibodies that recognize determinants of the Vβ8 gene subfamily[41,42] react with a large fraction (ca. 20%) of both Lyt-2$^+$ and L3T4$^+$ (largely Class I and Class II restricted, respectively) T cells.[44] Thus, the germline Vβ gene segment does not predict the Class I vs. Class II MHC specificity of T cells. Similarly the same Jβ and Dβ segments can be used by T cell clones with specificity for Class I or Class II MHC products.[33]

At present there is little comparable data concerning Vα and Jα usage in Class I vs. Class II restricted T cell clones. However, our recent analysis of V gene usage in T cell populations suggests that neither Vα nor Vβ gene germline segments by themselves determine Class I vs. Class II restriction.[45] Thus, we found that the frequencies of usage of three Vα gene segments (representing three distinct subfamilies), as well as three Vβ gene segments, were within two-fold in comparing Lyt-2$^+$ L3T4$^-$ (largely Class I restricted) and Lyt-2$^-$ L3T4$^+$ (largely Class II restricted) T cell populations. Thus, it appears that Class I vs. Class II MHC specificity is not a consequence of usage of nonoverlapping pools of Vβ, Jβ, Dβ, and Vα (germline gene segments).

Although a given Vα or Vβ gene segment can participate in receptors with either Class I or Class II specificity, it is valid to ask whether there is *preferential* usage of particular V segments by Class I vs. Class II restricted T cells, or by T cells restricted by different alleles of a given MHC locus. A critical issue which such data may bear on is whether one or the other chain is "more" specific for MHC recognition. As noted above, we found that the differences in Vα or Vβ usage were less than or equal to two-fold between Lyt-2$^-$ L3T4$^+$ cells and Lyt-2$^+$ L3T4$^-$ T cells which were not antigen-selected. Hence, there are no dramatic biases apparent in V gene usage in this analysis. The small biases observed may be significant, however. For example, as assessed by staining cells with the Vβ8-subfamily specific antibody KJ16, and analysis by flow cytometry, the Vβ8 subfamily is expressed by twice as many Lyt-2$^+$, L3T4$^-$ T cells than Lyt-2$^-$, L3T4$^+$ T cells,[44] a result confirmed by our RNA analysis. Such differences, though minor, may reflect a slightly greater compatibility of the Vβ8 gene segments for Class I vs. Class II recognition, although other possible explanations have not been ruled out. The present data, however, do not allow the conclusion that even such minor differences occur more frequently in Vβ usage than in Vα usage. Hence, such analyses have thus far *not* supported the point of view that the β chain is more critical in MHC recognition than the α chain, or vice versa.

### 3. V Gene Usage and Specificity for MHC Allele-Products

Analyses of many T cell clones indicate that the MHC restriction of a T cell cannot be generally predicted from the independent assessment of which Vβ gene, Dβ segment, or Jβ segment is used.[33] Furthermore, a recent study demonstrated that members of the same Vα gene subfamily are used by cytochrome C-specific T cells restricted by either IE$^k$ or IE$^s$.[46] A second approach to the question of V gene usage vs. H-2 restriction specificity is to analyze T cell populations which are not selected for antigen specificity, but are selected for MHC-restriction specificity. As an approach to this problem, we analyzed V gene usage in T cells of three H-2 congenic mouse strains, Balb/c (H-2$^d$), Balb.B (H-2$^b$) and Balb.K (H-2$^k$). The three strains have the same germ-line T cell receptor genes, but differ at the MHC locus. Because of thymus education, the T cells from the three strains are preferentially restricted to H-2$^d$, H-2$^b$, or H-2$^k$, respectively. Our analysis showed that the usage of three Vβ and three Vα gene segments is within two-fold in comparing T cells from these three strains.[45] Thus thymus education does not result in dramatic biases in usage of least the Vα and Vβ genes we analyzed, suggesting that specificity for allelic variants of MHC proteins cannot be generally correlated with particular germline V gene segments.

Note that the results discussed here do not rule out the possibility that particular α and/or β gene structures are dramatically more compatible with recognition of particular MHC molecules. This is because combinatorial diversity (provided by random V,D, and J joining), and junctional diversity (provided by variability in the exact recombination sites, and possible random nucleotide addition at junctions) may be critical in determining the MHC restriction specificity of a given receptor chain.

### 4. T Cell Receptor Gene Segment Usage and T Cell Fine Specificity

Several investigators have analyzed T cell receptor genes used by sets of clones specific for particular antigens, but with distinguishable antigen and MHC fine specificities. The advantage of this approach is that defined subtle differences in specificity may be correlated with defined differences in receptor chain structure. In terms of the more global questions (e.g., is one chain or the other more responsible for MHC vs. antigen specificity) the limitation of the approach is that a particular correlation in one antigen system may not hold in a different system (see below). However, by comparing the detailed results of many such analyses, with different antigen-MHC combinations, it is expected that a clear idea of the contribution of receptor structure to specificity will emerge. The results of the studies summarized below are depicted in Table 1.

The most detailed studies to date are in the cytochrome c system. The murine T cell response to pigeon cytochrome c is extremely restricted in that a given mouse strain often produces clones with only a very few distinguishable fine specificity patterns, and some strains are nonresponders altogether.[11,12] The contribution of particular amino acid residues in the immunogenic peptides of cytochrome c to T cell specificity have been analyzed in some detail. Furthermore, some clones but not others crossreact with cytochrome c in the context of a different MHC allele-product, allowing the possible determination of receptor features which result in such crossreactions.

Clones from B10.A mice fall into several groups based on MHC fine specificity. Some clones react with cytochrome c plus either IE$\beta^k$ or IE$\beta^b$ but not IE$\beta^s$. A distinct set of clones react with cytochrome c plus either IE$\beta^k$ or IE$\beta^s$ but not IE$\beta^b$. Three of three clones that crossreact between IE$^k$ and IE$^b$ were shown to use the V$\beta$3 gene segment and the J$\beta$1.2 or J$\beta$2.5 segments, whereas two of two clones that crossreact between IE$^k$ and IE$^s$ use the V$\beta$B10 gene segment and J$\beta$2.1[47](Table 1). All the clones analyzed use members of the V$\alpha$11 subfamily. Thus there is a correlation in these clones between the V$\beta$ and J$\beta$ segment used and the MHC-restriction fine specificity of the clones. Since all the clones use similar V$\alpha$ genes despite their different MHC fine specificities, the V$\alpha$ segment correlates with antigen specificity in this system.

An independent study of cytochrome c-specific T cell clones showed that eight of nine hybridomas specific for cytochrome c plus IE$^k$, and three of six hybridomas specific for cytochrome c plus IE$^s$, all use members of the V$\alpha$11 subfamily.[46] Based on these two studies, it appears that most cytochrome c specific T cells, including those restricted by two different Class II MHC proteins (and with different MHC and antigen fine specificities) use one or the other of the two members of the V$\alpha$11 gene subfamily. This striking correlation suggests that, at least in specific cases, the antigen specificity of T cells can be correlated with one of the two T cell receptor chains, with some independence from the MHC-restriction specificity. It will be interesting to determine whether the V$\alpha$11 chain contacts the cytochrome c peptide, as might be predicted from these results.

Studies of clones specific for ovalbumin from H-2$^d$ mice have yielded a mirror image of the cytochrome c results. In response to a particular ovalbumin peptide, two major fine specificity clonotypes are found. One set of clones reacts to antigen plus IA$^d$, cross-reacts variably with antigen plus IA$^b$, and weakly with IA$^b$ without antigen. A distinct set of clones reacts with IA$^d$ plus antigen but does not show the aforementioned cross-reactivities. Both types of clones use a member of the V$\beta$8 subfamily. They differ in that the cross-reactive clones all use the same V$\alpha$ segment (V$\alpha$ DO11), whereas the non-crossreactive clones usually use V$\alpha$ segments of distinct subfamilies.[48] Hence, in this system the MHC-fine specificity correlates with the V$\beta$ gene segment, and the antigen specificity correlates with the V$\alpha$ gene segment.

## D. Conclusions

A probably fair summation of the studies to date is that T cell specificity for MHC determinants vs. antigen is not generally determined by any one particular aspect of the $\alpha$ or $\beta$ chain sequence. Although more data will be required before a definitive statement can be made, it appears that the MHC and antigen specificity of a particular receptor can be influenced by both the $\alpha$ and $\beta$ chains sequences. It is possible that all documented means

## Table 1
## V GENE USAGE VS. FINE SPECIFICITY OF T CELL CLONES

| T cell specificity | | Crossreactivity | | T cell receptor[a] | | Ref. |
|---|---|---|---|---|---|---|
| **Immunogen** | | | | | | |
| **MHC** | **Antigen** | **MHC** | **Antigen** | **α chain** | **β chain** | |
| IEβ$^k$ | Pigeon cytochrome c | IEβ$^k$ | Moth cytochrome c | Vα11.1-Jα84 | Vβ3-Jβ1.2 | 47 |
| | | IEβ$^b$ | Moth cytochrome c | or Vα11.2-Jα2B4 | Vβ3-Jβ2.5 | |
| IEβ$^k$ | Pigeon cytochrome c | IEβ$^k$ | Moth cytochrome c | Vα11.1-JαC7 | Vβ3-Jβ1.2 | |
| | | IEβ$^b$ | Moth cytochrome c | | | |
| | | IA$^s$ | (alloreactive) | | | |
| IEβ$^k$ | Pigeon cytochrome c | IEβ$^k$ | Moth cytochrome c | Vα11.1-Jα84 | VβB10-Jβ2.1 | |
| | | IEβ$^s$ | Pigeon cytochrome c | | | |
| IE$^k$ | Pigeon cytochrome c | IE$^b$ | Pigeon cytochrome c | Vα11.1 or 11.2(8 of 9) | Vβ3(4 of 9) | 46 |
| IE$^s$ | Pigeon cytochrome c | IE$^v$ | Pigeon cytochrome c | Vα11(3 of 6) | Various | |
| IA$^d$ | Ovalbumin peptide | IA$^b$ | Ovalbumin peptide | VαDO11 | Vβ8 member | |
| | | IA$^b$ | (weak alloreactivity) | | | |
| IA$^d$ | Ovalbumin peptide | | (None documented) | Other Vαs | Vβ8 member | 48 |

[a] Where possible, a single nomenclature is used.[33] VβB10 and VαDO11 have not at present been assigned numbers.

of generating diversity in the sequences of both of these chains may influence the specificity for either antigen or MHC.

As has been pointed out elsewhere, this is not necessarily a surprising finding, considering the predicted structure of the α/β heterodimer. The primary sequences of the α and β genes are strikingly similar in some respects to those of the immunoglobulins, in that those residues most highly conserved in comparing different immunoglobulin heavy and light chains are also conserved in the α and β V gene sequences. Hence it is reasonable to predict that the rules governing the nature of the Ig and T cell receptor combining sites will be similar.[49] Many studies have suggested that the contributions of H and L chain sequences to Ig specificity cannot be generally separated, although in some specific cases it appears that either the H or L chain is more important in determining some particular aspect of Ig specificity.[50,51] Given that the three-dimensional structure of the combining site is influenced by both chains, it is perhaps not surprising that the contributions of each chain cannot be easily separated. It is important to note, however, that the reason for considering that T cell receptors might follow different rules than immunoglobulins was that T cell specificity apparently follows different rules than immunoglobulin specificity: i.e., T cells are MHC-restricted, whereas antibodies generally are not. If MHC and antigen were recognized by somewhat independent combining sites, one might indeed expect to find ascertainable differences not only in the structure of the receptors as compared to immunoglobulins, but also in the rules governing their specificity. The failure to do so, at least thus far, can thus be seen as supporting evidence for the concept that MHC and antigen are not recognized as independent entities but rather as a mutually interactive complex. This concept is embodied in the "altered-self" hypothesis of T cell recognition,[52] for which a plethora of other indirect evidence has been garnered over the years in the absence of any direct studies of the T cell receptor structure. Future structural studies will be necessary to corroborate this idea, and to provide a refined molecular model of T cell receptor-antigen-MHC interactions.

If T cell receptors and immunoglobulins are so similar, how is one to explain the overwhelming preoccupation of T cells with MHC proteins? *A priori,* this might be due to a germ-line predisposition of T cell receptors to react with MHC proteins, and/or it might be imposed somatically by selection during intrathymic T cell differentiation. The fact is that general predictable correlations between germline sequences and differences in specificity for MHC proteins are not obvious; it must be entertained that the specificity for MHC proteins is largely imposed somatically. In the extreme, it might be imagined that a random and unselected collection of T cell receptors would show no preoccupation with MHC recognition. This extreme scenario would appear unlikely, since the somatic selection process for MHC restricted T cells would be expected to result in the preservation in the germline of V gene segments preferentially reactive with MHC proteins over evolutionary time. Although further studies will be required to assess the relative germline vs. somatic contributions to T cell receptor specificity, it is important to note that an important somatic contribution has been demonstrated by the experiments showing that T cells are selected for MHC allele specificity during intrathymic differentiation. It is hoped that studies of this process will shed light on the means by which specificity for MHC is imposed.

## III. THE T CELL GAMMA GENE

### A. Introduction

This section will summarize the current state of studies of the murine T cell gamma gene family. The γ genes have an as-yet-unidentified function, but their similarities in many respects to the α and β genes is striking, suggesting a related function. Moreover, as noted below, the behavior of the genes, which are particularly actively expressed in immature thymocytes, raises the intriguing possibility that they function in selection of the T cell

```
              10            20            30            40            50
V1.2 4/203  G L G Q L E Q T E L S V T R E T D E N V Q I S C I V L P Y F S - N T A I H W Y R Q K I N Q Q F E Y L I Y V A
V2    17 γ  G H G K L E Q P E I S I S R P R D E T A Q I S C K V F I E S F R - S V T I H W Y R Q K P N Q G L E F L L Y V L
V3    13 γ  G D S W I S Q D Q L S F I R R P N K T V H I S C K L S G V P L H - N T I V H W Y Q L K E G P L R R I F Y G S
V4    11 γ  G S S L T S P L G S Y V I K R K G N T A F L K C Q I K T S V Q K P D A Y I H W Y Q E K P G Q R L Q R M L C S S


              60            70            80            90           100
V1.2 4/203  T N Y N Q R - P L G G K H K K I E A S K D F K S S T S T L E I N Y L K K E D E A T Y Y C A V W M  -  J - 1 0 . 5
V2    17 γ  A T P T H I - F L D K E Y K K M E A S K N P S A S T S I L T I Y S L E E E D E A I Y Y C S Y G  -  J - 1 3 . 4
V3    13 γ  V K T Y K Q - - - D K S H S R L E I D E K I D D G T F Y L I I N N V V T S D E A T Y Y C A C W D  -  J - 1 3 . 4
V4    11 γ  S K E N I V Y E K D F S D E R Y E A R T W Q S D L S S V L T I H Q V T E E D T G T Y Y C A C W D  -  J - 1 3 . 4
```

FIGURE 3. Comparison of four Vγ gene subfamilies. Homologies between V1.2,[6] V2, V3, and V4,[54] predicted amino acid sequences are boxed. (From Garman, R. D., Doherty, P., and Raulet, D. H., *Cell*, 45, 733, 1986. Copyright Cell Press. With permission.)

specificity repertoire. After summarizing the γ gene family and the expression and rearrangement patterns of the genes, I will summarize some speculations regarding their possible functions.

The first gamma cDNA clone, initially thought to encode the α chain, was isolated in Tonegawa's laboratory from a cloned CTL line by subtractive hybridization cloning and screening for T cell-specific gene rearrangement.[6] The overall structure of the γ-chain, predicted from the nucleotide sequence, is very similar to the α and β chains,[6,53] including a hydrophobic signal peptide, a ca. 100 amino acid variable region, a J segment, a constant region segment, a hydrophobic membrane domain, and a cytoplasmic domain slightly larger than those of the α and β chains. Cysteine residues in the V and C regions are placed appropriately for formation of the intrachain disulfide bridges of characteristic Ig-like domains, and an additional cysteine residue near the membrane domain is placed appropriately for an interchain disulfide linkage to an as-yet-unidentified putative partner chain. The original cDNA sequence predicts a subunit of 33 kDaltons which lacks asparagine-linked carbohydrates.

The overall homology of the deduced Vγ amino acid sequences with Vα and Vβ sequences is relatively low, as is the homology between Vα and Vβ sequences. However, the presence of residues highly conserved among all V sequences allows the unambiguous assignment of Vγ sequences as variable regions.[6,49,54] The conserved residues cluster near the expected framework regions neighboring the cysteine residues and the conserved tryptophan residue at position 39 (see Figure 3).

## B. Structure and Dynamics of the Gamma Gene Family

### 1. Structure and Diversity of Gamma Gene

The current status of the murine gamma gene family is summarized in Figure 4. Four gamma constant region genes have been identified, three of which (C1 to C3) are very similar in sequence,[53,54] and a fourth gene (C4) which does not crosshybridize.[56] the C3 gene appears to be nonfunctional by virtue of a defective 5' splice site bordering the second C exon.[53] Each C gene has a single associated J segment.

A total of six Vγ genes have been identified, three of which (V1.1 to V1.3) crosshybridize,[53] and three of which (V2 to 4) are very different than each other and the V1 subfamily.[54] The predicted amino acid sequences of V1.2, V2, V3, and V4 are compared in Figure 3. Although the four sequences have clear regions of homology, particularly near the predicted framework regions, they differ markedly from each other in overall amino acid sequence homology, ranging from 22% to 48% in pairwise comparisons. Hence the potential diversity of murine Vγ genes encompasses at least four distinct subfamilies, including six genes.

Combinatorial diversity in the γ genes appears to be very limited, as each V gene appears to rearrange to only a single J segment, and no D segments have been found as yet. The

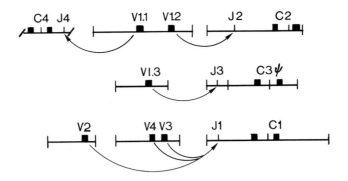

FIGURE 4.    The gamma gene family in Balb/c mice. Three gene clusters are shown. The C3 gene is defective,[53] and is deleted in C57B110 mice. The top cluster is from References 53 and 56, the bottom cluster from References 54 and 53.

**Table 2**
**REARRANGEMENT AND EXPRESSION OF GAMMA GENES**

| | Rearrangement/Expression[a] | | | | |
|---|---|---|---|---|---|
| **Gene combination** | **Fetal thymocytes[b]** | **Adult DN thymocytes** | **Adult thymocytes** | **Resting T cells** | **Activated T cells[d]** |
| V1.2-J2-C2 | +/+ | ++/++ | ++/± | ++/± | ++/++ |
| V2-J1-C1 | +/+ | ++/++ | ++/− | ++/− | ++/−[e] |
| V3-J1-C1 | +/+ | ±/± | −/− | −/− | −/− |
| V4-J1-C1 | +/+ | ±/± | −/− | −/− | −/− |

a    Approximate relative abundance of indicated gene rearrangement or mRNA from Reference 54.
b    Includes thymocytes from day 15 to day 17 of gestation.
c    DN thymocytes (double negative) are Lyt-2⁻, L3T4⁻ thymocytes from 4-week-old mice; approximately 3% of total thymocytes.
d    T cells activated with alloantigens in culture.
e    Although this mRNA is undetectable in our analysis of activated T cell populations, a corresponding cDNA was isolated from a CTL clone.[66]

V-J junctions of rearranged murine γ genes show only relatively limited diversity,[53,54,55] which may result from random nucleotide addition (N regions), variations in the site of recombination, and/or as yet undiscovered D segments. In sum, the potential diversity of the γ family is significant but limited compared to the α and β families.

Interestingly, comparisons of murine Vγ sequences with recently published human Vγ sequences[57] suggest that the Vγ genes have diverged rapidly between these species, although the Cγ genes are relatively conserved.[58] This observation suggests that Vγ proteins may be involved in recognition of intrinsic structures that also diverge rapidly between species (e.g., MHC proteins) or unpredictable extrinsic structures (e.g., antigens).

*2. Gamma Gene Rearrangements*

In Figure 3, the γ genes are organized in three clusters which represent the probable gene organization within a cluster; the organization of each cluster relative to the others is as of yet undetermined. In the following discussion each cluster will be considered independently (summarized in Table 2).

The V1.3 gene rearranges, albeit rarely, to the J3-C3 gene. Since the J3-C3 gene is defective,[53] the V1.3-J3-C3 rearranged gene is presumably nonfunctional, and will not be considered futher.

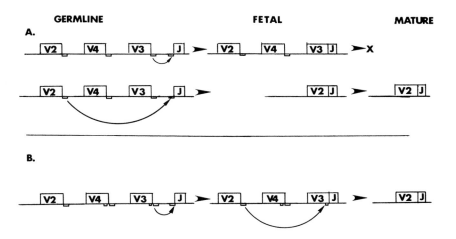

FIGURE 5.    Two mechanisms for dissappearance of rearranged γ genes as T cells mature. (A) Cells that make V3 (shown) or V4 (not shown) rearrangements do not mature, whereas cells that make V2 rearrangements do. (B) Cells that initially make V3 (shown) or V4 (not shown) rearrangements to J1 subsequently undergo secondary rearrangements of V2 to J1 that delete the rearranged V3 or V4 gene. Recombination signals are indicated by brackets and putative heptamer recombination signal in V coding sequences by a smaller bracket (in B).

The V1.2 gene rearranges to the J2-C2 gene.[53] This rearrangement is relatively rare in early fetal thymocytes, but accumulates to become a dominant rearrangement in mature T cells,[54] and is present in the large majority of CTL and helper T cell clones.[6,55,59] The transcript of this rearrangement corresponds to the original γ cDNA clone.

The V1.1 gene, which is closely linked but in the opposite transcriptional orientation to the V1.2 gene,[53] rearranges to the J4-C4 gene.[56] Although this rearrangement is present in some T cell clones, our analysis of V1 genes in T cell populations suggest it is rearranged rarely in fetal and adult thymocytes and T cells.[54].

The V2, V3, and V4 genes all rearrange to the J1-C1 gene, and thus on one chromosome only one of these genes can be rearranged at one time.[54] The V2 rearrangement is relatively rare in fetal thymocytes and accumulates later in ontogeny. In contrast, the V3 and V4 rearrangements are detectable in fetal thymocytes and diminish in representation at later times in development.[54] As the three genes all rearrange to J1, and the V2 gene is the most 5' of the three, at least two non-mutually exclusive explanations for this behavior can be considered (Figure 5). Cells that initially make V3 or V4 rearrangements may be at a selective disadvantage during the T cell differentiation process, so that cells that initially make V2 rearrangements predominate in mature T cells. Alternatively, the chromosomes in cells that initially make V3 or V4 rearrangements may undergo secondary rearrangements so that the rearranged V3 and V4 alleles are deleted by replacement with the V2 gene. The latter model appears at first glance unlikely, since the flanking heptamer-nonamer recombination signals will be deleted by the primary rearrangement. However, recent evidence suggest that a conserved heptamer sequence near the 3' end of most $V_H$ genes, may serve as a substrate for such secondary V-replacement recombination events in B cells. Such a heptamer (TACTGTG) is also present near the 3' end of the V3 and V4 coding sequences,[54] raising the possibility that such events may also occur in gamma gene rearrangements. Whether such a mechanism accounts for the disappearance of rearranged V3 and V4 genes during T cell differentiation remains to be tested experimentally. In any case, the phenomenon raises the possibility that the V3 and V4 genes serve a specific function in immature (fetal) thymocytes, and may be replaced in a given cell and its progeny by secondary rearrangements as T cells mature.

*3. Expression of Vγ Genes*

The expression of γ genes is particularly active in immature thymocytes,[60] a finding which led us to propose that the genes serve a critical function at this stage.[60] Detailed analysis of expression of different γ gene rearrangements has revealed some complexity, however, which is summarized below and in Table 2.

V1.2, V2, V3, and V4 mRNAs are all most abundant in immature thymocytes [fetal thymocytes or adult thymocytes with the immature Lyt-2$^-$, L3T4$^-$ ("double-negative") phenotype] and diminish thereafter to nearly undetectable levels in mature T cells.[54] The disappearance with fetal age of the V3 and V4 transcripts may result simply from the disappearance of the rearranged versions of the V3 and V4 genes noted above. However, the V1.2 and V2 rearrangements accumulate in the population as T cells develop,[54] and hence the disappearance of these mRNAs may reflect repression of transcription of the genes. In parallel, the level of Cγ-hybridizing transcripts decreases as T cells mature.[60]

In contrast to the V2-V4 transcripts, the V1.2 transcript accumulates in mature T cells following antigenic or mitogenic stimulation.[43,54] Although under some activation conditions the transcripts are confined to Lyt-2$^+$ L3T4$^-$ cells, activation in the presence of lymphokines leads to expression in Lyt-2$^-$ L3T4$^+$ T cells as well.[43] All Class I-specific clones thus far examined express V1.2-hybridizing transcripts,[6,55,56,61] as do some [62,63] but not all[59] Class II-specific L3T4$^+$ T cell clones.

*4. Productivity of γ Gene Rearrangements*

Like other rearranging gene families, the exact sites of V-J recombination joints of γ genes show some variability. Since some rearrangements will therefore generate joints in which the J-C segments are in the incorrect translational reading frame, analysis of recombination joints can be useful in evaluating the functional potential of particular rearranged genes. The first two published γ-cDNA sequences, from two independent CTL clones, had in-frame (functional) recombination joints,[6,55] consistent with a function for the gene in these cells. More recent analyses show, however, that cDNAs from several CTL clones are nonfunctional.[56,61] Since there are several gamma loci which often rearrange on both chromosomes, it is necessary in such studies to account for all the rearranged γ genes. In fact such analyses indicated that at least some CTL have no functional rearrangements of any of the known gamma loci.[61] Thus it can be concluded that function of at least the known gamma genes is not necessary for the specificity or function of at least some CTL. Since the known gamma genes are not expressed in many helper T cells, these genes are apparently not necessary for helper T cell function or specificity.[59] The overall significance of these observations is difficult to assess at present, however, since it is possible that there are gamma-like genes which do not hybridize with the existing probes, and which are functionally expressed in those cells that lack functional rearrangements of the known gamma genes.

The observation that several gamma loci are expressed at their highest levels in immature thymocytes raised the attractive possibility that the genes function during early T cell development, and perhaps exclusively at this time. Consistent with this possibility, we found that 5 of 6 rearranged gamma genes (corresponding to V2-J1, V3-J1, and V4-J1 rearrangements) isolated from a genomic library of DNA from day 17 fetal thymocytes are rearranged productively.[54] We conclude that many or most of the fetal thymocytes with these gamma rearrangments have productive rearrangements and thus the potential to produce a functional γ polypeptide. Interestingly, a discrepancy is apparent when comparing our data on genomic clones with the findings of others on cDNA clones from the fetal thymus. Thus, Heilig and Tonegawa[64] found that all of several γ cDNA clones analyzed from day 17 fetal thymus were nonproductive, including several V1.2-J2-C2 clones and several V2-J1-C1 clones. Barring technical differences between our studies and theirs, this finding suggests that transcripts of nonproductive alleles are overrepresented in day 17 fetal thymocytes. Several explanations can be considered including:

- The γ polypeptide down-regulates transcription of γ genes; those cells with only nonfunctional rearrangements might then have much higher γ-transcript levels than cells with productive rearrangements.
- A minor thymocyte subpopulation (e.g., differing in lineage or maturation state), which tends to have nonproductive γ rearrangements has higher levels of γ mRNA.
- Productive transcripts may have a shorter half-life than nonproductive transcripts.

*5. Current Questions*

The collctive data on the γ genes clearly presents a complex and confusing picture. Many unknowns prevent clear conclusions to be drawn. Several of the more important issues are summarized here.

**Is gamma gene function necessary for the functioning of effector (mature) T cells**? — The finding that the V1.2-J2-C2 gene is induced in mature T cells following T cell activation, and that all CTL have relatively abundant levels of this transcript, suggests that it may function in such cells. However, the observation that the transcripts from some CTL are nonproductive argues against an obligatory requirement for γ gene function in effector T cells. What is not known is whether there are additional non-cross-hybridizing gamma-like genes which may function in those cells which lack productive rearrangements of the known gamma genes. This will only be resolved by further studies.

**What is the nature of the gamma polypeptide**? — Thus far no protein has been identified, but it would be remarkable if such a complex gene family, which has no obvious defects at the nucleic acid level, were not functionally expressed. We have shown that V1.2-J2-C2 transcripts, produced by in-vitro transcription, can be translated in-vitro into a 33 kDalton polypeptide, demonstrating that the mRNA can be translated.[65] Intense efforts in several laboratories to identify the polypeptide in cells using antisera prepared against synthetic peptides and fusion proteins are now underway and should yield results in the near future. Of critical interest in the nature of the putative partner chain for the γ chain. The structure of the partner chain may yield important clues as to the function of the complex.

## C. Speculations

The γ gene family shows significant diversity, reinforcing the notion, based on its similarities to α, β, and Ig genes, that its product is involved in recognition of variable moities such as antigens or MHC proteins. The expression and rearrangement of the genes are particularly active in immature thymocytes, suggesting the genes may function there. Although the V1.2-J2-C2 gene is commonly expressed in mature CTL, many of the cells have only nonproductive rearrangements, raising the possibility that this expression does not reflect a function for the genes in these cells. In contrast, most day-17 fetal thymocyte γ gene rearrangements we sequenced are productive. Taken together, the available data are consistent with a function for γ gene products in immature thymocytes for recognition of variable moities. We proposed a speculative model in which the γ gene is involved in the events of thymus education.[60] Since β and γ, but not α, mRNA levels are high in immature thymocytes,[60] we proposed that cells bearing a heterodimer of the γ and β chains are initially subjected to selection for affinity for self-MHC antigens (Figure 6A). The role of the γ chain in the model is to recognize MHC molecules and thus focus the β chain for selection; γ chain variability might be necessary to accomodate recognition of the products of different MHC loci and/or alleles. Subsequently, as thymocytes mature, the γ genes are repressed and the α gene is expressed. The replacement of the γ chain with a random α chain might be expected to alter the structure and hence the affinity of the heterodimer for self-MHC proteins. If clones which retain a high affinity for self-MHC are deleted in a subsequent tolerization step, it might be imagined that the surviving clones would be those which have a low but significant affinity for self-MHC. Such clones would not be autoreactive, but

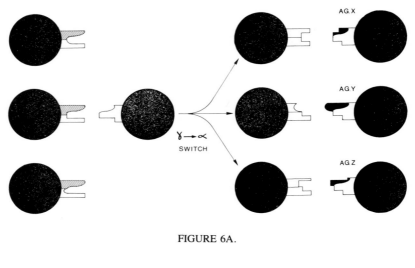

FIGURE 6A.

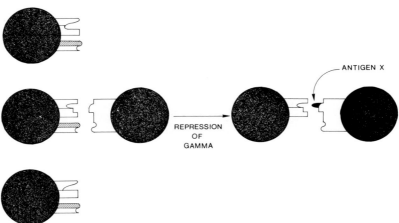

FIGURE 6.    Two models of γ chain function. (A) The γ/β → α/β switch model.[60] Immature thymocytes on the left express a heterodimer of a γ chain (hatched) and a β chain. Cells that express a β chain compatible with self-MHC recognition are allowed to mature. Random α chains replace the γ chain, yielding α/β heterodimers with low affinity for self-MHC but high affinity for antigen-modified self-MHC proteins. (B) In this model, a heterodimer of γ (hatched) and a partner chain acts as an accessory receptor to promote interaction of the α/β heterodimer with self-MHC antigens. In this way, cells with low affinity receptors for self-MHC are selected. Subsequently, γ is repressed and a presumptive tolerance step deletes cells with high-affinity anti-self receptors. The surviving cells have low affinity for self-MHC but high affinity for antigen modified self-MHC.

might react with high affinity with self-MHC proteins complexed with foreign antigens. The model suggests that the selected β chain retains a "memory" of self-MHC when paired with the α chain, and predicts that it is principally (though not necessarily exclusively) the β chain which contacts self-MHC during recognition by the α/β heterodimer. As of the present no definitive data allows either the acceptance or rejection of this model. The findings that Vβ gene usage does not generally correlate with the MHC restriction specificity of T cells raises some clear doubts about the model, but is not definitive evidence against it, since the contribution of combinatorial and junctional diversity to β chain specificity may be critically important.

An alternative model which circumvents the aforementioned difficulty is presented in Figure 6b. In this model the γ chain pairs with itself or another chain (call it δ) to form a receptor with affinity for MHC proteins on immature thymocytes. The interaction of this receptor serves to focus the newly expressed α/β heterodimer onto self MHC proteins, allowing positive selection of clones with even very low affinity receptors. Following repression of γ, clones with high affinity receptors for self-MHC are deleted in a tolerization step. The remaining clones have low affinity for self MHC alone, but may react if an antigen modifies the self-MHC molecule. The revised model, like the original model, is highly speculative, but can serve at least as a basis for additional experiments, since it makes testable predictions. Given the absence of crucial information about γ (e.g., the expressed form of the protein) it is perhaps perilous to propose any models at present. It is hoped that forthcoming information will soon provide the basis for a definitive understanding of the function of this very interesting gene family.

## NOTE ADDED IN PROOF

Since the submission of this manuscript, great progress has been made in analysis of the T-γ receptor. Antisera prepared against synthetic human and murine γ peptides have been shown to precipitate a second T cell receptor from a subset of CD4[-], CD8[-] fetal and adult thymocytes, and mature T cells which do not express the α/β T cell receptor.[67-70] The second receptor is disulfide-linked heterodimer of a γ-chain and a novel T cell receptor subunit called δ. The δ subunit is a glycosylated 40-50 kDalton chain. cDNA clones corresponding to the δ chain have been isolated, and a preliminary genomic organization of δ genes has been reported.[71-74] There is a single Cγ gene, at least two Jδ gene segments, and at least two Dδ gene segments. Strikingly, the D, J, and Cδ gene segments are localized within the α gene locus, just 5′ of the known Jα gene segments. While it is therefore possible that Vα gene segments rearrange to JδCδ genes, most Vδ segments so far characterized do not fall into the known Vα gene subfamilies, raising the possibility that Vα and Vδ genes are largely nonoverlapping.[71,72,74]

It appears that most adult muring thymic T cells that express γ/δ T cell receptors express one of a few Vδ genes.[74] In addition, most of these cells express a single Vγ-Jγ combination (Vγ2Jγ1Cγ1). Therefore the diversity of γ/δ receptors expressed by these cells appears to be relatively limited.

Other studies have shown that a small population of peripheral CD4[-], CD8[-] T cells express the γ/δ T cell receptors.[67] Furthermore, many of the γ/δ-T cell lines recently characterized carry out effector functions characteristic of ''conventional'' T cells, i.e., cytolysis and lymphokine production.[67,69] These findings have raised the possibility that γ/δ-T cells represent a separate lineage of T cells with a distinct immune function and/or specificity, rather than representing a stage in differentiation of α/β-T cells. The physiological ligands for γ/δ receptors are yet to be determined, however. Interestingly, a recent report indicates that some γ/δ-T cells can respond to allogeneic antigens encoded by MHC-linked genes.[75] With the current rate of progress, the physiological function of γ/δ T cells should be revealed in the near future.

# REFERENCES

1. **Kindred, B. and Schreffler, D. C.,** H-2 dependence of cooperation between T and B cells in vivo, *J. Immunol.,* 109, 940, 1972.
2. **Katz, D. H., Hamaoka, T., Dorf, M. E., Maurer, P. H., and Benacerraf, B.,** Cell interactions between histoincompatible T and B lymphocytes. IV. Involvement of the immune response (Ir) gene in control of lymphocyte interactions in responses controlled by the gene, *J. Exp. Med.,* 138, 734, 1973.
3. **Zinkernagel, G. D. and Doherty, P. C.,** Restriction of in vitro T-cell mediated cytotoxicity in lymphocytic choriomeningitis within a syngeneic or semi-allogenic system, *Nature,* 248, 701, 1974.
4. **Haskins, K., Kubo, R., White, J., Pigeon, M., Kappler, J., and Marrack, P.,** The major histocompatibility complex-restricted antigen receptor on T cells. I. Isolation with a monoclonal antibody, *J. Exp. Med.,* 157, 1149, 1983.
5. **Bevan, M. J.,** The major histocompatibility complex determines susceptibility to cytotoxic T cells directed against minor histocompatibility antigens, *J. Exp. Med.,* 142, 1349, 1975.
6. **Saito, H., Kranz, D. M., Takagaki, Y., Hayday, A. C., Eisen, H. N., and Tonegawa, S.,** Complete primary structure of a heterodimeric T-cell receptor deduced from cDNA sequences, *Nature,* 309, 757, 1984.
7. **Zinkernagel, R. M. and Doherty, P. C.,** H-2 compatibility requirement for T-cell-mediated lysis of targets infected with lymphocytic choriomeningitis virus. Different cytotoxic T-cell specificities are associated with structures coded in H-2K or H-2D, *J. Exp. Med.,* 141, 1427, 1975.
8. **Rosenthal, A. S., Barcinski, M. A., and Blake, J. T.,** Determinant selection is a macrophage dependent immune response gene function, *Nature,* 267, 156, 1977.
9. **Babbit, B. P., Allen, P. M., Matsueda, G., Haber, E., and Unanue, E. R.,** Binding of immunogenic peptides to Ia histocompatibility molecules, *Nature,* 317, 359, 1985.
10. **Hunig, T. R. and Bevan, M. J.,** Antigen recognition by cloned cytotoxic T lymphocytes follows rules predicted by the altered-self hypothesis, *J. Exp. Med.,* 155, 111, 1982.
11. **Heber-Katz, E., Schwartz, R. H., Matis, L. A., Hannum, C., Fairwell, T., Appella, E., and Hansburg, D.,** The contribution of antigen-presenting cell MHC-gene products to the specificity of antigen-induced T cell activation, *J. Exp. Med.,* 155, 1086, 1982.
12. **Hedrick, S. M., Matis, L. A., Hecht, T. T., Samelson, L. E., Longo, D. L., Herber-Katz, E., and Schwartz, R. H.,** The fine specificity of antigen and Ia determinant recognition by T cell hybridoma clones specific for pigeon cytochrome c, *Cell,* 30, 141, 1982.
13. **Bevan, M. J.,** Killer cells reactive to altered self antigens can also be alloreactive, *Proc. Natl. Acad. Sci. USA,* 74, 2094, 1977.
14. **Burakoff, S. J., Finberg, R., Glimcher, L., Lemonnier, F., Benacerraf, B., and Cantor, H.,** The biologic significance of alloreactivity. The ontongeny of T-cell sets specific for alloantigens or modified self antigens, *J. Exp. Med.,* 148, 1414, 1978.
15. **Sredni, B. and Schwartz, R. H.,** Alloreactivity of an antigen specific T-cell clone, *Nature,* 286, 855, 1980.
16. **Schwartz, R. H., Yano, A., and Paul, W. E.,** Interaction between antigen-presenting cells and primed T lymphocytes. An assessment of Ir gene expression in the antigen-presenting cell, *Immunol. Rev.,* 40, 153, 1978.
17. **Sprent, J.,** Role of H-2 gene products in the function of T helper cells from normal and chimeric mice *in vivo, Immunol. Rev.,* 42, 108, 1978.
18. **MacDonald, H. R., Glasebrook, A. L., and Cerottini, J.-C.,** Clonal heterogeneity in the functional requirement for Lyt-2/3 molecules on cytolytic T lymphocytes: Analysis by antibody blocking and selective trypsinization, *J. Exp. Med.,* 156, 1711, 1982.
19. **Swain, S. R., Dialynas, D., Fitch, F. W., and English, M.,** Monoclonal antibody to L3T4 blocks the function of T cells specific for Class II major histocompatibility complex antigens, *J. Immunol.,* 132, 1118, 1984.
20. **Marrack, P., Endres, R., Schimondevitz, R., Zlotnik, A., Dialynas, D., Fitch, F., and Kappler, J.,** The major histocompatibility complex restricted antigen receptor on T cells. II. Role of the L3T4 product, *J. Exp. Med.,* 158, 1077, 1983.
21. **Bevan, M. J. and Fink, P. J.,** The influence of thymus H-2 antigens on the specificity of maturing killer and helper cells, *Immunol. Rev.,* 42, 3, 1978.
22. **Zinkernagel, R. M., Callahan, G. N., Althage, A., Cooper, S., Klein, P. A., and Klein, J.,** On the thymus in the differentiation of H-2-self recognition by T cells: Evidence for dual recognition? *J. Exp. Med.,* 147, 882, 1978.
23. **Allison, J. R., McIntyre, B. W., and Bloch, D.,** Tumor-specific antigen of murine T lymphoma defined with monoclonal antibody, *J. Immunol.,* 129, 2293, 1982.

24. **Haskins, K., Kubo, R., White, J., Pigeon, M., Kappler, J., and Marrack, P.,** The major histocompatibility complex-restricted antigen receptor on T cells. I. Isolation with a monoclonal antibody, *J. Exp. Med.,* 157, 1149, 1983.

25. **Meuer, S. C., Fitzgerald, K. A., Hussey, R. E., Hodgdon, J. C., Schlossman, S. F., and Reinherz, E. L.,** Clonotypic structures involved in antigen-specific human T-cell function. Relationship to the T3 molecular complex, *J. Exp. Med.,* 157, 705, 1983.

26. **Hedrick, S. M., Cohen, D. I., Nielsen, E. A., and Davis, M. M.,** Isolation of cDNA clones encoding T cell-specific membrane-associated proteins, *Nature,* 308, 149, 1984.

27. **Hedrick, S. M., Nielsen, E. A., Kavaler, J., Cohen, D. I., and Davis, M. M.,** Sequence relationships between putative T-cell receptor polypeptides and immunoglobulins, *Nature,* 308, 153, 1984.

28. **Yanagi, Y., Yoshikai, Y., Leggett, K., Clark, S. P., Aleksander, I., and Mak, T.,** A human T cell-specific cDNA clone encodes a protein having extensive homology to immunoglobulin chains, *Nature,* 308, 145, 1984.

29. **Chien, Y., Becker, D., Lindsten, T., Okamura, M., Cohen, D., and Davis, M. M.,** A third type of murine T-cell receptor gene, *Nature,* 312, 31, 1984.

30. **Saito, H., Kranz, D. M., Takagaki, Y., Hayday, A. C., Eisen, H. N., and Tonegawa, S.,** A third rearranged and expressed gene in a clones of cytotoxic T lymphocytes, *Nature,* 312, 36, 1984.

31. **Gascoigne, N. R. J., Chien, Y.-H., Becker, D. M., Kavaler, J., and Davis, M. M.,** Genomic organization and sequence of T-cell receptor β-chain constant-and joining-region genes, *Nature,* 310, 387, 1984.

32. **Malisson, M., Minard, K., Mjolsness, S., Kronenberg, M., Goverman, J., Hunkapiller, T., Prystowsky, M. B., Yoshikai, Y., Fitch, F., Mak, T. W., and Hood, L.,** Mouse T-cell antigen receptor: Structure and organization of constant and joining gene segments encoding the β polypeptide, *Cell,* 37, 1101, 1984.

33. **Kronenberg, M., Siu, G., Hood, L. E., and Shastri, N.,** The molecular genetics of the T-cell antigen receptor and T-cell antigen recognition, *Ann. Rev. Immunol.,* 4, 529, 1986.

34. **Hayday, A., Diamond, D., Tanigawa, G., Heilig, J., Folsom, V., Saito, H., and Tonegawa, S.,** Unusual features of the organization and diversity of T-cell receptor α chain genes, *Nature,* 316, 828, 1985.

35. **Winoto, A., Mjolsness, S., Hood, L.,** Genomic organization of the genes encoding the mouse T-cell receptor α chain: 18 $J_\alpha$ gene segments map over 60 kilobases of DNA, *Nature,* 316, 832, 1985.

36. **Yoshikai, Y., Clark, S. P., Taylor, S., Sohn, U., Wilson, B., Minden, M., and Mak, T.,** Organization and sequences of the variable, joining and constant region genes of the human T-cell receptor α chain, *Nature,* 316, 837, 1985.

37. **Kappler, J. W., Skidmore, B., White, J., and Marrack, P.,** Antigen-inducible, H-2-restricted, interleukin-2-producing T cell hybridomas. Lack of independent antigen and H-2 recognition, *J. Exp. Med.,* 153, 1198, 1981.

38. **Marrack, P., Shimonkevitz, R., Hannum, C., Haskins, K., and Kappler, J.,** The major histocompatibility complex-restricted receptor on T cells. IV. An antiidiotypic antibody predicts both antigen and I-specificity, *J. Exp. Med.,* 158, 1635, 1983.

39. **Dembic, Z., Haas, W., Weiss, W., McCubrey, J., Kiefer, H., Von Boehmer, H., and Steinmetz, M.,** Transfer of specificity by murine α and β T-cell receptor genes, *Nature,* 320, 232, 1986.

40. **Rupp, F., Acha-Orbea, H., Hengartner, H., Zinkernagel, R., and Joho, R.,** Identical Vβ T-cell receptor genes used in alloreactive cytotoxic and antigen plus IA specific helper T cells, *Nature,* 315, 425, 1985.

41. **Sim, G. K. and Augustin, A.,** V gene polymorphism and a major polyclonal T cell receptor idiotype, *Cell,* 42, 89, 1985.

42. **Sim, G. K. and Augustin, A.,** personal communication, 1985.

43. **Garman, R. and Raulet, D. H.,** unpublished data, 1985.

44. **Roehm, N., Herron, L., Cambier, J., Di Giusto, D., Haskins, K., Kappler, J., and Marrack, P.,** The major histocompatibility complex-restricted antigen receptor on T cells: Distribution on thymus and peripheral T cells, *Cell,* 38, 577, 1984.

45. **Garman, R. D., Ko, J.-L., Vulpe, C. D., and Raulet, D. H.,** T cell receptor variable region gene usage in T-cell populations, *Proc. Natl. Acad. Sci. USA,* 83, in press.

46. **Winoto, A., Lan, N. C., Urban, J. L., Goverman, J., Hood, L., and Hansburg, D.,** Mouse T-cell receptors specific for cytochrome C: Predominant usage of a Vα gene segment, submitted.

47. **Fink, P. J., Matis, L. A., McElligott, D. L., Bookman, M., and Hedrick, S. M.,** Correlations between T cell specificity and the structure of the antigen receptor, *Nature,* in press.

48. **Kappler, J.,** personal communication, 1986.

49. **Novotny, J., Tonegawa, S., Saito, H., Kranz, D., and Eisen, H. N.,** Secondary, tertiary, and quaternary structures of T-cell-specific immunoglobulin-like polypeptide chains, *Proc. Natl. Acad. Sci. USA,* 83, 742, 1986.

50. **Clarke, S. H., Huppi, K., Ruezinsky, D., Standt, L., Gerhard, W., and Weigert, M.,** Inter- and intraclonal diversity in the antibody response to influenza hemagglutinin, *J. Exp. Med.,* 161, 687, 1985.

51. **Manser, T., Wysocki, L. H., Gridley, T., Near, R. I., and Gefter, M. L.,** The molecular evolution of the immune response, *Immunol. Today,* 6, 94, 1985.

52. **Bevan, M. J.,** Interaction antigens detected by cytotoxic T cells with the major histocompatibility complex as modifier, *Nature,* 256, 419, 1975.

53. **Hayday, A. C., Saito, H., Gillies, S. D., Kranz, D. M., Tanigawa, G., Eisen, H. N., and Tonegawa, S.,** Structure, organization, and somatic rearrangement of T cell gamma genes, *Cell,* 40, 259, 1985.

54. **Garman, R. D., Doherty, P., and Raulet, D. H.,** Diversity, rearrangement, and expression of murine T cell gamma genes, *Cell,* 45, 733, 1986.

55. **Kranz, D. M., Saito, H., Heller, M., Takagaki, Y., Haas, W., Eisen, H. N., and Tonegawa, S.,** Limited diversity of the rearranged T-cell gamma gene, *Nature,* 313, 752, 1985.

56. **Iwamoto, A., Rupp, F., Ohashi, P., Walker, C., Pircher, H., Joho, R., Hengarther, H., and Mak, T.,** T cell specific γ genes in C57B/10 mice. Sequence and expression of new constant and variable region genes, *J. Exp. Med.,* 163, 1203, 1986.

57. **LeFranc, M.-P., Forster, A., Baer, R., Stinston, M. A., and Rabbits, T. H.,** Diversity and rearrangement of the human T cell rearranging γ genes: Nine germ-line variable genes belonging to two subgroups, *Cell,* 45, 237, 1986.

58. **Dialynas, D., Murre, C., Quartermous, J., Boss, J. M., Leiden, J. M., Seidman, J. G., and Strominger, J. L.,** Cloning and sequence analysis of complementary DNA encoding an aberrantly rearranged human T-cell γ chain, *Proc. Natl. Acad. Sci. USA,* 83, 2619, 1986.

59. **Heilig, J. S., Glimcher, L. H., Kranz, D. M., Clayton, L. K., Greenstein, J. L., Saito, H., Maxam, A. M., Burakoff, S. J., Eisen, H. N., and Tonegawa, S.,** Expression of the T-cell-specific γ gene is unnecessary in T cells recognizing Class II MHC determinants, *Nature,* 317, 68, 1985.

60. **Raulet, D. H., Garman, R. D., Saito, H., and Tonegawa, S.,** Developmental regulation of T-cell receptor gene expression, *Nature,* 314, 103, 1985.

61. **Reilly, E. B., Kranz, D. M., Tonegawa, S., and Eisen, H. N.,** A functional γ gene formed by the known γ gene segments is not necessary for antigen-specific responses of some murine cytotoxic T lymphocytes, *Nature,* in press.

62. **Zauderer, M., Iwamoto, A., and Mak, T. W.,** Gene rearrangement and expression in autoreactive helper T cells, *J. Exp. Med.,* 163, 1314, 1986.

63. **Bluestone, J.,** personal communication, 1986.

64. **Heilig, J. and Tonegawa, S.,** personal communication, 1986.

65. **Ko, J.-L. and Raulet, D. H.,** unpublished data, 1986.

66. **Rupp, F.,** personal communication, 1986.

67. **Brenner, M. B., McLean, J., Dialynas, D., Strominger, J., Smith, J. A., Owen, F. L., Seidman, J., Ip, S., Rosen, F., and Krangel, M.,** Identification of a putative second T cell receptor, *Nature,* 322, 145, 1986.

68. **Lew, A., Pardoll, D., Maloy, W., Fowlkes, B., Kruisbeek, A., Cheng, S., Germain, R., Bluestone, J., Schwartz, R., and Coligan, J.,** Characterization of T cell receptor gamma chain expression in a subset of murine thymocytes, *Science,* 234, 1401, 1986.

69. **Pardoll, D., Fowlkes, B. J., Bluestone, J., Kruisbeek, A., Maloy, W., Coligan, J., and Schwartz, R.,** Differential expression of two distinct T cell receptors during thymocyte development, *Nature,* 326, 79, 1987.

70. **Nakanishi, N., Maeda, K., Ito, K., Heller, M., and Tonegawa, S.,** Tγ protein is expressed on murine fetal thymocytes as a disulphide-linked heterodimer, *Nature,* 325, 720, 1987.

71. **Chien, Y., Iwashima, M., Kaplan, K., Elliott, J., and Davis, M.,** A new T cell receptor gene located within the alpha locus and expressed early in T cell differentiation, *Nature,* 327, 677, 1987.

72. **Hata, S., Brenner, M., and Krangel, M.** Identification of putative human T cell receptor δ complementary DNA clones, *Science,* 238, 678, 1987.

73. **Band, H., Hochstenbach, F., McLean, J., Hata, S., Krangel, M., and Brenner, M.,** Immunochemical proof that a novel rearranging gene encodes the T cell δ subunit, *Science,* 238, 682, 1987.

74. **Korman, A., Marusic-Galesic, S., Kruisbeek, A., and Raulet, D. H.,** Limited diversity of expressed T cell receptor delta chains in the adult murine thymus, Submitted, 1987.

75. **Matis, L., Cron, R., and Bluestone, J. A.,** T lymphocytes expressing the T cell receptor gamma-delta heterodimer recognize a major histocompatibility complex-linked antigen, *Nature,* in press, 1987.

Chapter 6

# STRUCTURE AND FUNCTION OF A FAMILY OF LEUKOCYTE ADHESION MOLECULES (LEU-CAM) INVOLVED IN T CELL KILLING AND COMPLEMENT-MEDIATED PHAGOCYTOSIS*

## M. Amin Arnaout

## TABLE OF CONTENTS

*    Supported by US PH Grant AI-21963 and March of Dimes Grant 1011. Dr. Arnaout is an Established Investigator of the American Heart Association.

# I. INTRODUCTION

An understanding of the biochemical basis of cellular interactions has been steadily increasing over the past two decades. In several developmental systems, the basis of cellular recognition has been shown to be due, in large part, to the presence of unique proteins on the plasma membrane.[1-5] Several surface membrane proteins that mediate cell-cell adhesion have been isolated from neural or hepatic cells. These neural or hepatic cell adhesion molecules (N-CAM or L-CAM, respectively) appear to be of critical significance in embryonic development and morphogenesis.[6,7,8] In the immune system, understanding of the phenomenon of intercellular adhesion has been facilitated by development of monoclonal antibodies to leukocyte surface molecules and the identification of an inherited disorder of leukocyte adhesion in humans which underscored the essential role of intercellular adhesion in promoting such diverse leukocyte functions as phagocytosis and cytolytic T cell activity.

In this chapter, I will review the structure and function of a family of leukocyte adhesion molecules (Leu-CAM), their ontogeny, phylogeny, biosynthesis, the factors regulating their expression on the cell surface, and molecular cloning of the genes encoding for some of these molecules.

# II. IDENTIFICATION OF LEUKOCYTE SURFACE MOLECULES THAT PROMOTE CELL ADHESION

Two different lines of investigation have converged in identifying leukocyte surface molecules involved in adhesion-dependent functions. On the one hand, the monoclonal antibody technology introduced by Kohler and Milstein[9] has allowed the development, by a number of groups, of monoclonal antibodies that defined a macrophage-monocyte surface antigen named Mac-1, OKM1, or Mol.[10-12] Monoclonal antibodies were developed by immunizing rats or mice with mouse peritoneal macrophages,[10] or with human monocytes,[11,12] respectively. Immunoprecipitation from [125]I-labeled cells revealed that the Mac-1/Mol antigen is a heterodimer consisting of two noncovalently linked glycoproteins with an alpha subunit that is slightly larger in the mouse (apparent molecular mass 185 kDalton vs. 155 to 165 kDalton in the human) and a beta subunit of apparent molecular mass of 94 to 95 kDalton in both species.[10-12]

Trowbridge and Omary showed that Mac-1 belongs to a family of antigenically and structurally related murine glycoproteins analogous to the T200 glycoprotein family.[13] Using a rat monoclonal antibody directed against the murine T cell line, BW5147, they immunoprecipitated from cytolytic T cells another antigen with a slightly larger alpha subunit that was distinct from the alpha subunit of Mac-1, as determined by peptide mapping, but associated with the same beta subunit. Interestingly, this monoclonal antibody blocked cytolytic activity of murine cytotoxic T cell lines.[13] This T lymphocyte function-associated antigen (LFA-1) or (TA-1) was also independently identified in humans by Lebien and Kersey[14] and Kurzinger et al.[15] Additional monoclonal antibodies directed against the beta subunit were developed.[16-18] These beta-chain-specific monoclonal antibodies confirmed that in man, as in mouse, Mol and LFA-1 have distinct alpha subunits noncovalently linked to an identical beta subunit. These beta-specific antibodies also unravelled the existence of a third alpha chain (apparent molecular mass 130 to 150 kDalton) that is also noncovalently associated with the same beta subunit and is immunoprecipitated by anti-beta antibodies together with the other two alpha subunits of Mol and LFA-1. This third heterodimer was named P150, 95[18] and later shown to be identical with LeuM5, an antigen defined by a monoclonal antibody raised against a human hairy cell leukemia cell line[19] (Figure 1). That Mol, LFA-1, and Leu M5 antigens exist in a 1:1 alpha/beta heterodimeric form is shown in experiments in which radiolabelled and detergent solubilized monocyte lysate were sub-

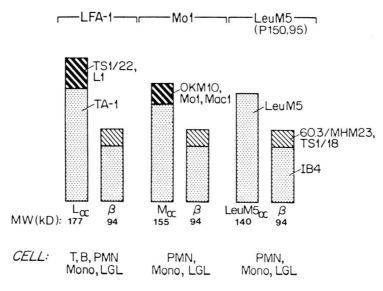

FIGURE 1. Schematic diagram showing the structure and cell disribution of Mol/LFA-1/Leu M5 family of leukocyte adhesion molecules (Leu-CAM). The distinct alpha subunits of LFA-1 (L$_a$), Mol (M$_a$), and Leu M5 (p150, 95) (Leu M5$_a$) are associated non-covalently on a one-to-one basis with an apparently identical beta ($\beta$) subunit. The shaded and stippled areas represent, respectively, functionally active and nonactive portions of these molecules. Letters refer to epitopes on these molecules defined by monoclonal antibodies. T, B, PMN, Mono., and LGL represent T and B lymphocytes, granulocytes, monocytes, and large granular lymphocytes, respectively. (Adapted from Todd and Arnaout.[109])

jected to cross-linking with a cleavable reagent (such as dithio-bis-succinimidyl propionate) and immunoprecipitated with alpha or beta specific antibodies. The cross-linked products were separated in the first dimension on SDS polyacrylamide tube gels followed by cleavage of the cross linker with dithiothreitol. Gel electrophoresis in the second dimension, resolved the cross-linked Mol/LFA-1/Leu M5 into their basic polypeptide alpha and beta subunits.[18]

On another front, an experiment of nature suggested an association between certain leukocyte surface molecules and cell adhesion. In 1980, Crowley et al. found a patient with recurrent bacterial infections whose granulocytes were deficient in a surface glycoprotein of 110 kDalton (gp110). Granulocytes from this patient did not spread on glass or plastic surfaces nor migrate normally in a chemotactic gradient.[20] Arnaout et al. described a similar patient whose granulocytes were deficient in a surface glycoprotein of 150 kDalton (gp150) associated with severe impairment in phagocytosis of serum opsonized particles.[21] A monoclonal antibody developed against gp150 immunoprecipitated a heterodimeric molecule with an alpha subunit of 150 to 155 kDalton and a beta subunit of 94 kDalton from normal granulocytes but not from cells deficient in gp150.[22] Sequential immunoprecipitation using this monoclonal antibody as well as a polyclonal antibody to gp150 revealed that gp150 is in fact identical with the alpha subunit of Mol and that the patient described has Mol/Mac-1 deficiency.[23] Identical results were obtained upon analysis of leukocytes obtained from the patient described by Crowely et al.[24] Flow cytometric analysis, as well as immunoprecipitation using monoclonal antibodies previously developed against LFA-1, Leu M5, and the beta subunit that is common to all three antigens, showed that these two patients are deficient in all members of the Mol/LFA-1/Leu M5 (Leu-CAM) family of surface molecules.[22-25] Similar results were obtained in a third patient using the monoclonal antibody 60.3, that is directed against the common beta subunit.[26]

## III. CELL DISTRIBUTION, ONTOGENY, AND PHYLOGENY OF Mol/LFA-1/Leu M5 (Leu-CAM) ANTIGENS

Both Mol and Leu M5 are present on the surface of mature granulocytes, monocytes, and LGL cells,[27,28] with Mol being the more abundant surface antigen. LeuM5 is barely detectable on nonactivated granulocytes and is more abundant on monocytes (Figure 2). LFA-1 is expressed on a broader spectrum of cell types, including both T and B lymphocytes, granulocytes, monocytes, LGL cells, and thymocytes.[13,18,29]

Mol is found on 21% of human adult bone marrow cells.[30] Fetal bone marrow (15 to 17 week gestation) contains about 27% Mol$^+$ cells. This proportion decreases with increasing gestational age until it reaches the adult value. The Mol epitope is not detected on the surface of normal colony-forming unit-mixed granulocyte/erythrocyte (CFU-mix) or on granulocyte/ monocyte progenitor cells (CFU-GM) and begins to be detected at the blast cell stage of differentiation.[31] Human myeloid cell lines, like undifferentiated HL60 or U937, express little or no Mol surface antigen and small amounts of surface LFA-1 and LeuM5 antigens.[32] Induction of HL60 cells to differentiate along the monocytic pathway (using tumor-promoting phorbol esters or retinoic acid) leads to a concomitant increase in surface expression of Mol, LFA-1 and Leu M5. Differentiation of HL60 cells along the granulocytic pathway (using dimethyl sulfoxide) results in a marked increase in Mol and minimal increases in LFA-1 and Leu M5.[32,33]

Mol is conserved throughout the order primates. Surface analysis of granulocytes obtained from species as distinct phylogenetically as the slow loris and man showed both cells to express the Mol antigen. Of interest is the finding that whereas human granulocytes expressed two epitopes present on Mol (designated 44 and 904), cells from other primates, such as the dog, expressed the 904 epitope only.[34]

## IV. ROLE OF Mol/LFA-1/LeuM5 (Leu-CAM) IN LEUKOCYTE ADHESION-DEPENDENT FUNCTIONS

Knowledge on the role of this family of cell surface molecules in leukocyte functions was derived primarily from experiments in which the effects of monoclonal antibodies on normal cell function was determined. The availability of leukocytes genetically deficient in this glycoprotein family helped to establish the connection between the deficiency state and abnormal leukocyte adhesion and the biologic role of these surface molecules in immunity against pyogenic infections. Certain monoclonal antibodies directed against LFA-1 inhibited cytolytic T cell activity (CTL).[13,35] Further studies of mouse and human LFA-1 have suggested a role for LFA-1 in the initial Mg$^{++}$-dependent recognition-adhesion step between the cytolytic T cell (CTL) and the target cell.[15,29,36,37] LFA-1 appears to increase the avidity of effector cells to their targets, a property also shared by other lymphocyte surface antigens like T4, T8, and possibly T11.[38] Anti-LFA-1 monoclonal antibodies (directed against the alpha or beta subunits) also inhibit natural killing (NK), and killer (K) activities,[29,39,40] and the proliferative response to antigen (e.g., tetanus toxoid), mitogen (e.g., phytohemagglutinin (PHA), Concanavalin A (Con A)), or alloantigens,[24,40] presumably by impeding cell to cell contact.[37] Epstein-Barr virus (EBV)-transformed B cell lines established from patients with inherited Mol/LFA-1/Leu M5 deficiency do not aggregate spontaneously in culture or when exposed to PMA.[41,42] Monoclonal antibodies directed against epitopes on the alpha subunit of LFA-1 or the common beta subunit inhibit homotypic adhesion of human B lymphocytes and tetradecanoyl phorbol ester (TPA)-induced adhesion between mononuclear leukocytes.[43,44] Monoclonal antibodies directed against the alpha subunit of Mol (syn. OKM1, Mac-1) inhibit binding of granulocytes and monocytes to particles coated with iC3b, a fragment of the third complement component C3.[17,45,46] These data suggested that Mol is a

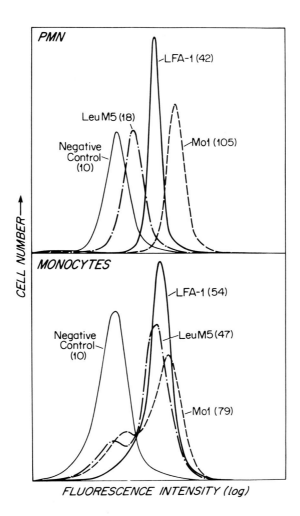

FIGURE 2.   Immunofluorescence analysis of human granulocytes (PMN) and monocytes using monoclonal antibodies directed against the alpha subunits of LFA-1 ($L_a$), Mol ($M_a$), and Leu M5 (Leu $M5_a$). Quantitative expression of these antigens was performed using a FACS IV flow cytometer (Becton Dickinson). The mean peak channel fluorescence (log · scale) was converted to a linear scale (in parentheses). A nonreactive monoclonal antibody was used as negative control.

receptor for iC3b (so-called complement receptor type 3, CR3), a finding confirmed by demonstrating that patients who totally lack Mol surface expression do not bind to iC3b-coated particles.[47] Further proof of the identity of Mol with CR3 was obtained recently by demonstrating direct binding of detergent-soluble and [125]I-labeled Mol to iC3b covalently linked to sepharose.[48,49] Binding of Mol, on intact cells or in the detergent soluble form to iC3b requires divalent cations and is totally inhibited in the presence of EDTA.[17,48-50] Removal of sialic acid residues from CR3, does not significantly reduce its binding to iC3b.[49] Trypsin treatment (1 mg/m$\ell$, 30 min, 37°C) on the other hand, abrogates the CR3 activity.[49] Inhibition of phagocytosis (and degranulation) of serum opsonized particles by anti-Mol monoclonal antibodies may be secondary to interference with the CR3 activity of Mol.[46,51] In addition to its function as a complement receptor, Mol appears to have a role in a number of granulocyte adhesion-related functions. Monoclonal antibodies directed against certain epitopes on the alpha subunit of Mol ($M_a$), even in their monovalent Fab form, inhibit F-met-leu-phe-, complement C5a- or PMA-induced granulocyte aggregation,[52] as well as granulocyte spreading on plastic surfaces[25,52] Other monoclonal antibodies directed against different epitopes on Mol$_a$, only inhibit CR3 activity but not aggregation, spreading, or chemotaxis.[52] The monoclonal antibody, 60.3, that is directed against the beta subunit common to Mol/LFA-1/Leu M5 inhibits CR3 activity, chemotaxis, leukoaggregation, spreading, and adherence of granulocytes stimulated with PMA or calcium ionophore A23187 to endothelial cell monolayers.[26,53] These findings suggest that Mol not only functions as CR3 but may also have a more general role in promoting adhesion of granulocytes to a number of substrates and to each other. Whether this adhesion-promoting activity is located in the alpha subunit or in the beta subunit common to Mol/LFA-1/Leu M5 is unclear at present.

Following up on the finding that Leu-CAM deficient granulocytes do not bind or metabolically respond to unopsonized zymosan, Ross et al.[54] found that certain monoclonal antibodies to Mol inhibited binding of granulocytes to unopsonized zymosan and rabbit erythrocytes, two surfaces that are known activators of the alternative complement pathway. These antibodies also inhibited superoxide generation by granulocytes exposed to unopsonized zymosan but did not block binding of granulocytes to sheep erythrocytes coated with iC3b (EiC3b).[54] These authors concluded that Mol has two binding sites, one of which acts as a receptor for activators of the alternative complement pathway and is presumably identical with the beta glucan phagocytic receptor described by Czop and Austen.[55] Chakravarti and colleagues, however, found that ingestion of activators of the alternative complement pathway by human monocytes is induced by a cytokine, is not inhibited by anti-Mol, but is blocked by beta glucan.[56] Another group provided data that enough C3 is deposited on unopsonized zymosan by monocytes to allow ingestion to proceed via the iC3b binding site in CR3 without the need to incriminate an independent binding site in the molecule.[57] It remains unclear, therefore, whether inhibition of zymosan binding by certain antibodies directed against M$_a$ is due to inhibition of a distinct functional domain in Mol or is secondary to steric inhibition of another molecule in the Leu-CAM protein complex.

Recently, work by Wright and colleagues have shown that binding of iC3b to Mol on monocytes is not sufficient to trigger phagocytosis of iC3b-coated erythrocytes.[58] Additional signals, such as those provided by substrate-bound fibronectin, serum amyloid P component (SAP) or PMA are necessary to render Mol competent to generate a phagocytic signal.[58] Of interest is the finding that even the binding of Mol to EiC3b can be modulated. Recombinant gamma interferon, for example, causes a 5- to 10-fold depression in binding of cultivated human monocytes to EiC3b.[59]. This effect is maximal in 48 hr, is reversed by fibronectin and is not due to a reduction in the number of surface receptors.[59] Furthermore, the myelocytic cell line, KG1, expresses normal amounts of Mol on the plasma membrane, yet they fail to bind to EiC3b or to adhere to plastic coverslips.[60] These findings suggest constitutive or inducible qualitative changes in Mol that prevent it from interacting with ligand and could involve alterations in receptor mobility in the plasma membrane. Of interest in this regard is the recognition that some patients with Leu-CAM deficiency have defects in actin polymerization,[61] suggesting an association between Mol and the cytoskeleton.

Conflicting data exist as to whether binding of iC3b to phagocytic cells is sufficient to trigger superoxide production.[62,63,64] Soluble iC3b was shown to induce chemiluminescence in granulocytes.[62] Cultivated human monocytes did not produce superoxide in response to EiC3b.[63] iC3b deposited on zymosan particles however, induced superoxide production by granulocytes.[52] These data probably reflect the complex nature of interaction between iC3b and leukocytes. iC3b has been shown to interact with more than one C3 receptor on granulocytes.[54] It is also possible that the metabolic responses elicited in phagocytes by iC3b depend on the nature of the surface on which iC3b is deposited (e.g. sheep erythrocytes vs zymosan particles). The surface could affect the density of iC3b deposited or present additional ligands acting as cofactors in certain CR3 dependent metabolic responses.

Interaction of target cell associated iC3b with Mol present on granulocytes, monocytes, or K cells has also been shown to enhance the antibody dependent cell-mediated cytotoxicity towards the target.[65,66]

Little information is available regarding the functional significance of Leu M5 (p150, 95), the third member of the glycoprotein family. An initial report suggested that it is the CR4 receptor of human phagocytes.[67] This conclusion was based on the finding that adherence of monocytes to coverslips precoated with IB4, a monoclonal antibody directed against a nonfunctional epitope on the beta subunit, inhibits binding of monocytes to sheep erythrocytes coated with the C3d fragment of C3 (EC3d), presumably through depletion of the Leu-CAM complex from the apical portion of the cell membrane.

More recently, Micklem and Sim have shown that LeuM5 contains an iC3b binding site. Detergent-soluble Leu M5 derived from TPA-induced U937 cells bound directly to iC3b-coated sepharose.[48] Binding of LeuM5 to its ligand was divalent cation dependent, a characteristic shared by LFA-1 and Mol. Since iC3b contains the C3dg fragment of C3, it is likely that Leu M5 may be interacting with this fragment in the iC3b molecule consistent with the data by Wright et al.[67] In addition to this C3 binding activity, Leu M5 also promotes adhesion of granulocytes and monocytes to endothelium.[68] Baseline adherence of human monocytes to umbilical vein endothelial cell monolayers is inhibited by a monoclonal antibody directed against the alpha subunit of Leu M5. The role of Leu M5 in adhesion of granulocytes to endothelium by is stimulus-specific. No inhibition is observed when adhesion is induced by phorbol esters. Adhesion in this circumstance is primarily mediated by Mol. Pretreatment of endothelium with recombinant IL-1 induces adhesion of granulocytes that is inhibited by anti-Leu M5 monoclonal antibodies.[68] The degree of inhibition under these conditions is comparable to that seen with monoclonal antibodies directed against the alpha subunits of LFA-1 or Mol. Moreover, the inhibition produced by the simultaneous use of all anti-alpha subunit specific antibodies is additive and approaches the 80% inhibition observed when anti-beta subunit antibodies are used. These data suggest that all three alpha subunits contribute to leukocyte-endothelium interactions and that the relative contribution of each subunit is stimulus-specific. The nature of the ligands that mediate this interaction at the endothelial cell level are unknown.

## V. FUNCTIONAL ABERRATIONS IN Leu-CAM DEFICIENCY

Patients suffering from genetic deficiency of Mol/LFA-1/Leu M5 and their common beta subunit (Leu-CAM deficiency) present clinically with recurrent and severe bacterial infections starting in the first few weeks of life.[25] Both males and females are affected. Infections most commonly involve the skin and mucous membranes. Gingivitis, otitis media, pneumonias, tracheo-bronchitis, vaginitis, perianal abcesses, and septicemias are common. Staphylococci, Pseudomonas species, Klebsiella, and enterococci are common pathogens. In some patients, delayed separation of the umbilical cord was noted.[69-71] Quantitation of Mol antigen on the surface of cells revealed that an incomplete form of the disease also exists.[24,25] In most patients, trace amounts of surface Mol (5 to 10% of normal) are detected. These patients usually have the milder form of the disease and may reach 40 years of age.[25] A minority of patients have no detectable surface Mol, have more severe functional abnormalities and clinical course, and may die in the first few years of life from overwhelming sepsis.[47] Interestingly, no predisposition to viral infections is present in the majority of cases. In addition delayed hypersensitivity, and skin-testing using antigens (i.e., tetanus toxoid) or mitogens (PHA) are normal.[20,21,47,69-71] All the patients described have persistent leukocytosis, even during infection-free periods, and normal serum immunoglobulin levels. Inheritance is most frequently on an autosomal recessive basis.[21,25] In some families only the mother is a carrier, suggesting some heterogeneity in the inheritance of this disorder.[20,25,72] Table 1

**Table 1**
## IN VITRO LEUKOCYTE ABNORMALITIES IN PATIENTS WITH LEU-CAM DEFICIENCY

Defects in phagocyte functions
1.  Phagocytosis of particles coated with complement C3- or limited amounts of IgG
2.  Chemotaxis and random migration
3.  Spreading on glass, nylon wool, plastic, lipopolysaccharide- or fibronectin-coated surfaces
4.  Stimulated adherence to endothelial cell monolayers
5.  C3-induced respiratory burst and degranulation
6.  Unopsonized zymosan-induced respiratory burst and degranulation
7.  Granulocyte aggregation in response to chemotactic peptides PMA or calcium ionophore A23187
8.  Antibody-dependent granulocyte mediated cytotoxicity (ADCC) to certain target cells
9.  Abnormal actin polymerization in some patients
10. Binding of phagocytes to particles coated with complement iC3b

Defects in lymphocyte functions
1.  Mitogen-, antigen- and alloantigen-induced proliferation
2.  CTL and NK cytotoxicity
3.  Spontaneous or induced B cell aggregation
4.  Helper activity for Ig production by B cells
5.  Alpha and gamma interferon production

summarizes the adhesion defects detected in phagocytes and lymphocytes from patients with Leu-CAM deficiency. The defects observed in granulocyte/monocyte functions span a spectrum of adhesion-related phenomena such as phagocytosis, superoxide generation, and degranulation induced by serum opsonized particles; adhesion to glass, plastic, nylon wool, or endothelial cell monolayers; spreading; chemotaxis; granulocyte aggregation; binding to iC3b-coated particles; and antibody-dependent granulocyte-mediated cytotoxicity (ADCC).[20,21,24,26,47,69-73] Membrane fluidity, electrophoretic mobility, and membrane depolarization in response to F-met-leu-phe are normal.[69-74] The observed functional defects can easily explain the predisposition of these patients to recurrent bacterial infections. Monoclonal antibodies directed against the alpha subunit of Mol LFA-1 and Leu M5 or against the beta subunit common to LFA-1/Mol/Leu M5 can reproduce most of these defects in normal cells.[24-26] In some patients, there is a marked abnormality in the ability of granulocyte actin to form filaments in vitro in response to potassium chloride, suggesting that the Leu-CAM complex may be associated with the cytoplasmic actin.[61] The prevalance of this abnormality in other patients with Leu-CAM deficiency is under investigation. Granulocytes from one patient did not bind to erythrocytes coated with C3dg, a further cleavage product derived from iC3b,[75] suggesting that these cells were also deficient in the C3dg receptor.[76] These data are consistent with the hypothesis that Leu M5 is identical with the C3dg receptor.[67,48]

The functional abnormalities in Leu-CAM deficient lymphocytes are more difficult to demonstrate. Initial studies of lymphocyte functions in all the patients showed no detectable defects in lymphoproliferation, both in vivo and in vitro, and positive delayed hypersensitivity skin testing suggesting normal T helper cell-macrophage interactions.[20,21,70-75] Defects in lymphoproliferation in response to PHA or ConA were more readily demonstrable, however, when the mitogen concentration used to elicit proliferation was low.[25,26] Cytolytic T cells (generated by mitogen or alloantigen stimulation) killed their targets normally.[24,72] Natural killing (NK) of certain targets (e.g., K562 cell line) was normal in some patients,[24,72] but absent in others.[77] It is important to note that in all patients with measurable T cell or NK responses, detectable amounts of LFA-1 were present (5 to 10%), and lymphocyte proliferation, CTL, and NK activities by the patients' cells were more sensitive to inhibition by anti-LFA-1 monoclonal antibodies.

EBV transformed B cell lines established from Leu-CAM deficient B lymphocytes do not aggregate either spontaneously in culture or in response to PMA.[41,42] In some cases, B cells failed to produce immunoglobulins (Ig) in the presence of syngeneic or allogeneic T cells and pokeweed mitogen in vitro,[72] or the patients had no antibody response after vaccination with polio virus, diphtheria, or tetanus toxoid.[75] A monoclonal antibody directed against LFA-1 inhibited in vitro antibody response by normal lymphocytes to influenza virus as well as the helper activity for in vitro Ig production by normal B cells.[71,75] In three patients, a profound impairment in alpha and gamma interferon production by deficient cells was observed.[71,78,75] These defects could not be reproduced in normal cells by monoclonal antibodies against LFA-1 and are therefore uncertain. The preponderance of bacterial infections in patients with Leu-CAM deficiency reflects a more pronounced phagocytic rather than a lymphocytic disorder. The small amounts of LFA-1 detected on lymphocytes from deficient patients may be sufficient to normalize the function of these cells. Alternatively, other lymphocyte surface molecules involved in effector-target cell interactions such as T4, T8, T11 and the T3/Ti cell receptor complex, which are normally expressed on these patients' lymphocytes, may compensate for the LFA-1 deficiency and thus prevent any clinically important sequelae to the deficiency of LFA-1 on lymphocytes.

## VI. MODULATION OF EXPRESSION OF Leu-CAM ON LEUKOCYTES

Stimuli that enhance granulocyte adhesiveness, such as the chemotactic peptides F-met-leu-phe and C5a, leukotrien B4, tumor-promoting phorbol esters, calcium ionophore A 23187, and phagocytosis per se, all increase the expression of Mol on the surface of granulocytes by 3 to 10-fold, as determined by fluorocytometry and direct binding studies with radiolabeled antibody.[24,79,80] Calcium ionophore ($1 \mu M$) increases the number of Mol receptors on granulocytes from $6 \times 10^4$ to $6 \times 10^5$ per cell.[24] Increased Mol surface expression by various stimuli is rapid, occurring within minutes, is complete by 20 min at 37°C, and does not require protein synthesis. Augumented surface expression of Mol can also be demonstrated in vivo. Patients hemodialyzed with a new cuprophane membrane increase the expression of Mol on the surface of circulating granulocytes by five-fold. This rise in surface Mol may contribute to the C5a-induced leukoaggregation and the leukopenia characteristically seen in these patients during first use of the complement-activating cuprophane dialysis membranes.[81]

Optimal expression of Mol by F-met-leu-phe, leukotrein B4, or PMA requires release of calcium from intracellular stores as well as an influx of extracellular calcium. Calmodulin antagonists (e. g., phenothiazines) and drugs that block release of calcium from intracellular stores, both inhibit augmented Mol surface expression when induced by a variety of stimuli.[82] Increased expression of Mol on the granulocyte surface appears to be due to a translocation of this antigen from an intracellular pool to the plasma membrane. This intracellular pool is present in the subcellular fraction containing both specific and tertiary granules on percoll gradients.[24,79,83,84] PMA has a biphasic effect on Mol surface expression. At 0.5 ng/mℓ, PMA increases surface Mol by 7.5-fold above baseline. At higher concentrations, Mol expression is reduced to 58% of its peak value, probably secondary to receptor-mediated endocytosis induced by high concentrations of PMA.[83]

Most patients with Leu-CAM deficiency significantly increase Mol expression on the granulocyte surface following stimulation with calcium ionophore A23187, although the total amount expressed is still ten times less than that expressed on activated normal cells.[24] Granulocytes from patients with specific granule deficiency can not augment the expression of Mol on the cell surface following stimulation.[83] This relative Mol deficiency state may explain the adhesion defects seen in specific granule disease as well as the increased susceptibility of these patients to recurrent bacterial infections.

Recently, the monokine, tumor necrosis factor, was found to increase Mol surface expression in association with its enhancing effect on the adhesion of granulocytes to endothelial cell monolayers.[85] The lymphokine, granulocyte/monocyte colony stimulating factor, has also been shown to promote granulocyte adhesion and increase the expression of Mol and Leu M5 on the surface of granulocytes.[86] It appears likely, therefore, that release of these cytokines can increase the adhesiveness and cytotoxicity of granulocytes at local sites of inflammation and thus be biologically important in host defense mechanisms. Systemic production of these cytokines may, as in the case of systemic C5a generation (during dialysis or sepsis), lead to leukoaggregation and to impaired granulocyte migration across endothelial cells, thus predisposing the host to pyogenic infections.

The same stimuli that increase Mol surface expression also increase the expression of Leu M5 on the granulocyte surface,[19] suggesting that these antigens may be present in the same intracellular pool. Interestingly, none of these stimuli significantly increase LFA-1 expression on the granulocyte surface.[24]

Human monocytes isolated by elutriation (but not by adherence) also increase their surface expression of Mol by 1.5- to 2-fold in response to F-met-leu-phe or C5a.[87,88] The intracellular source of Mol in monocytes is yet undetermined. In murine macrophages, $\beta$ interferon (INF) derived from fibroblasts down-regulates the cellular expression of Mac 1 with a 50% decrease of Mac-1 positive cells effected at an INF concentration of 0.1 IU/m$\ell$.[89] Human monocytes adherent to polystyrene plastic surfaces also progressively lose surface Mol during the first 2 weeks in culture.[90] The mechanism for this loss is not determined.

LFA-1 expression on the surface of lymphocytes is also affected by the state of cell activation.[24] A ten-fold increase in the surface expression of LFA-1 is seen on lymphoblasts generated in response to a 6-day culture with mitogens or alloantigens.[24] Patients with Leu-CAM deficiency also increase LFA-1 expression on their lymphoblasts, but the amount expressed remains approximately 5 to 10% of normal. The mechanism for this increase of LFA-1 during blastogenesis is undetermined, but may involve protein neosynthesis.

## VII. BIOSYNTHESIS OF Mol/LFA-1/Leu M5 AND THE MOLECULAR BASIS FOR Leu-CAM DEFICIENCY

The biosynthesis of the three members of this family of molecules and their common beta subunit has been studied using mouse peritoneal macrophages, a murine T cell line, freshly isolated human monocytes, established human EBV cell lines, and U937, a human myelomonocytic cell line.[18,91,92,93] Various cell types were pulsed with $^{35}$S methionine, chased with unlabeled methionine, and immunoprecipitation was carried out using monoclonal or polyclonal antibodies to the various subunits. LFA-1 is synthesized as a precursor with an apparent molecular mass of 170 kDalton that "matures" to the 177 kDalton form expressed on the cell surface by 4 hr. The biosynthesis of Mol appears to be similar. An Endo-H sensitive precursor form of 150 kDalton is chased to the mature form with a $t_{1/2}$ of 2 hr. Both precursor forms can be seen associating with a precursor beta chain, suggesting that association of the alpha and beta subunits precedes the processing of these molecules to their mature forms.[18] Biosynthesis of Leu M5 was studied indirectly by using a monoclonal antibody directed against the common beta subunit. In PMA-induced U937, Leu M5$_a$ precursor was seen after two hr of pulsing with $^{35}$S methionine, was distinct from the M$_a$ precursor, did not change in molecular mass during 22 hr of chase, and was identical in size to the surface expressed molecule.[18] Biosynthesis of the beta subunit was more complex. A precursor form (apparent molecular mass 85 kDalton) is detected after a two hr pulse. This form is already glycosylated, as evidenced by its Endo-H sensitivity which reduces its molecular mass by approximately 10 kDalton.[93] The 85 kDalton form matures to the surface-expressed 94 kDalton species by 24 hr. Significant amounts of the precursor are still detected, even at that time, in established EBV cell lines.[93]

Since patients with Leu-CAM deficiency lack or have severely reduced levels of the three alpha subunits and of the common beta subunit, it appeared reasonable to suggest that the basic defect may lie in the lack or deficiency of the common beta subunit.[23] To examine this question, biosynthesis studies were carried out on EBV cell lines or PHA blasts derived from one patient who totally lacks surface LFA-1[47] and on two others with partial deficiency (surface LFA-1 less than 10% of normal).[94] The authors found, in all three patients, normal amounts of $L_a$ precursor that never matured. In addition, they found no evidence of a precursor or a mature form of the beta subunit.[94] They concluded that all three patients lack normal beta precursors and therefore are unable to process the alpha precursors and transport them to the cell surface. We reexamined the biosynthesis of the beta subunit in the same patient that totally lacks surface LFA-1 expression,[47] using a polyclonal antibody to the beta subunit.[93] We found that this patient's EBV cells synthesize normal amounts of the beta precursor that did not mature to the 94 kDalton form expressed on the cell surface. In two other patients with partial deficiency,[21,22] only about 5 to 10% of the precursor matured.[93] This apparent discrepancy in the results obtained in the same patient may be explained by the fact that the beta-specific monoclonal antibody used in the first study[94] did not recognize the normal precursor form of human beta subunit.

Biosynthesis studies in two additional patients studied recently showed that leukocytes from one patient synthesized no detectable beta subunit precursor, and the other patient had reduced amounts of a precursor that appeared degraded. Both patients synthesized normal amounts of alpha precursors.[95] These data indicate that heterogenous defects in the beta gene underlie lack of, or reduced, surface expression of the Leu-CAM heterodimers. In patients who synthesize a normal-sized beta precursor, the defect could prevent the alpha and beta subunits from associating, thus interfering with the transport of the heterodimer across the golgi apparatus and its surface expression.

## III. N-TERMINAL AMINO ACID SEQUENCING AND MOLECULAR BIOLOGY OF Leu-CAM

Enough quantities of the alpha subunits of murine LFA-1 and Mac-1 were purified to allow N-terminal amino acid sequencing.[96] The N-terminal sequences of LFA-1 and Mac-1 alpha subunits were 33% homologous with four contiguous amino acids (positions 2 to 5) being identical in both. In addition, analysis of the N-terminal 19 amino acids in LFA-1 showed a statistically significant 20 to 27% homology with mouse alpha interferons. These data therefore indicate the presence of structural similarities between LFA-1 and Mac-1, although the functional significance of LFA-1 homology to alpha interferons is less obvious. The N-terminal sequence of the alpha subunit of human and guinea pig Mol have also been obtained.[97,98]

Among the N-terminal 15 amino acids, 13 residues were identical in man, mouse, and guinea pigs; and two represented conserved substitutions.[97,98] Of equal significance is the finding that the N-terminus of Mol was significantly homologous to the N-terminus of the alpha subunit in the platelet adhesion receptor IIb/IIIa.[97,98,99] The platelet heterodimer IIb/IIIa is a member of a family of receptors which recognize the tetrapeptide Arg-Gly-Asp-Ser. Other members in this family include the fibronectin and vitronectin receptors.[100] Homology among these glycoproteins also extend to their beta subunits. The beta subunit of Mol has been cloned, and the deduced amino acid sequence bears an overall amino acid identity of 47% to the corresponding structure in the chicken fibronectin receptor (Integrin).[101-102] Like chicken integrin,[103] the beta subunit of Mol has a cohesive structure with extensive disulfide bonding (a total of 57 cysteine residues with 42 found within a stretch of 256 amino acids at identical positions in both glycopeptides). These data led to the hypothesis that Leu-CAM, platelet IIb/IIa, fibronectin — and vitronectin receptors belong to a family of adhesion receptors (Integrins) that play major roles in cell-cell and cell-matrix interactions.[100]

Recent data suggest that the gene encoding for the beta subunit is located on chromosome 21 in man.[104] Mouse-human hybridomas containing specific human chromosomes were analyzed by fluorocytometry using a beta-specific monoclonal antibody. Cell lines that expressed the beta subunit on the cell surface, presumably in association with mouse alpha subunit, were always shown to contain human chromosome 21. Confirmation of these data using probes derived from cDNA in the beta subunit will be needed.

cDNA probes specific for the beta subunit of Mol were used to further characterize the molecular basis of Leu-CAM deficiency. Patients with the complete or partial deficiency were studied. Included in this group are patients who synthesized a normal-sized beta precursor, a degraded precursor, or no precursor[93,95] Leukocytes from all these patients contained normal amounts of a normal-sized beta subunit mRNA (3.4 kilo-base) consistent with the biosynthesis data mentioned above and suggesting that small mutations, rather than large deletions or rearrangements in the beta subunit gene, may underlie defective leukocyte adhesion in these patients.

Attempts by several groups are being made to obtain cDNA or genomic clones that encode for the various alpha subunits of the Leu-CAM family. Recently, Cosgrove and colleages reported on the isolation of a 20 kilo-base (kb) genomic clone encoding the alpha chains of Mol, LFA-1, and platelet glycoprotein IIb-IIIa.[98] This clone was isolated by transfecting TK$^-$ L cells with human DNA cloned into lambda phage and selection of transfectants that surface express Mol/LFA-1/platelet gpIIb-IIIa, using antigen-specific monoclonal antibodies. Transfection with the purified recombinant phage DNA yielded a transfectant that reacted with monoclonal antibodies directed against OKM1, LFA-1 and platelet glycoprotein IIb-IIIa. No nucleotide sequence data were reported in this study.

Sastre et al. identified a partial genomic clone coding for an N-terminal region in the alpha subunit of mouse Mac-1 (Mac-1$_a$).[106] Partial sequencing of this clone revealed that it contained an exon coding for 28 amino acids from the N terminus of Mac-1 followed by an intron of undetermined size. This precluded further characterization of the gene. The size of Mac-1$_a$ mRNA was 6 kb. We identified cDNA clones coding for the alpha subunit of Mol in both humans and guinea pigs.[107] Sequencing of a partial cDNA human clone encoded a 126 amino acid peptide which contained a tryptic peptide derived from the purified antigen. The 126 amino acid stretch contained a carboxy-terminal region of Mol that bears significant homology to a region that spans the junction between the large and small subunits of the alpha chains of platelet IIb/IIIa, fibronectin receptor, and vitronectin receptor. All four glycoproteins contained the consensus sequence CXXXXCXXXXC, where C stands for cysteine and X stands for any other amino acid. The Mol alpha subunit mRNA was approximately 5 kb in size in both humans and guinea pigs. The single copy Mol$_a$ gene in humans was mapped to chromosome 16 by analysis of human-hamster hybrids.[107] The alpha subunit of LFA-1 has also been mapped to this chromosome by immunochemical analysis of mouse-human hybrid cells.[108] These data suggest that the genes coding the alpha subunits of Mol and LFA-1 and possibly of Leu M5 have probably arisen by gene duplication and divergence from a primordial gene. It remains to be seen if the alpha subunits of other adhesion receptors are also located on chromosome 16.

Despite the significant degrees of homology of Leu-CAM to other adhesion receptors on platelets and fibroblasts, Leu-CAM are distinct immunochemically, biochemically, and functionally. Within the Leu-CAM sub-family, differences exist in the function, surface regulation, cell distribution, and gene expression during leukocyte differentiation. Although available data conclusively show that Leu-CAM mediate leukocyte adhesion functions, the underlying mechanisms involved are not yet adequately defined. The availability of cDNA probes encoding for this family of adhesion receptors should now permit detailed studies of the structure as it relates to the specific and unique functions mediated by these molecules. Furthermore, studies on the organization and regulation of the genes encoding these molecules are now possible. The results of these studies should lead to better understanding of the processes controlling such diverse functions as wound healing, cell mediated cytotoxicity, and embryogenesis.

## ACKNOWLEDGMENTS

I wish to thank Ms. Toni Condangelo for secretarial assistance.

## REFERENCES

1. **Oseroff, A. R., Robbins, P. W., and Burger, M. M.,** The cell surface membrane: biochemical aspects and biophysical probes, *Ann. Rev. Biochem.*, 42, 647, 1973.
2. **Humphreys, T.,** Chemical dissolution and in vitro reconstruction of sponge cell adhesions. I. Isolation and functional demonstration of the components involved, *Dev. Biol.*, 8, 27, 1963.
3. **Weise, L. and Weise, W.,** On sexual agglutination and mating type substances in isogamous dioecious Chlamydomonads, *Dev. Biol.*, 43, 264, 1975.
4. **Burger, M. M. and Jumblatt, J.,** Membrane involvement in cell-cell interactions. 2-Component model system for cellular recognition that does not require live cells, in *Cell and Tissue*, Lash, J. W. and Burger, M. M., Eds., Raven Press, New York, 155, 1977.
5. **Ray, J. and Lerner, R. A.,** A biologically active receptor for the carbohydrate-binding protein(s) of dictyostelium discoideum, *Cell*, 28, 91, 1982.
6. **Hoffman, S., Sorkin, B. C., White, P. C., Brackenbury, R., Mailhammer, R., Rutishauser, U., Cunningham, B. A., and Edelman, G. M.,** Chemical characterization of aneural cell adhesion molecule purified from embryonic brain membranes, *J. Biol. Chem.*, 257, 7720, 1982.
7. **Thiery, J. P., Delouvee, A., Gallin, W. J., Cunningham, B. A., and Edelman, G. M.,** Ontogenic expression of cell adhesion molecules: L-CAM is found in epithelia derived from the three primary germ layers, *Dev. Biol.*, 102, 61, 1984.
8. **Edelman, G. M.,** Cell adhesion molecules, *Science*, Wash, DC., 219, 450, 1983.
9. **Milstein, C. and Lennox, E.,** The use of monoclonal antibody techniques in the study of developing cell surfaces, *Curr. Top. Dev. Biol.*, 14, 1, 1980.
10. **Springer, T., Galfre, G., Secher, D. S., and Milstein, C.,** Mac-1: a macrophage differentiation antigen identified by monoclonal antibody, *Eur. J. Immunol.*, 9, 301, 1979.
11. **Breard, J., Reinherz, E. L., Kung, P. C., Goldstein, G., and Schlossman, S. F.,** A monoclonal antibody reactive with human peripheral blood monocytes, *J. Immunol.*, 124, 1943, 1980.
12. **Todd, R. F. III, Nadler, L. M., and Schlossman, S. F.,** Antigens on human monocytes identified by monoclonal antibodies, *J. Immunol.*, 126, 1435, 1981.
13. **Towbridge, I. S. and Omary, M. B.,** Molecular complexity of leukocyte surface glycoproteins related to the macrophage differentiation antigen Mac-1, 154, 1517, 1981.
14. **LeBien, T. W. and Kersey, J. H.,** A monoclonal antibody (TA-1) reactive with human T lymphocytes and nonocytes, *J. Immunol.*, 125, 2208, 1980.
15. **Kurzinger, K., Reynolds, T., Germain, R. N., Davignon, D., Martz, E., and Springer, T. A.,** A novel lymphocyte function-associated antigen (LFA-1): cellular distribution, quantitative expression and structure, *J. Immunol.*, 127, 596, 1981.
16. **Beatty, P. G., Ledbetter, J. A., Martin, P. J., Price, T. H., and Hansen, J. A.,** Definition of a common leukocyte cell-surface antigen (LP95-150) associated with diverse cell-mediated immune functions, *J. Immunol.*, 131, 2913, 1983.
17. **Wright, S. D., Rao, P. E., Wesley, C., Van Voorhis, W. C., Craigmyle, L. S., Iida, K., Talle, M. A., Westberg, E. F., Goldstein, G., and Silverstein, S. C.,** Identification of the C3bi receptor of human monocytes and macrophages with monoclonal antibodies, *Proc. Natl. Acad. Sci. USA.*, 80, 5699, 1983.
18. **Sanchez-Madrid, F., Nagy, J. A., Robbins, E., Simon, P., and Springer, T. A.,** A human leukocyte differentiation antigen family with distinct alpha subunits and a common beta subunit: the lymphocyte-function associated antigen (LFA-1) the C3bi complement receptor (OKM1/Mac-1), and the p150, 95 molecule, *J. Exp. Med.*, 158, 1785, 1983.
19. **Lanier, L. L., Arnaout, M. A., Schwarting, R., Warner, N. L., and Ross, G. D.,** p150/95, third member of the LFA-1/CR3 polypeptide family identified by anti-Leu M5 monoclonal antibody, *Eur. J. Immunol.*, 15, 713, 1985.

20. **Crowley, C. A., Curnutte, J. T., Rosin, R. E., Andre-Schwartz, J., Gallin, J. I., Klempner, M., Snyderman, R., Southwick, F. S., Stossel, T. P., and Babior, B. M.,** An inherited abnormality of neutrophil adhesion: its genetic transmission and its association with a missing protein, *N. Eng. J. Med.,* 302, 1163, 1980.
21. **Arnaout, M. A., Pitt, J., Cohen, H. J., Melamed, J., Rosen, F. S., and Colten, H. R.,** Deficiency of a granulocyte-membrane glycoprotein (gp 150) in a boy with recurrent bacterial infections, *N. Eng. J. Med.,* 306, 693, 1982.
22. **Dana, N., Pitt, J., Todd, F. F. III, Melamed, J., Colten, H. R., and Arnaout, M. A.,** Deficiency of a monocyte-granulocyte surface glycoprotein (Mol) in man, *Clin. Res.,* 31, 489, 1983.
23. **Dana, N., Todd, R. F. III, Pitt, J., Springer, T. A., and Arnaout, M. A.,** Deficiency of a surface membrane glycoprotein (Mol) in man, *J. Clin. Invest.,* 73, 153, 1983.
24. **Arnaout, M. A., Spits, H., Terhorst, C., Pitt, J., and Todd, R. F. III,** Deficiency of a leukocyte surface glycoprotein (LFA-1) in two patients with Mol deficiency: effects of cell activation on Mol/LFA-1 surface expression in normal and deficient leukocytes, *J. Clin. Invest.,* 74, 1291, 1984.
25. **Arnaout, M. A., Dana, N., Pitt, J., and Todd, R. F. III,** Deficiency of two human leukocyte surface membrane glycoproteins (Mol and LFA-1), *Fed. Proc.,* 44, 2664, 1985.
26. **Beatty, P. G., Harlan, J. M., Rosen, H., Hansen, J. A., Ochs, H. D., Price, T. H., Taylor, R. F., and Klebanoff, S. J.,** Absence of monoclonal-antibody-defined protein complex in boy with abnormal leukocyte function, *Lancet,* 1, 535, 1984.
27. **Todd, R. F. III, van Agthovan, A., Schlossman, S. F., and Terhorst, C.,** Structural analysis of differentiation antigen Mol and Mo2 on human monocytes, *Hybridoma,* 1, 329, 1982.
28. **Schwarting, R., Stein, H., and Wang, C. Y.,** The monoclonal antibodies anti-HCL (anti-Leu-14) and anti-S-HCL (anti-Leu M5) allow the diagnosis of hairy cell leukemia, *Blood,* 65, 974, 1985.
29. **Hildreth, J. E. K., Gotch, F. M., Hildreth, P. D. K., and McMichael, A. J.,** A human lymphocyte-associated antigen involved in cell-mediated lympholysis, *Eur. J. Immunol.,* 13, 202, 1983.
30. **Rosenthal, P., Rimm, I. J., Umiel, T., Griffin, J. D., Osathanondh, R., Schlossman, S. F., and Nadler, L. M.,** Ontogeny of human hematopoietic cells: analysis utilizing monoclonal antibodies, *J. Immunol.,* 31, 232, 1983.
31. **Sabbath, K. D., Ball, E. D., Larcom, P., Davis, R. B., and Griffin, J. D.,** Heterogeneity of Clonogenic Cells in Acute Myeloblastic Leukemia, *J. Clin. Invest.,* 75, 746, 1985.
32. **Hickstein, D. D., Smith, A., Fisher, W., Beaty, P. G., Schwartz, B. R., Harlan, J. M., Root, R. K., and Locksley, R. M.,** Expression of leukocyte adherence-related glycoproteins during differentiation of HL-60 promyelocytic leukemia cells, *J. Immunol.,* 138, 513, 1987.
33. **Schreiber, R. D.,** The chemistry and biology of complement receptors, *Springer Semin. Immunopathol.,* 7, 221, 1984.
34. **Letvin, N. L., Todd, R. F. III, Palley, L. S., Schlossman, S. F., and Griffin, J. D.,** Conservation of myeloid surface antigens on primate granulocytes, *Blood,* 61, 408, 1983.
35. **Springer, T., Kurzinger, K., Germain, R., Davignon, D., and Martz, E.,** Monoclonal antibody to a novel lymphocyte function-associated antigen LFA-1, *Fed. Proc.,* 40, 1171, 1981.
36. **Sarimento, M., Dialynas, D. P., Lancki, D. W., et al.,** Cloned T lymphocytes and monoclonal antibodies as probes for cell surface molecules active in T cell-mediated cytolysis, *Immunol. Rev.,* 68, 135, 1982.
37. **Pierres, M., Goridis, C., and Goldstein, P.,** Inhibition of murine T cell-mediated cytolysis and T-cell proliferation by a rat monoclonal antibody immunoprecipitating two lymphoid cell surface polypeptides of 94,000 and 180,000 molecular weight, *Eur. J. Immunol.,* 12, 60, 1982.
38. **Reinherz, E. L., Meuer, S. C., and Schlossman, S. F.,** The delineation of antigen receptors on L human T Lymphocytes, *Immunol. Today,* 4, 5, 1983.
39. **Miedema, F., Teteroo, P. A. T., Hesselink, W. G., Werner, G., Spits, H., and Melief, C. J. M.,** Both Fc receptors and lymphocyte function associated antigen 1 are required for the effector cell function in antibody-dependent cellular cytotoxicity (K-cell activity) mediated by T cells, *Eur. J. Immunol.,* 14, 518, 1984.
40. **Krensky, A. M., Sanchez-Madrid, F., Robbins, E., Nagy, J. A., Springer, T. A., and Burakoff, S. J.,** The functional significance, distribution, and structure of LFA-1, LFA-2, and LFA-3: cell surface antigens associated with CTL-target interactions, *J. Immunol.,* 131, 611, 1983.
41. **Buescher, E. K., Gaither, T., Nath, J., and Gallin, J. I.,** Abnormal adherence-related functions of neutrophils, monocytes, and Epstein-Barr virus-transformed B cells in a patient with C3bi receptor deficiency, *Blood,* 65, 1382, 1985.
42. **Rothlein, R., and Springer, T. A.,** The requirement for lymphocyte function-associated antigen 1 in homotypic leukocyte adhesion stimulated by phorbol ester, *J. Exp. Med.,* 163, 1132, 1986.
43. **Patarroyo, M., Beatty, P. G., Fabre, J. W., and Gahmberg, C. G.,** Identification of a cell surface protein complex mediating phorbol ester-induced adhesion (binding) among human mononuclear leukocytes, *Scand. J. Immunol.,* 22, 171, 1985.

44. **Mentzer, S. J., Gromkowski, S. H., Krensky, A. M., Burakoff, S. J., and Martz, E.,** LFA-1 membrane molecule in the regulation of homotypic adhesions of human B lymphocytes, *J. Immunol.,* 135, 9, 1985.

45. **Beller, D. I., Springer, T. A., and Schreiber, R. D.,** Anti-Mac-1 selectively inhibits the mouse and human type three complement receptor, *J. Exp. Med.,* 56, 1000, 1982.

46. **Arnaout, M. A., Todd, R. F. III, Dana, N., Melamed, J., Schlossman, S. F., and Colten, H. R.,** Inhibition of phagocytosis of complement C3 or immunoglobulin G-coated particles and of C3bi binding by monoclonal antibodies to a monocyte-granulocyte membrane glycoprotein (Mol), *J. Clin. Invest.,* 72, 171, 1983.

47. **Anderson, D. C., Schmalstieg, F. C., Arnaout, M. A., Kohl, S., Tosi, M. F., Dana, N., Buffone, G. J., Hughes, B. J., Brinkley, B. R., Dickey, W. D., Abramson, J. S., Springer, T., Boxer, L. A., Hollers, J. M., and Smith, C. W.,** Abnormalities in polymorphonuclear leukocyte function associated with a heritable deficiency of a high molecular weight surface glycoproteins (GP 138): common relationship to dismissed cell adherence, *J. Clin. Invest.,* 74, 536, 1984.

48. **Micklem, K. J., and Sim, R. B.,** Isolation of complement-fragment-iC3b-binding proteins by affinity chromatography, *Biochem. J.,* 231, 233, 1985.

49. **Arnaout, M. A. and Cole, J. L.,** Binding Properties of the leukocyte surface proteins, Mol and Leu M5 (P150,95), *Clin. Res.,* 34 (Abstr.), 667, 1986.

50. **Lay, W. H. and Nussenzweig, V.,** Receptors for complement on leukocytes, *J. Exp. Med.,* 128, 991, 1968.

51. **Klebanoff, S. J., Beatty, P. G., Schreiber, R. D., Ochs, H. D., and Waltersdorph, A. M.,** Effect of antibodies directed against complement receptors on phagocytosis by polymorphonuclear leukocytes: use of iodination as a convenient measure of phagocytosis, *J. Immunol.,* 134, 1153, 1985.

52. **Dana, N., Styrt, B., Griffin, J. D., Todd, R. F. III, Klempner, M. S., and Arnaout, M. A.,** Two functional domains in the phagocyte membrane glycoprotein Mol indentified with monoclonal antibodies, *J. Immunol.,* 137, 3259, 1986.

53. **Harlan, J. M., Killen, P. D., Senecal, F. M., Schwartz, B. R., Yee, E. K., Taylor, R. F., Beatty, P. G., Price, T. H., and Ochs, H. D.,** The role of neutrophil membrane glycoprotein GP-150 in neutrophil adherence to endothelium in vitro, *Blood,* 66, 167, 1985.

54. **Ross, G. D., Cain, J. A., and Lachmann, P. J.,** Membrane complement receptor type three (CR₃) has lectin-like properties analogous to bovine conglutinin and functions as a receptor for zymosan and rabbit erythrocytes as well as a receptor of iC3b, *J. Immunol.,* 134, 3307, 1985.

55. **Czop, J. K. and Austen, K. F.,** A B-glucan inhibitable receptor on human monocytes: Its identity with the phagocytic receptor for particulate activators of the alternative complement pathway, *J. Immunol.,* 134, 2588, 1985.

56. **Chakravarti, B., Schreiber, R. D., and Muller-Eberhard, H. J.,** Phagocytosis by human monocytes of unopsonized particulate activators of the human alternative complement pathway: Induction by cytokine, *Fed. Proc.,* 45 (Abstr.), 1106, 1986.

57. **Ezekowitz, R. A. B., Sim, R. B., Hill, H., and Gordon, S.,** Local opsonization by secreted macrophage complement components. Role of receptors for complement in uptake of zymosan, *J. Exp. Med.,* 159, 244.

58. **Wright, S. D., Craigmyle, L. S., and Silverstein, S. C.,** Fibronectin and serum amyloid P component stimulate C3b- and C3bi-mediated phagocytosis in cultured human monocytes, *J. Exp. Med.,* 158, 1338, 1983.

59. **Wright, S. D., Detmers, P. A., and Jong, M. T. C.,** Interferon gamma (IFN) causes monocytes to express C3b and C3bi receptors that do not bind ligand, an effect reversed by fibroconectin, *Fed. Proc.,* 45 (Abstr.), 1106, 1986.

60. **Dana, N., todd, R. F. III, Colten, H. R., and Arnaout, M. A.,** A dysfunctional Mol glycoprotein is present on a subline of the KG1 acute myelogenous leukemia cell line, *J. Immunol.,* 138, 3549, 1987.

61. **Southwick, F. S., Holbrook, T., Howard, T., Springer, T., Stossel, T. P., and Arnaout, M. A.,** Neutrophil actin dysfunction is associated with a deficiency of Mol, *Clin. Res.,* 34 (Abstr.), 533, 1986.

62. **Schreiber, R. D., Pangburn, M. K., Bjornson, A. B., Brothers, M. A., and Muller-Eberhard, H. J.,** The role of C3 fragments in endocytosis and extracellular cytotoxic reactions by polymorphonuclear leukocytes, *Clin. Immunol. Immunopathol.,* 23, 335, 1982.

63. **Wright, S. D. and Silverstein, S. C.,** Receptors for C3b and C3bi promote phagocytosis but not the release of toxic oxygen from human phagocytes, *J. Exp. Med.,* 158, 2016, 1983.

64. **Cain, J. A., Newman, S. L., and Ross, G. D.,** Role of fixed C3 fragments versus yeast (Y) cell wall components in the superoxide (O₂) burst response of human neutrophils (PMN), *Fed. Proc.,* 44 (Abstr.), 1877, 1985.

65. **Perlmann, H., Perlmann, P., Schreiber, R. D., and Muller-Eberhard, H. J.,** Interaction of target cell-bound C3bi and C3d with human lymphocyte receptors. Enhancement of antibody-mediated cellular cytotoxicity, *J. Exp. Med.,* 153, 1592, 1981.

66. **Wahlin, B., Perlmann, H., Perlmann, P., Schreiber, R. D., and Muller-Eberhard, H. J.,** C3 receptors on human lymphocyte subsets and recruitment of ADCC effector cells by C3 fragments, *J. Immunol.*, 130, 2831, 1983.

67. **Wright, S. D., Licht, M. R., Silverstein, S. C.,** The receptor for C3d (CR2) is a homologue of CR3 and LFA-1, *Fed. Proc.*, 43 (Abstr.), 1487, 1984.

68. **Arnaout, M. A. and Faller, D. V.,** Contribution of the leukocyte Mol/LFA-1/Leu M5 glycoprotein family to granulocyte-monocyte endothelial cell adhesion, *Kidney Int.*, 31, 312 (abstr.), 1987.

69. **Bowen, T. J., Ochs, H. D., Altman, L. C., Price, T. H., Van Epps, D. E., Brautigan, D. L., Rosin, R. E., Perkins, W. D., Babior, B. M., Klebanoff, S. J., and Wedgwood, R. J.,** Severe recurrent bacterial infections associated with defective adherence and chemotaxis in two patients with neutrophils deficient in a cell-associated glycoprotein, *J. Pediatr.*, 101, 932, 1982.

70. **Hayward, A. R., Leonard, J., Wood, C. B. S., Harvey, B. A. M., Greenwood, M. C., and Soothill, J. F.,** Delayed separation of the umbilical cord, widespread infections, and defective neutrophil mobility, *Lancet,* 1, 1326 1979.

71. **Davies, G. G., Isaacs, D., and Levinsky, R. J.,** Defective immune interferon production and natural killer activity associated with poor neutrophil mobility and delayed umbilical cord separation, *Clin. Exp. Immunol.*, 50, 454, 1982.

72. **Miedema, F., Tetteroo, P. A. T., Terpstra, F. G., Keizer, G., Roos, M., Weening, R. S., Weemaes, C. M. R., Roos, D., and Melief, C. J. M.,** Immunologic studies with LFA-1 and Mol-deficient lymphocytes from a patient with recurrent bacterial infections, *J. Immunol.*, 134, 3075, 1985.

73. **Abramson, J. S., Mills, E. L., Sawyer, M. K., Regelmann, W. R., Nelson, J. D., and Quie, P. G.,** Recurrent infections and delayed separation of the umbilical cord in an infant with abnormal phagocytic cell locomotion and oxidative response during partial phagocytosis, *J. Pediatr.*, 99, 887, 1981.

74. **Weisman, S., Berkow, R. L., Coates, T. D., Plantz, G., Torres, M., McGuire, W. A., Haak, R., Jersild, R., and Baehner, R. L.,** Glycoprotein-180 deficient neutrophils (PMN): genetics and abnormal activation, *Clin. Res.*, 32, (Abstr.), 500, 1984.

75. **Fisher, A., Seger, R., Durandy, A., Grospierre, B., Virelizier, J. L., Grischelli, C., Fisher, E., Kazatchkine, M., Bohler, M., Descamps-Latscha, B., Trung, P. H., Olive, D., Springer, T. A., and Mawas, C.,** Deficiency of the adhesive protein complex LFA-1, C3bi complement receptor, p 150, 95 in a girl with recurrent bacterial infections, *J. Clin. Invest.*, 76, 2385, 1985.

76. **Ross, G. D., Thompson, R. A., Walport, M. J., Springer, T. A., Watson, J. V., Ward, R. H. R., Lida, J., Newman, S. L., Harrison, R. A., and Lachmann, P. J.,** Characterization of patients with an increased susceptibility to bacterial infections and a genetic deficiency of leukocyte membrane complement receptor type 3 and the related membrane antigen LFA-1, *Blood*, 66, 882, 1985.

77. **Ross, G. D.,** Clinical and laboratory features of patients with an inherited deficiency of neutrophil membrane complement receptor type 3 (CR3) and the related membrane antigens LFA-1 and p150, 95, *J. Clin. Immunol.*, 6, 107, 1986.

78. **Fischer, A., Descamps-Latscha, B., Gerota, I., Scheinmetzier, C., Virelizner, J. I., Trung, P., Grospierri, B. L., Perez, N., Druandy, A., and Grischeili, C.,** Bone marrow transplantation for inborn error of phagocytic cells associated with defective adherence, chemotaxis, and oxidative response during opsonized particle phagocytosis, *Lancet*, 2, 473, 1983.

79. **Todd, R. F. III, Arnaout, M. A., Rosin, R. E., Crowley, C. A., Peters, W. A., and Babior, B. M.,** Subcellular localization of the large subunit of Mol (Mol: formerly, gp 110), surface glycoprotein associated with neutrophil adhesion, *J. Clin. Invest.*, 74, 1280, 1984.

80. **Berger, M., O'Shea, J., Cross, A. S., Folks, T. M., Chused, T. M., Brown, E. J., and Frank, M. M.,** Human neutrophils increase expression of C3bi as well as C3b receptors upon activation, *J. Clin. Invest.*, 74, 1566, 1984.

81. **Arnaout, M. A., Hakim, R. M., Todd, R. F. III, Dana, N., and Colton, H. R.,** Increased expression of an adhesion promoting surface glycoprotein in the granulocytopenia of hemodialysis, *New. Engl. J. Med.*, 312, 457, 1985.

82. **Berger, M., Birx, D. L., Wetzler, E. M., O'Shea, J. J., Brown, E. J., and Cross, A. S.,** Calcium requirements for increased complement receptor expression during neutrophil activation, *J. Immunol.*, 135, 1342, 1985.

83. **O'Shea, J. J., Brown, E. J., Seligmann, B. E., Metcalf, J. A., Frank, M. M., and Gallin, J. I.,** Evidence for distinct intracellular pools of receptors for C3b and C3bi in human neutrophils, *J. Immunol.*, 134, 2580, 1985.

84. **Petrequin, P. R., Todd, R. F. III, Devall, L. J., Boxer, L. A., and Curnutte, J. T.,** Association between tertiary granule release and increased plasma membrane expression of the Mol glycoprotein, *Blood*, 66, Suppl. 1, Abstr. 249, 1985.

85. **Gamble, J. R., Harlan, J. M., Klebanoff, S. J., and Vadas, M. A.,** Stimulation of the adherence of neutrophils to umbilical vein endothelium by human recombinant tumor necrosis factor, *Proc. Natl. Acad. Sci. USA.*, 82, 8667, 1985.

86. **Arnaout, M. A., Wang, E. A., Clark, S. C., and Sieff, C. A.,** Human recombinant GM-CSF increases cell to cell adhesion and surface expression of adhesion-promoting surface glycoproteins on mature granulocytes, *J. Clin. Invest.,* 78, 597, 1986.

87. **Arnaout, M. A., Todd, R. R. III, and Dana, N.,** Increased surface expression of Mol on human granulocytes by chemical and phagocytic stimuli, *Fed. Proc.,* 43 (Abstr.), 1665, 1984.

88. **Yancey, K. B., O'Shea, J., Cushed, T., Brown, E., Takahashi, T., Frank, M. M., and Lawley, T. J.,** Human C5a modulates monocyte Fc and C3 receptor expression, *J. Immunol.,* 135, 465, 1985.

89. **Vogel, S. N., English, K. E., Fertsch, D., and Fultz, M. J.,** Differential modulation of macrophage membrane markers by inter-term: analysis of Fc and C3b receptors, Mac-1 and Ia antigen expression, *J. Interferon. Res.,* 3, 153, 1983.

90. **Todd, R. F. III and Schlossman, S. F.,** Analysis of antigenic determinants on human monocytes and macrophages, *Blood,* 59, 775, 1982.

91. **Dahms, N. M. and Hart, G. W.,** Lymphocyte function-associated antigen 1 (LFA-1) contains sulfated N-linked oligosaccharides, *J. Immunol.,* 134, 3978, 1985.

92. **Ho, M. K. and Springer, T. A.,** Tissue distribution, structural characterization and biosynthesis of Mac-3, a macrophage surface glycoprotein exhibiting molecular weight heterogeneity, *J. Biol. Chem.,* 258, 636, 1983.

93. **Dana, N. Clayton, L. K., Tenen, D. G., Pierce, M. W., Lachmann, P. J., Law, S. A., and Arnaout, M. A.,** Leukocytes from four patients with complete or partial Leu-CAM deficiency contain the common beta-subunit precursor and beta-subunit messenger RNA, *J. Clin. Invest.,* 79, 1010, 1987.

94. **Springer, T. A., Thompson, W. S., Miller, L. J., Schmalstieg, F. C., and Anderson, D. C.,** Inherited deficiency of the Mac-1, LFA-1, P150, 95 glycoprotein family and its molecular basis, *J. Exp. Med.,* 160, 1901, 1985.

95. **Dimanche, M. T., Le Deist, F., Fischer, A., Arnaout, M. A., Griscelli, C., and Lisowska-Grospierre, B.,** LFA-1 beta-chain synthesis and degradation in patients with leukocyte-adhesive proteins deficiency, *Eur. J. Immunol.,* 17, 417, 1987.

96. **Springer, T. A., Teplow, D. B., and Dreyer, W. J.,** Sequence homology of the LFA-1 and Mac-1 leukocyte adhesion glycoproteins and unexpected relation to leukocyte interferon, *Nature,* 314, 540, 1985.

97. **Arnaout, M. A., Pierce, M. W., Dana, N., and Clayton, L. K.,** Human complement receptor type 3, in *Methods in Enzymology,* DiSabato, G., Langone, J. J., and Van Vanakis, H., Eds., Academic Press, Orlando, Fla., 150, 602, 1987.

98. **Pierce, M. W., Remold-O'Donnell, E., Todd, R. F. III, and Arnaout, M. A.,** N-terminal sequence of human leukocyte glycoprotein Mol: conservation across species and homology to platelet II/IIIa, *Biochem. Biophys. Acta,* 874, 368, 1986.

99. **Charo, I. F., Fitzgerald, L. A., Steiner, B., Rall, S. C. Jr., Bekeart, L. S., and Philips, D. R.,** Platlet glycoproteins IIb and IIIa: evidence for a family of immunologically and structurally related glycoproteins in mammalian cells, *Proc. Natl. Acad. Sci. U.S.A.,* 83, 8351, 1986.

100. **Hynes, R. O.,** Integrin receptors, *Cell,* 48, 549, 1987.

101. **Law, S. K. A., Gagnon, J., Hildreth, J. E. K., Wells, C. E., Willis, A. C., and Wong, A. J.,** The primary structure of the beta subunit of cell surface adhesion glycoproteins LFA-1, CR3 and p150, 95 and its relationship to the fibronectin receptor, *EMBO J.,* 4, 915, 1987.

102. **Kishimoto, T. K., O-Connor, K., Lee, A., Roberts, T. M., and Springer, T. A.,** Cloning of the beta subunit of the leukocyte adhesion proteins: homology to an extracellular matrix receptor defines a novel supergene family, *Cell,* 48, 681, 1987.

103. **Tamkun, J. W., DeSimone, D. W., Fonda, D., Patel, R. S., Buck, C., Horwitz, A. F., and Hynes, R. O.,** Structure of integrin, a glycoprotein involved in the transmembrane linkage between fibronectin and actin, *Cell,* 46, 271, 1986.

104. **Soumalainen, H. A., Gahmberg, C. G., Patarroyo, M., Beatty, P. G., and Schroder, J.,** Genetic assignment of GP90, leukocyte adhesion glycoprotein, to human chromosome 21, *Somat. Cell. Genet.,* 12, 297, 1986.

105. **Cosgrove, L. J., Sandrin, M. S., Rajasekariah, P., and McKenzie, I. F. C.,** A genomic clone encoding the chain of the OKMI, LFA-1, and platelet glycoprotein IIb-IIIa molecules, *Proc. Natl. Acad. Sci. USA.,* 83, 752, 1986.

106. **Sastre, L., Roman, J. M., Teplow, D. B., Dreyer, W. J., Gee, C. E., Larson, R. S., Roberts, T., and Springer, T. A.,** A partial genomic DNA clone for the alpha subunit of the mouse complement receptor type 3 and cellular adhesion molecule Mac-1, *Proc. Natl. Acad. Sci. U.S.A.,* 84, 5644, 1986.

107. **Arnaout, M. A., Remold-O'Donnell, E., Pierce, M. W., Harris, P., and Tenen, D. G.,** Molecular cloning of the alpha subunit of human and guinea pig leukocyte adhesion glycoprotein Mol: Homology to the alpha subunits of Integrins, Submitted, 1987.

108. **Marlin, S. D., Morton, C. C., Anderson, D. C., and Springer, T. A.,** LFA-1 immunodeficiency disease: definition of the genetic defect and chromosomal mapping of the alpha and beta subunits of the lymphocyte function-associated-antigen 1 (LFA-1) by complementation in hybrid cells, *J. Exp. Med.,* 164, 855, 1986.
109. **Todd, R. F. III and Arnaout, M. A.,** Monoclonal antibodies that identify Mol and LFA-1, two human leukocyte membrane glycoproteins: A review, in *Leukocyte Typing* II: vol. 3, Reinherz, E. L., Haynes, B. F., Nadler, L. M., and Bernstein, I. D., Eds., Springer-Verlag, New York, 1986, chap. 8.

Chapter 7

# THE ROLE OF ACCESSORY MOLECULES IN T CELL RECOGNITION

**Julia L. Greenstein, Steven J. Mentzer, and Steven J. Burakoff**

## TABLE OF CONTENTS

# I. INTRODUCTION

A traditional approach for the cellular immunologist has been the definition of cellular heterogeneity by the use of antibodies directed against cell surface proteins. Over many years this approach has been refined by the advent of tumor cell models, functional T cell clones and hybridomas, and monoclonal antibody (MAb) technology. The combination of these approaches has resulted in an expansive literature which examines the role of various T cell surface molecules in T cell function. Our goal, for this review, is to examine the role of a subset of these T cell surface molecules. We have been interested in the study of the surface molecules which demonstrate evidence of direct participation in T cell function, as defined by the ability of specific MAb to block T cell function. This review will address the role of some of these T cell surface molecules in the activation of mouse and human T cells.

T cell activation and effector function has been studied for many years. Only recently has the antigen-specific major histocompatibility complex (MHC) restricted T cell receptor (TcR) been isolated and demonstrated to be a disulfide-linked heterodimer composed of an α and β chain with variable and constant regions on both chains.[1] Much has been learned about the structure and genetics of this molecule, which is part of the immunoglobulin super-gene family.[2-6] On the cell surface, this heterodimer has been shown to be associated with the three polypeptide chains of T3, another T cell surface molecule[7-9] based on comodulation, immunoprecipitation, and cross-linking experiments. It has also been demonstrated that a defect in TcR expression leads to a loss of T3 surface expression.[10] Some MAb specific for T3 and for the TcR have the ability to stimulate various T cell functions in the absence of antigen.[9,11-15] It appears that T cell activation occurs via a TcR/T3 signalling process, related in some way to cross-linking and modulation of these receptors. It has been proposed that T3 is responsible for the triggering of T cell activation, possibly via the formation of a $Ca^{++}$ ion channel.[16-18]

The emphasis of our research has been to study the relationship of other functionally relevant T cell surface molecules in T cell activation. Functionally relevant cell surface molecules have been defined by the ability of specific MAb to block T cell function.[19] Recently, the human T cell molecules have been classified so that all MAb that appear to define a single marker have been grouped into distinct subsets called clusters of differentiation (CD).[20] We will use this nomenclature for this review and will designate the murine equivalent by mCD when a distinction between them is required. These molecules include the mouse and human markers in the CD2, CD3, CD4, and CD8 T cell antigen groups as well as the lymphocyte functional antigens: LFA-1 and LFA-3. Other T cell molecules have also been shown to be involved in T cell function but will not be addressed here.

Interaction of a MAb with a T cell surface molecule may affect the T cell in many ways. The basic premise for their functional role involves the observation that MAb to these surface molecules block various T cell functions. The ability of MAb specific for the TcR to block T cell activation can be obviously understood. The interaction of a T cell with antigen leading to T cell activation is a demonstration of the inherent specificity of immune responses. However, the ability of MAb directed toward nonclonally distributed T cell surface molecules suggests a requirement for that surface molecule in the pathway of T cell activation. It is important to note that many MAb which bind T cells do not affect T cell function. This implies that the MAb which do block T cell function are defining antigens which may in some way be relevant to T cell function or associated with molecules which are relevant.

There are many steps involved in the T cell interaction with a stimulator or target cell which bears the appropriate antigen. Therefore, the ability of a MAb to block effector T cell function may reflect the disruption of activation at different stages of T cell activation. The inability to demonstrate direct antigen binding to the antigen specific TcR has been

**Table 1**
**CELL SURFACE MOLECULES ASSOCIATED WITH T CELL FUNCTION**

| Molecule | Cell distribution | Effect of MAb binding | Proposed function |
|---|---|---|---|
| Ti/CD3 complex | T cells | Stimulates and/or blocks effector function | Antigen receptor and activation signal |
| CD4/CD8 | Generally, mutually exclusive expression by T cells | Blocks effector function | Accessory molecule interacts with nonpolymorphic MHC |
| CD2 | T cells | Stimulates and/or blocks effector function | Accessory molecule, may bypass Ti activation by antigen |
| LFA-1 | Lymphoid cells | Blocks effector function | Adhesion molecule |
| MHC molecules | All nucleated cells | Blocks function at the target cell level | Sites for MHC restriction of Ti and accessory molecule interaction; ligand for CD2 |
| LFA-3 | All human cells (no murine equivalent has been defined) | Blocks function at the target cell level | Involved in T cell/target interaction; ligand for CD2 |

proposed to reflect a low affinity of the TcR for antigen. Since a direct binding assay has not been developed, "affinity" of the TcR interaction with antigen can not be assessed. Affinity has been indirectly assessed by relative sensitivity to blocking with some MAb and by the concentration of antigen needed to trigger T cell activation. For the purpose of discussion, we will use instead the term "functional avidity" to define the strength of interaction of a T cell with its stimulator or target cell.

T cell activation has been demonstrated to be an ordered event. Following the T cell interaction with the appropriate antigen and MHC determinants, the T cell is induced to produce receptors for various growth factors,[21-24] such as IL-2. The T cell can then respond to the growth and differentiation factors made by itself or by other responding T cells. These signals result in the proliferation and differentiation to effector T cells; helper, cytotoxic or suppressor T cells.

The avidity of a T cell for its appropriate antigen bearing cell must be high enough to trigger T cell activation. The ability of MAb to T cell surface molecules to inhibit T cell activation may reflect a decrease in avidity between the T cell and its antigen-bearing cells due to blocking of a receptor ligand interaction. This implies the presence of a ligand on the antigen-bearing cell which interacts with the T cell surface molecules and contributes to the avidity of the cell-cell interaction. There are several other possible mechanisms by which MAb binding to the T cell surface might effect T cell activation. These include: steric inhibition of a physically associated T cell surface molecule, or the delivering of an "off signal" to the cell by MAb binding to a cell surface antigen. We plan to address the role of several T cell surface molecules in T cell activation and to discuss the mechanism(s) whereby MAb might inhibit T cell activation. Table 1 summarizes the cell surface molecules to be discussed.

## II. CD4/CD8

Initially, the aim of many investigators was to define T cell surface molecules which separate the functional subsets of T cells. The T cell molecules that were thought, until recently, to best fulfill these criteria were the CD4 and CD8 molecules.[25-47] CD4 (most commonly defined by the MAb OKT4 and Leu3) and mCD4 (the murine L3T4 molecule, described by MAb, GK1.5) have been shown to be glycoproteins of 55,000 to 62,000 Dalton. CD8 (most commonly defined by MAb OKT8 and Leu2) and mCD8 (the murine Lyt2 molecule) have been demonstrated to be disulfide-linked homodimers, composed of a complex of 30,000 to 32,000 Dalton glycoproteins for CD8 and 30,000 to 34,000 Dalton glycoproteins for mCD8. The protein and nucleotide sequences of these molecules place them in the family of immunoglobulin-like molecules, implying that these molecules may have a receptor-like function.[48-51]

This group of molecules have been used to separate functional groups of T cells and T cells at various stages of differentiation.[25,32,33,34,37-40] Pre-thymic T cells do not express these molecules. Following entry into the thymic environment pre-T cells co-express CD4 and CD8. It appears that early in thymic development T cells segregate for expression of either CD4 or CD8. Mature functional T cells exclusively express one or the other of these molecules.

The original descriptions of MAb which defined these groups in both human and mouse concluded that these molecules separated T cells into functional subpopulations. It was concluded that CD4 expressing T cells served as helper T cells for both antibody and cytolytic responses, while CD8 expressing T cells functioned as cytotoxic/suppressor T cells. This hypothesis was first challenged by Swain and collaborators when they examined the phenotype of mouse alloantigen specific help.[41] They found that helper cells specific for class I MHC antigens expressed mCD8 ($Lyt2^+$) antigens and that helper cells specific for class I MHC antigens were $mCD8^-$ and $Lyt1^+$. These data led to the hypothesis that these molecules were related in some way to the ability of the TcR to recognize class I vs. class II MHC antigens. Our laboratory isolated a novel population of $CD4^+$ cytotoxic T lymphocytes (CTL) that were shown to be specific for DR6, and the function of these CTLs was blocked by the addition of anti-CD4 MAb.[26] We presented the hypothesis that CD4 might serve a receptor-like function and interact directly with the DR molecule. Subsequently, several other laboratories have shown that most $CD4^+$ CTL are specific for class II MHC antigens while most $CD8^+$ CTL are specific for class I MHC antigens.[27-32,35,36,41-46] However, exceptions to the CD4/class II, CD8/class I rule have been described.[52-55] It should remain clear throughout this discussion that the proposed ability of CD4/CD8 molecules to interact with MHC molecules via a receptor-like interaction is not responsible for the specificity of the TcR, i.e., the MHC specificity of the TcR is independent of the MHC specificity of the CD4/CD8 molecules. The nonpolymorphic nature of the CD4/CD8 molecules suggests that the CD4/CD8 molecules would interact with a relatively nonpolymorphic determinant of the class II or class I molecules. This is in contrast to the TcR, which recognizes or is restricted by polymorphic MHC determinants. The general correlation of the CD4/CD8 phenotype with MHC restriction of the TcR is not a result of physical association between CD4/CD8 and the TcR, and perhaps results from developmental selection.

Initially, it was difficult to test the hypothesis that CD4 and CD8 directly interacted with class I or class II molecules, because most class II restricted T cells were $CD4^+$ and most class I restricted T cells were $CD8^+$; thus, both the TcR and the CD4/CD8 receptor interacted with epitopes on the same MHC molecule. A mouse cytotoxic and IL-2 producing T cell hybridoma which is specific for $H-2D^d$, a class I MHC molecule and is $mCD4^+$, allowed us to test the hypothesis that CD4/CD8 were receptors whose ligands were MHC encoded determinants.[56] This hybridoma allowed the investigation of the role of mCD4 in the absence of a class II restricted TcR.[57] The cytolytic activity of the hybridoma and its ability to produce IL-2 was stimulated by both $Ia^+$ and $Ia^-$, $H-2D^d$ target or stimulator cells. The stimulation or lysis of both $Ia^+$ and $Ia^-$ cells was blocked by anti-$H-2D^d$ and anti-TcR MAb. These results, along with the ability to stimulate this hybridoma with mouse L cells transfected with the $H-2D^d$ gene demonstrated the specificity of its TcR to be for the $H-2D^d$ gene product. Anti-L3T4 (mCD4) and anti-Ia MAb only blocked stimulation by or lysis of the $Ia^+$ antigen bearing cell. These data suggest that the ligand for the TcR is on the class I molecule, while the ligand for the mCD4 is on Ia. We also used this hybridoma to show that the proposed mCD4/Ia interaction involved a nonpolymorphic Ia determinant; as demonstrated by the ability of spleen cells from various congeneic mouse strains that expressed H-2D$^d$ but varied Ia haplotypes to stimulate this hybridoma. We also demonstrated that L3T4 could interact with either Ia haplotype on an F$_1$ stimulator.

Golding et al. have recently suggested that the ligand for mCD4 may reside in the β$_1$ domain of Ia.[58] Using class II specific, mCD4$^+$ CTL, they have shown that a transfected target cell which expresses a hybrid MHC molecule with the class I β$_1$ domain linked to a class I molecule can be recognized and blocked by the addition of anti-mCD4 MAb. Though β$_1$ is the polymorphic domain of Ia, it is possible that the Ia determinant which interacts with mCD4 is nonpolymorphic. Data from many other laboratories have reported the hypothesis of a receptor-ligand interaction involving CD4/DR, mCD4/Ia, CD8/HLA, and mCD8/H-2K/D interactions.[59-63] In fact, it has been suggested that mCD4 and mCD8 can interact with the appropriate human MHC antigens during a xenogeneic T cell response.[32]

Though it appeared that the CD4/CD8 group of T cell molecules could interact with MHC antigens, it remained unclear why these T cell molecules seemed to be involved in T cell activation under some conditions of activation but were not always required. A spontaneous variant of the hybridoma we have discussed, which lacked expression of mCD4, was shown to retain activity, but was not inhibited by the addition of either anti-mCD4 or anti-Ia MAb even if the target cell expressed Ia.[57] This adds to the evidence suggesting that mCD4 interacts with Ia but also suggests that the mCD4/Ia interaction was not absolutely required for T cell function but plays an accessory role in cell interactions. This L3T4$^-$ variant appeared to compensate for its lack of L3T4 by an increase in the number of TcR expressed on its surface. These results suggest that, when required, the L3T4/Ia interaction adds to the avidity required for T cell activation. The first experiments to directly address the accessory function of the L3T4/Ia interaction involved studying a panel of T cell hybridomas specific for antigen and class II MHC.[47] Although all the hybridomas expressed mCD4, the sensitivity to blocking by anti-mCD4 correlated with the sensitivity of the responses to anti-Ia MAb and inversely correlated with the dose of antigen required to stimulate the hybrids. Similarly, it has been shown that mCD8$^+$ T cell clones could not be blocked by anti-mCD8 when the clone was lysing a target that expressed the antigen which the clone was immunized against, yet was sensitive to anti-mCD8 when the clone was lysing a target which expressed a cross-reacting antigen, suggesting a relationship to avidity of the TcR.[42] These experiments suggested that the CD4/Ia and CD8/H-2K/D interactions were needed during suboptimal stimulation; i.e., when the avidity of the TcR/antigen interaction was insufficient to trigger T cell activation.[61,62]

To test this hypothesis we studied the requirement for a mCD4/Ia interaction in activation of the H-2D$^d$ specific, mCD4$^+$ T cell hybridoma discussed above.[64] Initially, we selected stimulator and target cells that expressed high amounts of H-2D$^d$ and were either Ia$^-$ (P815) or Ia$^+$ (A20). The Ia$^-$ cells were demonstrated to express at least five-times more H-2D$^d$, compared to the Ia$^+$ cells. Both P815 and A20 could stimulate the T cell hybridoma, suggesting than an mCD4/Ia interaction was required for activation under conditions of limiting amounts of antigen. This was directly tested by stimulation of the T cell hybridoma with L cells that had been transfected with the gene for H-2D$^d$ ± the genes for I-A$^k$. These cell lines expressed high and equal levels of H-2D$^d$. Stimulation of the mCD4$^+$ T cell hybridoma with these cell lines did not require a CD4/Ia interaction (i.e., was not blocked by either anti-mCD4 or anti-Ia MAb) unless a suboptimal number of stimulator cells were added to the culture, or the density of available H-2D$^d$ on the stimulator cell was decreased by the addition of a subsaturating concentration of anti-H-2D$^d$ MAb. Therefore, the accessory role of CD4 appears to increase the avidity, such that the threshold for T cell activation is reached. Similar conclusions have been made by examining the avidity of interaction of CD4$^+$ CTL with target cells by cold target inhibition of conjugate formation and the relative sensitivity of those clones to blocking by anti-CD4 MAb.[61] There appears to be a direct correlation of the ability to block a clone with anti-CD4 and the relatively lower number of cold target cells that are required to inhibit conjugate formation. Evidence for a mCD8/class I interaction which serves a similar function for T cell activation has been proposed.[62] These experiments have shown that anti-mCD8 MAb block activation of CTL on cross-reacting or lower avidity antigen interactions, but not when CTL interact with target cells bearing the immunizing antigen.

Recently, data from several laboratories have suggested that MAb to CD4 might deliver an "off signal" to the T cell rather than block a CD4/class II interaction.[63,65-67] Several approaches have resulted in the ability of anti-CD4 MAb to block T cell activation of CD4$^+$ T cells in the apparent absence of an Ia ligand. The ability to stimulate T cells with the lectin, Concanavalin A (Con A) has been shown to be sensitive to blocking by anti-mCD4 at both a functional level and by the ability to decrease the Con A stimulated flux of Ca$^{++}$. This was interpreted as the ability of anti-CD4 to deliver a negative or off signal to the responding cell[63]. However, these results may also reflect the ability of Con A to interact directly with mCD4 (Greenstein and Sitkovsky, preliminary data) and replace Ia as the ligand for mCD4. Similar experiments have demonstrated the ability of mCD8 to be involved in lectin mediated activation.[68] Recent data have also suggested that some anti-CD4 MAb can deliver a negative signal in the absence of lectins.[67] Anti-CD3 stimulation of peripheral T cells was shown to be blocked by some anti-CD4 MAb (OKT4c) in the apparent absence of Ia$^+$ cells. We have similar data which shows that the same T cell hybridoma for which a mCD4/Ia interaction can function as an accessory interaction for activation, can be affected by a negative signal via an anti-mCD4/mCD4 interaction, depending on the type of activation signal (unpublished data).

We have shown that stimulation of IL-2 production of this hybridoma by MAb specific for the TcR idiotype of this hybridoma can be blocked by anti-mCD4 MAb. We propose that the mCD4/Ia interaction can augment T cell activation when the avidity between the TcR and its antigen is lower than the threshold for activation. Ia provides the physiological ligand for mCD4, which may be replaced by Con A. Anti-CD4 may inhibit binding of CD4 to its ligand, but may also transmit a negative signal for T cell activation. Delivery of one signal or the other may be associated with the kinetics of cross-linking the TcR/CD3 complex relative to the interaction of CD4 with a ligand.

## III. CD2

CD2 is the earliest known T cell specific cell surface molecule expressed on human T lymphocytes.[33,70] The CD2 molecule is occasionally expressed in the bone marrow of children, but it is found on all thymocytes. The molecule is also expressed on peripheral blood T cells. Although the CD2 molecule is expressed throughout T cell development, initial biochemical characterization of the molecule suggests that it can exist at a variety of molecular weights.[72-74] Gel electrophoresis has generally shown a diffuse band at approximately 49,000 Daltons, but the apparent molecular weight can vary between cell lines. Whether this structural heterogeneity is due to amino acid sequence or glycosylation differences is unknown. An homologous structure on mouse T cell has not been identified. A putative ligand for CD2 has been described as a 42,000 Dalton glycoprotein, which is present on sheep erythrocytes and human white blood cells.[75] Work from our laboratory has suggested conservation of this ligand structure on monkey cells, but not mouse cells.[76]

The initial functional characterization of the CD2 molecule was the unlikely finding that the molecule mediated human T cell binding to sheep erythocytes.[70] Although this observation suggests a receptor function for CD2, the functional relevance of a sheep erythrocyte receptor on human T cells is obscure. An indication that the CD2 molecule was involved in normal T cell function was the finding that anti-CD2 MAb were able to inhibit virtually all T cell functions.[71-74,77] The CD2 epitope defined by the anti-LFA-2 MAb was identified by screening MAb hybridomas for the inhibition of CTL-mediated cytolysis. In addition to inhibiting cytolysis, the anti-LFA-2 MAb was found to inhibit both allostimulated and lectin-dependent T cell proliferation.[71,73] The anti-LFA-2 MAb appears to inhibit T cell function at several levels. Anti-LFA-2 MAb has been shown to inhibit CTL-target cell adhesion as well as PHA-induced $Ca^{++}$ mobilization.[78,79] These findings suggest an important role for the CD2 molecule in T cell activation.

Further evidence for the involvement of the CD2 molecule in T cell activation has been provided by MAb which recognize other functional epitopes on the CD2 molecule. Meuer et al. have shown that a combination of MAb ($T11_2$ and $T11_3$) can trigger T cell mitogenesis and IL-2 secretion.[80] These MAb do not inhibit T cell mitogenesis or cytotoxicity, suggesting that these epitopes are functionally distinct from the epitope recognized by the anti-LFA-2 MAb. T cell activation by the $T11_2$ and $T11_3$ MAb appears to depend on co-expression of the TCR-T3 complex. This finding suggests an important and as yet undefined functional relationship between the CD2 molecule and the TCR-T3 complex. Although these MAb have contributed to our understanding of CD2 function, further work will be required to clarify the relevance of these MAb epitopes to normal T cell activation.

## IV. LFA-1

Monoclonal antibodies have also identified functional T cell surface molecules that do not appear to be directly involved in the transduction of an activation signal. The molecule termed LFA-1 was initially identified by screening hybridoma supernatants for the ability to inhibit CTL-mediated cytotoxicity in the absence of complement. In both the human and mouse systems, MAb to the LFA-1 membrane molecule inhibited CTL-mediated cytotoxicity.[71,73,81-86] In addition to CTL-mediated cytotoxicity, anti-LFA-1 MAb has been shown to inhibit both NK-mediated killing and T cell proliferation.[73,86] The ability of anti-LFA-1 MAb to inhibit a variety of T cell functions, irrespective of antigen specificity, has led to the suggestion that LFA-1 regulates T cell adhesion.

LFA-1 is a membrane glycoprotein consisting of a noncovalently associated 177 kDalton heavy chain and a 95 kDalton light chain. In addition to its surface expression on all T cells, LFA-1 is expressed on B cells, monocytes, granulocytes, most thymocytes, and a third of bone marrow cells.[73] LFA-1 is a member of a family of at least three structurally related membrane molecules.[87-89] The three molecules have different heavy chains that are associated with a common 95 kDalton light chain. Mol, a MAb to one of the other members of this family, inhibits C3bi-dependent phagocytosis by neutrophils and monocytes.[90] Because of this finding, the molecule is termed complement receptor type 3 (CR3). The third known member of this structural family, p150,95, has also been implicated in the specific binding of the C3bi molecule.[91] Neither CR3 or p150,95 are expressed on T cells; both appear to be primarily expressed on monocytes and granulocytes.

The involvement of LFA-1 in T cell adhesion has been investigated using MAb. We have screened a variety of MAb to T cell surface molecules for their ability to inhibit T cell adhesion. MAb to most cell surface molecules, even those present at high cell surface density, do not affect cell-cell adhesion. Anti-LFA-1 MAb have been shown to inhibit CTL adhesion to target cells[92] and T cell adhesion to endothelial cells.[93] The adhesions are inhibited regardless of T cell subset or antigen specificity.

The broad distribution of LFA-1 has permitted the study of LFA-1 in a variety of cell-cell adhesion reactions. Using a B lymphoblast cell line, we have shown that B cell-B cell adhesions were markedly inhibited by anti-LFA-1 MAb[94] After exposure to gamma-interferon, monocytes also form homotypic adhesions. We have been able to show that gamma-interferon induced adhesions correlated with an induction of LFA-1 surface expression. The direct involvement of LFA-1 in monocyte-monocyte adhesion was again suggested by MAb inhibition. Two different anti-LFA-1 MAb were able to completely inhibit homotypic adhesion.[95]

The ability of anti-LFA-1 MAb to inhibit cell-cell adhesion in several different systems is good evidence that the LFA-1 molecule directly participates in T cell adhesion reactions. It remains equally possible, however, that the LFA-1 molecule is only indirectly involved in cell-cell adhesion. Anti-LFA-1 MAb may inhibit adhesion by other mechanisms. For example, anti-LFA-1 MAb may hinder a physically associated molecule responsible for T cell adhesion. Alternatively, anti-LFA-1 MAb may have disruptive membrane effects or trigger an intracellular "off signal." These effects are illustrated by MAb binding to the epidermal growth factor (EGF) receptor. Anti-EGF receptor MAb can trigger a change in the membrane morphology and a decrease in cell-substratum adhesion.[96]

Because of these uncertainties, alternative experimental approaches have been used to investigate the function of LFA-1. One approach has been to develop a panel of MAb which recognize functionally distinct epitopes on the LFA-1 membrane molecule. We have developed a panel of MAb to both the heavy and light chains of LFA-1. Based on cross-blocking studies, these MAb recognize five functionally distinct epitopes on the LFA-1 molecule.[97] Detailed comparison of CTL- and natural killer-mediated cytolysis has suggested identical utilization of functional epitopes on the LFA-1 molecule.[98] Similarly, studies of LFA-1 mediated adhesion of human monocytes has suggested that the panel of LFA-1 MAb blocks adhesion in a hierarchy identical to that observed in cell-mediated cytotoxicity.[95] Thus, using a panel of MAb to both the heavy and light chain of LFA-1, we have demonstrated identical utilization of five functional epitopes to LFA-1.

A complementary approach to MAb inhibition is the study of a T cell population genetically deficient in the molecule of interest. For example, in the mouse we have used spontaneous loss variants of T cell hybridomas to investigate the function of cell surface molecules such as mCD4[57]. The rarity of spontaneous mutants in human T cell clones has hindered the isolation of human genetic variants. Given the difficulties of in vitro isolation of mutant human T cells, an important finding was a naturally occurring genetic deficiency of LFA-1. Several kindred with a genetic deficiency of LFA-1 cll surface expression have been described.[99-110] The clinical syndrome is characterized by recurrent life-threatening bacterial infections, severe periodontal disease and poor wound healing.[102]

Serologic and biochemical evaluation of these patients indicate that their T cells exhibit less than 5% of the normal amount of LFA-1. Functional analysis demonstrates several T cell abnormalities. Peripheral blood mononuclear cells from LFA-1 deficient patients demonstrate abnormal proliferation to both alloantigen and lectin stimulation.[110] CTL clones deficient in LFA-1, but expressing normal levels of other serologically detectable cell surface molecules, also have significantly diminished cytolytic activity.[111]

The decreased cytolytic capacity of LFA-1 deficient CTL clones is consistent with earlier work using MAb inhibition. MAb pretreatment experiments show marked inhibition when the CTL was pretreated with anti-LFA-1 MAb, but little or no inhibition with MAb pretreatment of the target cell.[73] A role for LFA-1 on the CTL was confirmed in studies using target cells that did not express LFA-1. CTL-mediated cytolysis of fibroblasts and endothelial cells was significantly inhibited with anti-LFA-1 MAb, despite the absence of LFA-1 on the target cell surface.[112]

Given the importance of LFA-1 expressed on the CTL, an interesting finding was the ability of LFA-1 deficient CTL clones to effectively lyse a variety of lymphoid target cells. Although the lytic activity of the LFA-1 deficient CTL clones was significantly decreased, the level of cytolysis was consistently 50% of control CTL clones. The ability of the LFA-1 deficient CTL clones to partially compensate for their deficiency may reflect several potential mechanisms. The most important mechanism is clonal expansion. Polyclonal populations of LFA-1 deficient CTL have demonstrated significant improvement in cytolytic activity with repetitive antigen stimulation in vitro. The basis for the improvement in cytolytic activity is unknown. One possibility is that the clonal expansion of antigen reactive T cells selects for CTL with an increase in the number and/or avidity of functional cell surface molecules. Although no significant differences in the number of known cell surface molecules has yet been demonstrated, this possiblity cannot be excluded. Another possiblity is that LFA-1 deficient CTL compensate by utilizing LFA-1 expressed on lymphoid target cells. This compensation mechanism has been demonstrated using MAb pretreatment experiments; that is, in contrast to normal CTL, LFA-1 deficient CTL can be inhibited by anti-LFA-1 MAb pretreatment of the target cell.[110] Confirmatory experiments have been done with lymphoid target cells from patients genetically deficient in LFA-1. When both the CTL and the target cell were deficient in LFA-1, the level of cytolysis was less than 10% of normal CTL clones.[111] These results demonstrate one mechanism by which human T cells may compensate for a significant genetic deficiency. In addition, these findings suggest an essential role of LFA-1 in lymphoid cell-cell interactions.

## V. LFA-3

LFA-3 is a membrane molecule that was also identified by screening for MAb that inhibit CTL-mediated cytolysis.[71] LFA-3 is a 60kDalton membrane glycoprotein that is expressed on virtually all human cells.[73] The molecular weight of the LFA-3 molecule varies in different tissues. The reason for this heterogeneity is unknown. The tissue polymorphism may reflect differences in tissue glycosylation, but possible structural differences in the protein have not been excluded.

The surface expressions of LFA-3 on virtually all human cells initially implied that the LFA-3 might participate in the CTL-target cell interactions at the level of either the CTL or the target cell. However, MAb pretreatment of the effector and target cells have demonstrated the involvement of LFA-3 at the level of the target cell.[73] This novel observation makes LFA-3 the only non MHC encoded cell surface molecule implicated in CTL function at the level of the target cell. The broad tissue distribution of LFA-3 and the ability of anti-LFA-3 to inhibit T cells at the level of the target cell required evidence that the molecule was not a product of the major histocompatibility complex (MHC). To address this possibility, we used somatic cell hybrids to localize the chromosome encoding LFA-3. Mouse cells were found to be serologically negative for LFA-3 and were therefore used as recipient cells for the transfer of whole genomic human DNA. After DNA transfer, the "hybrid" mouse cells were positively and negatively sorted for the surface expression of the LFA-3 molecule. This approach permitted the mapping of the LFA-3 gene to chromosome 1 and provided definitive evidence that LFA-3 was not an MHC gene product.[113]

The functional role of LFA-3, with the availability of HLA-A2 CTL clones, was studied using HLA-A2+, LFA-3+ or HLA-A2+, LFA-3− somatic cell hybrids.[113] When human HLA-A2 specific CTL clones were used to lyse the hybrid cells expressing HLA-A2, the LFA-3+ and LFA-3− hybrids were lysed equally well. When anti-LFA-3 MAb was added, however, the MAb inhibited cytolysis of the target cell line coexpressing HLA-A2 and LFA-3 but did not affect lysis of LFA-3− target cells.[113] The finding that LFA-3 was only relevant to CTL function in the context of MAb inhibition was supported by experiments that used trypsin to cleave the LFA-3 molecule. Although anti-LFA-3 MAb no longer inhibited killing, the human target cell line JY was still effectively lysed by human CTL after trypsin cleavage of the LFA-3 molecule.[114]

The finding that LFA-3 is nonessential to CTL function, yet anti-LFA-3 MAb inhibits CTL function, suggests that the MAb may have effects that are only indirectly relevant to immunologic recognition. For example, anti-LFA-3 MAb may effect changes in membrane

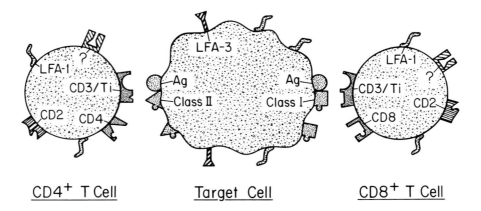

**CD4⁺ T Cell**          **Target Cell**          **CD8⁺ T Cell**

FIGURE 1.   A proposed interaction model for T cell activation. This diagram depicts the interaction molecules and their ligands as proposed in this review. The CD3/Ti complex interacts with antigen (Ag) in the context of self-MHC molecules as a restriction element. The CD8/CD4 molecules are proposed to interact with a nonpolymorphic determinant of self-MHC class I or class II molecules, respectively. CD2 may interact with an undefined ligand on the target cell and may be directly linked to T cell activation. LFA-1 may have an undefined ligand and can act at the level of the effector or target call. In contrast, LFA-3 may have an undefined ligand (pictured), yet acts only at the level of the target cell.

fluidity, thereby disrupting the CTL-target cell conjugate. Alternatively, anti-LFA-3 MAb may influence the mobility of target cell surface molecules. Changes in the mobility of cell surface molecules may be particularly relevant to T cell recognition of membrane-bound antigens. The membrane effects of MAb that inhibit T cell function is currently an active area of investigation in our laboratory.

## VI. CONCLUSIONS

It is evident that T cell activation is a complicated pathway which involves the cooperative interaction of many cell surface molecules. (Figure 1) It appears that the cooperative involvement of several T cell surface molecules is required for the generation of effector T cell function. It seems clear that the key to T cell specificity is the TcR/CD3 complex. This complex defines the antigen and MHC restriction specificity for T cell activation and has been postulated to form an ion channel for the transport of $Ca^{++}$, which may be directly involved in T cell activation. Therefore, the TcR/T3 complex serves to define the T cell specificity and provide an activation signal. Why then do other T cell surface molecules appear to be associated with T cell activation?

A large body of data suggests that T cells do not bind free antigen. This may reflect a low affinity of the TcR for antigen. It is probable that the requirement for a T cell to interact with an antigen bearing cell as a stimulator of T cell function or as a target for T cell effector function may reflect a requirement for multivalent binding, but suggests a dependence on molecules other than the TcR/CD3 complex.

The ability of MAb to CD4, CD8, CD2, LFA-1 and LFA-3 to block T cell activation and function imply a role for these molecules in a pathway of T cell activation. The characteristics of the blocking by MAb to these surface markers suggest that they act at distinct levels of T cell activation and that the same molecule can have differential effects depending on the kinetics of the activation versus blocking signals. Data from many experiments have suggested that the CD4/CD8 molecules may be involved in the generation of either a positive or negative signal that influences T cell activation. These molecules appear to have the capacity to interact with nonpolymorphic determinants of class II or Class

I MHC molecules, respectively. It appears that this interaction can promote T cell activation when the antigenic signal to the TCR is suboptimal. In contrast, CD4 (and perhaps CD8, although it has not been directly assessed) may also transduce a negative signal inhibiting T cell activation. This may reflect the kinetics of interaction of the antigenic signal with the TcR relative to MAb binding to CD4. These experiments demonstrate the range of effects that MAb can demonstrate and underscore the importance of careful interpretation of MAb blocking studies. A similar finding for positive and negative influences by a single MAb can be seen from the experiments to determine the role of CD2 in T cell activation. Therefore the CD4, CD8, and CD2 molecules may fit into a group of activation-related accessory molecules whose role is dependent on the expression of the TcR/CD3 complex. They may serve to focus the T cell toward the proper antigen bearing cell and to increase the general avidity of interaction between these cells, with a selective capacity for the relevant cell type.

In contrast, other cell surface molecules such as LFA-1 and LFA-3, with a wider tissue distribution appear to promote general cell-cell adhesions and may serve to cause the T cell to interact with any cell, without an obvious selectivity. These molecules appear to be relevant to T cell activation unrelated to the functional avidity of the T cell and have not been demonstrated to be directly involved in the activation process.

It remains evident that our knowledge of T cell activation is in no way complete. The approach of understanding the role of T cell accessory molecules by manipulating T cell activation with MAb has provided insight into the activation process. It is our expectation that further experimentation with this approach will continue to enlighten our understanding of T cell activation.

## NOTE ADDED IN PROOF

Many groups have presented evidence for LFA-3 to act as a ligand for CD2.

## REFERENCES

1. **Moller, G., Ed.,** T cell receptors and genes, *Immunol. Rev.,* Vol. 81, 1984.
2. **Hedrick, S. M., Nielsen, E. A., Kavaler, J., Cohen, D. I., and Davis, M. M.,** Sequence relationships between punative T cell receptor polypeptides and immunoglobulins, *Nature,* 308, 153, 1984.
3. **Yanagi, Y., Yoshikai, Y., Legget, K., Clark, S. P., Aleksandra, I., and Mak, T.,** A human T cell specific cDNA clone encodes a protein having extensive homology to immunolgobulin chains, *Nature,* 308, 415, 1984.
4. **Chien, Y., Becker, D., Lindsten, T., Okamura, M., Cohen, D., and Davis, M.,** A third type of murine T-cell receptor gene, *Nature,* 312, 31, 1984.
5. **Saito, H., Kranz, D., Takagaki, Y., Hayday, A., Eisen, H., and Tonegawa, S.,** A third rearranged and expressed gene in a clone of cytotoxic T lymphocytes, *Nature,* 312, 36, 1984.
6. **Sim, G., Yague, J., Nelson, J., Marrack, P., Palmer, E., Augustin, A., and Kappler, J.,** Primary sequence of human T-cell receptor α-chain, *Nature,* 312, 771, 1984.
7. **Brenner, M. B., Trowbridge, I. S., and Strominger, J. L.,** Cross-linking of human T cell receptor proteins: Association between the T cell idiotype subunit and the T3 glycoprotein heavy subunit, *Cell,* 40, 183, 1985.
8. **Elsen, P. V. D., Shepley, B., Cho, M., and Terhorst, C.,** Isolation and characterization of a cDNA clone encoding the murine homologue of the human 20K T3/T-cell receptor glycoprotein, *Nature,* 314, 542, 1985.
9. **Reinherz, E. L., Meurer, S., Fitzgerald, K. A., Hussey, R. E., Levine, H., and Schlossman, S. F.,** Antigen recognition by human T lymphocytes is linked to surface expression of the T3 molecular complex, *Cell,* 30, 735, 1982.
10. **Weiss, A. and Stobo, J.,** Requirement for the co-expression of T3 and the T cell antigen receptor on a malignant human T cell line, *J. Exp. Med.,* 161, 1284, 1984.

11. **Van Wauwe, J., DeMey, J., and Goossens, J.,** OKT3: a monoclonal anti-human T lymphocyte antibody with potent mitogenic properties, *J. Immunol.,* 124, 2708, 1980.

12. **Reinherz, E. L., Hussey, R. E., and Schlossman, S. F.,** A monoclonal antibody blocking human T cell function, *Eur. J. Immunol.,* 10, 758, 1980.

13. **Kappler, J., Kubo, R., Haskins, K., White, J., and Marrack, P.,** The mouse T cell receptor: comparison of MHC-restricted receptors in two T cell hybridomas, *Cell,* 34, 727, 1983.

14. **Meuer, S. C., Acuto, O., Hussey, R. E., Hodgdon, J. C., Fitzgerald, K. A., Schlossman, S. F., and Reinherz, E. L.,** Antigen-like effects of monoclonal antibodies directed at receptors on human T cell clones, *J. Exp. Med.,* 158, 988, 1983.

15. **Kaye, J. and Janeway, C. A., Jr.,** The Fab fragment of a directly activating monoclonal antibody that precipitates a disulfide linked heterodimer from a helper T cell clone blocks activation by either allogeneic Ia or antigen and self-Ia, *J. Exp. Med.,* 159, 1397, 1984.

16. **Weiss, A., Imboden, J., Shoback, D., and Stobo, J.,** Role of T3 molecules in human T cell activation: T3 dependent activation results in an increase in cytoplasmic free calcium, *Proc. Natl. Acad. Sci. USA,* 81, 4169, 1984.

17. **Oettgen, H. C., Terhorst, C., Cantley, L. C., and Rosoff, P. M.,** Stimulation of the T3-T cell receptor complex induces a membrane-potential-sensitive calcium influx, *Cell,* 40, 583, 1985.

18. **Imboden, J. B. and Stobo, J. D.,** Transmembrane signalling by the T cell antigen receptor. Perturbation of the T3-antigen receptor complex generates inositol phosphates and releases calcium ions from intracellular stores, *J. Exp. Med.,* 161, 446, 1985.

19. **Martz, E., Heagy, W., and Gromkowski, S. H.,** The mechanism of CTL-mediated killing: monoclonal antibody analysis of the roles of killer and target-cell membrane proteins, *Immunol. Rev.,* 72, 73, 1983.

20. **IUIS-WHO Nomenclature Subcommittee,** Nomenclature for clusters of differentiation (CD) of antigens defined on human leukocyte populations, Bull. *WHO,* 62, 809, 1984.

21. **Andrew, M. E., Braciale, V. L., and Braciale, T. J.,** Regulation of interleukin 2 receptor expression on murine cytotoxic T lymphocyte clones, *J. Immunol.,* 132, 839, 1984.

22. **Hemler, M. E., Brenner, M. B., McLean, J. M., and Strominger, J. L.,** Antigen stimulation regulates the level of expression of interleukin 2 receptor on human T cells, *Proc. Natl. Acad. Sci. USA,* 81, 2172, 1984.

23. **Raulet, D. H. and Bevan, M. J.,** A differentiation factor required for the expression of cytotoxic T cell function, *Nature (London),* 296, 754, 1982.

24. **Erard, F., Corthesy, P., Smith, K. A., Fiers, W., Conzelmann, A., and Nabholz, M.,** Characterization of soluble factors that induce the cytolytic activity and the expression of T cell growth factor receptor of a T cell hybrid, *J. Exp. Med.,* 160, 584, 1984.

25. **Engleman, E. G., Benike, C. G., Glickman, E., and Evans, R. L.** Antibodies to membrane structures that distinguish suppressor/cytotoxic and helper T lymphocyte subpopulations block the mixed leucocyte reaction in man, *J. Exp. Med.,* 154, 193, 1981.

26. **Krensky, A. M., Reiss, C. S., Mier, J. W., Strominger, J. L., and Burakoff, S. J.,** Long-term human cytolytic T cell lines allospecific for HLA-DR6 antigen are OKT4[+], *Proc. Natl. Acad. Sci. USA,* 79, 2365, 1982.

27. **Spits, H., Borst, J., Terhorst, C., and deVries, J. E.,** The role of T cell differentiation markers in antigen-specific and lectin-dependent cellular cytotoxicity mediated by T8[+] and T4[+] human cytotoxic T cell clones directed at class I and class II MHC antigens, *J. Immunol.,* 129, 1563, 1982.

28. **Krensky, A. M., Clayberger, C., Reiss, C. S., Strominger, J. L., and Burakoff, S. J.,** Specificity of OKT4[+] cytotoxic T lymphocyte clones, *J. Immunol.,* 129, 2001, 1982.

29. **Meuer, S. C., Schlossman, S. F., and Reinherz, E. L.,** Clonal analysis of human cytotoxic T lymphocytes: T4[+] and T8[+] effector T cells recognize products of different major histocompatibility complex regions, *Proc. Natl. Acad. Sci. USA,* 79, 4395, 1982.

30. **Biddison, W. E., Rao, P. E., Talle, M. A., Goldstein, G., and Shaw, S.,** Possible involvement of the OKT4 molecule in T cell recognition of class II HLA antigens. Evidence from studies of cytotoxic T lymphocytes specific for SB antigens, *J. Exp. Med.,* 156, 1065, 1982.

31. **Meuer, S. C., Hussey, R. E., Hodgdon, J. C., Hercend, T., Schlossman, S. F., and Reinherz, E. L.,** Surface structures involved in target recognition by human cytotoxic T lymphocytes, *Science,* 218, 471, 1982.

32. **Swain, S. L., Dutton, R. W., Schwab, R., and Yamamoto, J.,** Xenogeneic human anti-mouse T cell responses are due to the activity of the same functional T cell subsets responsible for allospecific and major histocompatibility complex-restricted responses, *J. Exp. Med.,* 157, 720, 1983.

33. **Reinherz, E. L. and Schlossman, S. F.,** Differentiation and function of human T lymphocytes, *Cell,* 19, 821, 1980.

34. **Evans, R. L., Wall, D. W., Platsoucas, C. D., Siegal, F. P., Fikrig, S. H., Testa, C. M., and Good, R. A.,** Thymus-dependent membrane antigen in man: inhibition of cell-mediated lympholysis by monoclonal antibodies to the TH2 antigen, *Proc. Natl. Acad. Sci. USA,* 78, 544, 1981.

35. **Platsoucas, C. D.,** Human T cell antigens involved in cytotoxicity against allogeneic or autologous chemically modified targets. Association of the Leu 2a/T8 antigen with effector-target cell binding and the T3/Leu4 antigen with triggering, *Eur. J. Immunol.,* 14, 566, 1984.

36. **Spits, H., Yssel, H., Voordouw, A., and deVries, J. E.,** The role of T8 in the cytotoxic activity of cloned cytotoxic T lymphocyte lines specific for class II and class I major histocompatibility complex antigens, *J. Immunol.,* 134, 2294, 1985.

37. **Snow, P. M. and Terhorst, C.,** The T8 antigen is a multimeric complex of two distinct subunits on human thymocytes but consists of homomultimeric forms of peripheral blood T lymphocytes, *J. Biol. Chem.,* 258, 14675, 1983.

38. **Nakayama, E., Shiku, H., Stockett, E., Oettgen, H. F., and Old, L. J.,** Cytotoxic T cells: Lyt phenotype and blocking of killing activity by Lyt antisera, *Proc. Natl. Acad. Sci. USA,* 76, 1977, 1979.

39. **Hollander, N., Pillemer, E., and Weissman, I. L.,** Blocking effect of Lyt-2 antibodies on T cell functions, *J. Exp. Med.,* 152, 674, 1980.

40. **Shinohara, N., Hammerling, U., and Sachs, D.,** Mouse alloantibodies capable of blocking cytotoxic T cell function. II. Further study on the relationship beween the blocking antibodies and the products of the Lyt-2 locus, *Eur. J. Immunol.,* 10, 589, 1980.

41. **Swain, S. L.,** Significance of Lyt phenotypes: Lyt-2 antibodies block activities of T cells that recognize class I major histocompatibility complex antigens regardless of their function, *Proc. Natl. Acad. Sci. USA,* 78, 7101, 1981.

42. **MacDonald, H. R., Glasebrook, A. L., Bron, C., Kelso, A., and Cerrotini, J. C.,** Clonal heterogeneity in the functional requirement for Lyt-2/3 molecules on cytotoxic T lymphocytes (CTL): possible implications for the affinity of CTL antigen receptors, *Immunol. Rev.,* 68, 89, 1982.

43. **Dialynas, D. P., Wilde, D. B., Marrack, P., Pierres, A., Wall, K. A., Havran, W., Otten, G., Loken, M. R., Pierres, M., Kappler, J., and Fitch, F. W.,** Characterization of the murine antigenic determinant, designated L3T4a, recognized by monoclonal antibody GK1.5: expression of L3T4a by functional T cell clones appears to correlate primarily with class II MHC antigen-reactivity, *Immunol. Rev.,* 74, 29, 1983.

44. **Dialynas, D. P., Quan, Z. S., Wall, K. A., Pierres, A., Quintans, J., Loken, M. R., Pierres, M., Fitch, F. W.,** Characterization of the murine T cell surface molecule, designated L3T4, identified by monoclonal antibody GK1.5: similarity of L3T4 to the human Leu3/T4 molecule, *J. Immunol.,* 131, 2445, 1984.

45. **Wilde, D. B., Marrack, P., Kappler, J., Dialynas, D. P., and Fitch, F. W.,** Evidence implicating L3T4 in class II MHC antigen reactivity: monoclonal antibody GK1.5 (anti-L3T4a) blocks class II MHC antigen-specific proliferation, release of lymphokines, and binding by cloned murine helper T lymphocyte lines, *J. Immunol.,* 131, 2178, 1983.

46. **Swain, S. L., Dialynas, D., Fitch, F. W., and English, M.,** Monoclonal antibody to L3T4 blocks the function of T cells specific for class 2 major histocompatibility complex antigens, *J. Immunol.,* 132, 1118, 1984.

47. **Marrack, P., Endres, R., Shimonkevitz, R., Zlotnik, A., Dialynas, D., Fitch, F., and Kappler, J.,** The major histocompatibility complex-restricted antigen receptor on T cells. II. Role of the L3T4 product, *J. Exp. Med.,* 158, 1077, 1983.

48. **Littman, D. R., Thomas, Y., Maddon, P. J., Chess, L., and Axel, R.,** The isolation and sequence of the gene encoding T8: A molecule defining functional classes of T lymphocytes, *Cell,* 40, 237, 1985.

49. **Kavathas, P., Sukhatme, V. P., Herzenberg, L. A., and Parnes, J. R.,** Isolation of the gene coding for the human T lymphocyte differentiation antigen Leu2 (T8) by gene transfer and cDNA subtraction, *Proc. Natl. Acad. Sci. USA,* 81, 7688, 1984.

50. **Nakauchi, H., Nolan, G. P., Hsu, C., Huang, H. S., Kavathas, P., and Herzenberg, L. A.,** Molecular cloning of Lyt-2, a membrane glycoprotein marking a subset of mouse T lymphocytes: molecular homology to its human counterpart, Leu-2/T8, and to immunoglobulin variable regions, *Proc. Natl. Acad. Sci. USA,* 82, 5126, 1985.

51. **Maddon, P. J., Littman, D. R., Godfrey, M., Maddon, D. E., Chess, L., and Axel, R.,** The isolation and nucleotide sequence of a cDNA encoding the T cell surface protein T4: A new member of the immunoglobulin gene family, *Cell,* 42, 93, 1985.

52. **Krensky, A. M., Clayberger, C., Greenstein, J., Crimmins, M., Burakoff, S. J.,** A DC-specific cytolytic T lymphocyte is OKT8[+], *J. Immunol.,* 131, 2777, 1983.

53. **Spits, H. H., Yssl, H., Thompson, A., and DeVries, J. E.,** Human T4[+] and T8[+] cytotoxic T lymphocyte clones directed at products of different class II MHC loci, *J. Immunol.,* 131, 678, 1983.

54. **Flomenberg, N., Naito, K., Duffy, E., Knowles, R. W., Evans, R. L., and Dupont, B.,** Allocytotoxic T cell clones: both Leu2[+]3[−] and Leu2[−]3[+] T cells recognize class I histocompatibility antigens, *Eur. J. Immunol.,* 13, 905, 1983.

55. **Strassman, G. and Bach, F. H.,** OKT4[+] cytotoxic T cells can lyse targets via class I molecules and can be blocked by monoclonal antibody against T4 molecules, *J. Immunol.,* 133, 1705, 1984.

56. **Endres, R., Marrack, P., and Kappler, J. W.,** An IL-2 secreting T cell hybridoma that responds to a self class I histocompatibility antigen in the H-2D region, *J. Immunol.,* 131, 1656, 1983.

57. **Greenstein, J. L., Kappler, J., Marrack, P., and Burakoff, S. J.,** The role of L3T4 in recognition of Ia by a cytotoxic H-2D$^d$-specific T cell hybridoma, *J. Exp. Med.,* 159, 1213, 1984.

58. **Golding, H., McCluskey, J., Munitz, T. I., Germain, R. N., Margulies, D. H., and Singer, A.,** T-cell recognition of a chimeric class II/class I MHC molecule and the role of L3T4, *Nature,* 317, 425, 1985.

59. **Biddison, W. M., Rao, P. E., Talle, M. A., Goldstein, G., Shaw, S.,** Possible involvement of the T4 molecule in T cell recognition of class II HLA antigens: evidence from studies of CTL-target cell binding, *J. Exp. Med.,* 159, 783, 1984.

60. **Watts, T. H., Brian, A. B., Kappler, J. W., Marrack, P., and McConnell, H. M.,** Antigen presentation by supported planar membranes containing affinity purified I-A$^d$, *Proc. Natl. Acad. Sci. USA,* 81, 7564, 1984.

61. **Shaw, S., Goldstein, G., Springer, T. A., and Biddison, W. E.,** Susceptibility of cytotoxic T lymphocyte (CTL) clones to inhibition by anti-T3 and anti-T4 (but not anti-LFA-1) monoclonal antibodies varies with the "avidity" of the CTL-target interaction, *J. Immunol.,* 134, 3019, 1985.

62. **Shimonkevitz, R., Luescher, B., Cerottini, J. C., and MacDonald, H. R.,** Clonal analysis of cytolytic T lymphocyte-mediated lysis of target cells with inducible antigen expression: correlation between antigen density and requirement for Lyt-2/3 function, *J. Immunol.,* 135, 892, 1985.

63. **Tite, J. P., Sloan, A. and Janeway, C. A., Jr.,** The role of L3T4 in T cell activation: L3T4 may be both an Ia-binding protein and a receptor that transduces a negative signal, *J. Cell Mol. Immunol.,* 2, 179, 1986.

64. **Greenstein, J. L., Malissen, B. and Burakoff, S. J.,** Role of L3T4 in antigen-driven activation of a class I-specific T cell hybridoma, *J. Exp. Med.,* 162, 369, 1985.

65. **Bekoff, M., Kakiuchi, T., and Grey, H. M.,** Accessory cell function in the Con A response: Role of Ia-positive and Ia-negative accessory cells, *J. Immunol.,* 134, 1337, 1985.

66. **Wassmer, P., Chan, C., Logdberg, L., and Shevach, E. M.,** Role of the L3T4 antigen in T cell activation. II. Inhibition of T cell activation by monoclonal anti-L3T4 antibodies in the absence of accessory cells, *J. Immunol.,* 135, 2237, 1985.

67. **Bank, I. and Chess, L.,** Perturbation of the T4 molecule transmits a negative signal to T cells, *J. Exp. Med.,* 162, 1294, 1985.

68. **Hunig, T.,** Monoclonal anti-Lyt-2.2 antibody blocks lectin-dependent cellular cytotoxicity of H-2-negative target cells, *J. Exp. Med.,* 159, 551, 1984.

69. **Kamoun, M. P., Martin, P. J., Hasen, J. A., Brown, M. A., Siadek, A. W., and Nowinski, R. A.,** Identification of a human T lymphocyte surface protein associated with the E rosette receptor, *J. Exp. Med.,* 153, 207, 1981.

70. **Howard, F. D., Ledbetter, J. A., Wong, J., Bieber, C. P., Stinson, E. B., and Herzenberg, L. A.,** A human T lymphocyte differentiation marker defined by monoclonal antibodies that block E rosette formation, *J. Immunol.,* 126, 2117, 1981.

71. **Sanchez-Madrid, F., Krensky, A. M., Ware, C. F., Robbins, E., Strominger, J. L., Burakoff, S. J., and Springer, T. A.,** Three distinct antigens associated with human T lymphocyte-mediated cytolysis: LFA-1, LFA-2, and LFA-3, *Proc. Natl. Acad. Sci. USA,* 79, 7489, 1982.

72. **Palacios, R. and Martinez-Maza, J.,** Is the E receptor on human T lymphocytes a "negative signal receptor?" *J. Immunol.,* 129, 2479, 1982.

73. **Krensky, A. M., Sanchez-Madrid, F., Robbins, E., Nagy, J., Springer, T. A., and Burakoff, S. J.,** The functional significance distribution, and structure of LFA-1, LFA-2, and LFA-3: cell surface antigens involved with the CTL-target interaction, *J. Immunol.,* 131, 611, 1983.

74. **Martin, P. J., Longton, G., and Ledbetter, J. A., et al.,** Identification and functional characterization of two distinct epitopes on the human T cell surface protein Tp50, *J. Immunol.,* 131, 180 1983.

75. **Hunig, T.,** The cell surface molecule recognized by the erythrocyte receptor of T lymphocytes. Identification and partial characterization using a monoclonal antibody, *J. Exp. Med.,* 162, 890, 1985.

76. **Mentzer, S. J., Barbosa, J. A., Strominger, J. L., Biro, P. A., and Burakoff, S. J.,** Species-restricted recognition of transfected HLA-A2 and HLA-B7 by human CTL clones, *J. Immunol.,* 137, 408, 1986.

77. **Wilkinson, M. and Morris, A.,** The E receptor regulates interferon-gamma production: four-receptor model for human lymphocyte activation, *Eur. J. Immunol.,* 14, 708, 1984.

78. **Weiss, M. J., Daley, J. F., Hodgdon, J. C., and Reinherz, E. L.,** Calcium dependency of antigen-specific (T3-Ti) and alternative (T11) pathways of human T-cell activation, *Proc. Natl. Acad. Sci. USA,* 81, 6836, 1984.

79. **O'Flynn, K., Krensky, A. M., Beverly, P. C. L., Burakoff, S. J., and Linch, D. C.,** Phytohaemag-glutinin activation of T cells through the sheep red blood cell receptor, *Nature,* 313, 686, 1985.

80. **Meuer, S. C., Hussey, R. E., and Fabbi, M., et al.,** An alternative pathway of T cell activation: a functional role for the 50 kd T11 sheep erythrocyte receptor protein, *Cell,* 36, 897, 1984.

81. **Springer, T. A., Davignon, D., Ho, M. K., Kurzinger, K., Martz, E., and Sanchez-Madrid, F.,** LFA-1 and Lyt-2,3 molecules associated with T lymphocyte-mediated killing: and Mac-1, and LFA-1 homologue associated with complement receptor function, *Immunol. Rev.*, 68, 111, 1982.

82. **Davignon, D., Martz, E., Reynolds, T., Kurzinger, K., and Springer, T. A.,** Lymphocyte function-associated antigen 1 (LFA-1): a surface antigen distinct from Lyt-2,3 that participates in T lymphocyte-mediated killing, *Proc. Natl. Acad. Sci. USA*, 78, 4535, 1981.

83. **Kaufman, Y., Golstein, P., Pierres, M., Springer, T. A., and Eshhar, Z.,** LFA-1 but not Lyt-2 is associated with killing activity of cytotoxic T lymphocyte hybridomas, *Nature*, 300, 357, 1982.

84. **Pierres, M., Coridis, C., and Golstein, P.,** Inhibition of murine T cell-mediated cytolysis and T cell proliferations by a rat monoclonal antibody immunoprecipitating two lymphoid cell surface polypeptides of 94,000 and 180,000 molecular weights, *Eur. J. Immunol.*, 12, 60, 1982.

85. **Hildreth, J. E., Gotch, F. M., Hildreth, D. K., and McMichael, A. J.,** A human lymphocyte-associated antigen involved in cell-mediated lympholysis, *Eur. J. Immunol.*, 13, 202, 1983.

86. **Krensky, A. M., Mentzer, S. J., Greenstein, J. L., Crimmins, M., Clayberger, C., Springer, T. A., and Burakoff, S. J.,** Human cytolytic T lymphocyte clones and their function-associated cell surface molecules, in *Hybridoma Technology in the Biosciences and Medicine*, Springer, T. A., Ed., Plenum Press, New York, 1985.

87. **Kurzinger, K., Ho, M. K., and Springer, T. A.,** Structural homology of a macrophage differentiation antigen and an antigen involved in T lymphocyte mediated killing, *Nature*, 296, 688, 1982.

88. **Sanchez-Madrid, F., Simon, P., Thompson, S. and Springer, T. A.,** Mapping of antigenic and functional epitopes on the α and β subunits of two related mouse glycoproteins involved in cell interactions LFA-1 and Mac-1, *J. Exp. Med.*, 158, 586, 1983.

89. **Springer, T. A., Davignon, D., Ho, M. K., Kurzinger, K., Martz, E., and Sanchez-Madrid, F.,** LFA-1 and Lyt 2,3, molecules associated with T lymphocyte-mediated killing and Mac-1, an LFA-1 homologue associated with complement receptor function, *Immunol. Rev.*, 68, 111, 1982.

90. **Beller, D. L., Springer, T. A., and Schreiber, R. D.,** Anti-Mac-1 selectively inhibits the mouse and human type three complement receptor, *J. Exp. Med.*, 156, 1000, 1982.

91. **Micklem, K. J. and Sim, R. B.,** Isolation of complement fragment-iC3b-binding proteins by affinity chromatography, *Biochem J.*, 231, 233, 1985.

92. **Krensky, A. M., Robbins, E., Springer, T. A., and Burakoff, S. J.,** LFA-1, LFA-2, and LFA-3 are involved in CTL-target cell conjugation, *J. Immunol.*, 132, 2180, 1984.

93. **Mentzer, S. J., Burakoff, S. J., and Faller, D. V.,** T cell adhesion to endothelial cells is regulated by the LFA-1 membrane molecule, *J. Cell Physiol.*, 126, 285, 1986.

94. **Mentzer, S. J., Gromkowski, S. H., Krensky, A. M., Burakoff, S. J., and Martz, E.,** LFA-1 membrane molecule in the regulation of homotypic adhesion of human B lymphocytes, *J. Immunol.*, 135, 15, 1985.

95. **Mentzer, S. J., Faller, D. V., and Burakoff, S. J.,** Interferon-gamma induction of LFA-1 mediated homotypic adhesions of human monocytes, *J. Immunol.*, 137, 108, 1986.

96. **Schreiber, A. B., Lax, I., Yarden, Y., Eshhar, Z., and Schlessinger, J.,** Monoclonal antibodies against receptor for epidermal growth factor induce early and delayed effects of epidermal growth factor, *Proc. Natl. Acad. Sci. USA*, 78, 7535, 1981.

97. **Ware, C. F., Sanchez-Madrid, F., Krensky, A. M., Burakoff, S. J., Stronminger, J. L., and Springer, T. A.,** Human lymphocyte function associated antigen-1 (LFA-1): identification of multiple antigenic epitopes and their relationship to CTL-mediated cytoxicity, *J. Immunol.*, 131, 1182, 1983.

98. **Mentzer, S. J., Krensky, A. M., and Burakoff, S. J.,** Mapping functional epitopes of the human LFA-1 glycoprotein: Inhibition of CTL and NK-mediated cytolysis, *Human Immunol.*, 17, 288, 1986.

99. **Fischer, A., Seger, R., Durandy, A., Grospierre, B., Virelizier, J. L., LeDeist, F., Griscelli, C., Fischer, E., Kazatchkine, M., Bohler, M. C., Descamps-Latscha, B., Trung, P. H., Springer, T. A., Olive, D., and Mawas, C.,** Deficiency of the adhesive protein complex lymphocyte function associated antigen 1, complement receptor type 3, glycoprotein, p150,95 in a girl with recurrent bacterial infections. Effects on phagocyte cells and lymphocyte functions, *J. Clin. Invest.*, 76, 2385, 1985.

100. **Springer, T. A., Rothlein, R., Anderson, D. C., Burakoff, S. J., and Krensky, A. M.,** The function of LFA-1 in cell-mediated killing and adhesion: studies on heritable LFA-1, Mac-1 deficiency and on lymphoid cell self-aggregation, in *Mechanisms of Cell-Mediated Cytotoxicity*, Vol. 2, Plenum Press, New York, 1985.

101. **Miedema, F. P., Tetteroo, A. F., Terpstra, F. G., Keizer, G., Roos, M., Weening, R. S., Weemaes, M. R., Roos, D., and Melief, C. J. M.,** Immunologic studies with LFA-1 and Mol-deficient lymphocytes from a patient with recurrent bacterial infections, *J. Immunol.*, 134, 3075, 1985.

102. **Anderson, D. C., Schmalstieg, F. C., Finegold, M. J., Hughes, B. J., Rothlein, R., Miller, L. J., Kohl, S., Tosi, M. F., Jacobs, R. L., Goldman, A., Shearer, W. T., and Springer, T. A.,** The severe and moderate phenotypes of heritable Mac-1, LFA-1 deficiency: their quantitative definition and relation to leukocyte dysfunction and clinical features, *J. Inf. Dis.*, 152, 668, 1985.

103. **Springer, T. A., Thompson, W. S., Miller, L. J., Schmalstieg, F. C., and Anderson, D. C.,** Inherited deficiency of the Mac-1, LFA-1. p150.95 glycoprotein family and its molecular basis, *J. Exp. Med.,* 160, 1901, 1984.

104. **Anderson, D. C., Schmalstieg, F. C., Arnaout, M. A., Kohl, S., Tosi, M. F., Dana, N., Buffone, G. J., Hughes, B. J., Brinkley, B. R., Dickey, W. D., Abramson, J. S., Springer, T. A., Boxer, L. A., Hollers, J. M., and Smith, C. W.,** Abnormalities of polymorphonuclear leukocyte functions associated with a heritable deficiency of high molecular weight surface glycoproteins (GP138): common relationship to diminished cell adherence, *J. Clin. Invest.,* 74, 536, 1984.

105. **Dana, N., Todd, R. R., Pitt, J., Springer, T. A., and Arnaout, M. A.,** Deficiency of a surface membrane glycoprotein (Mol) in man, *J. Clin. Invest.,* 73, 153, 1984.

106. **Arnaout, M. A., Spits, H., Terhorst, C., Pitt, J., and Todd, R. F. I.,** Deficiency of a leukocyte surface glycoprotein (LFA-1) in two patients with Mol deficiency, *J. Clin. Invest.,* 74, 1291, 1984.

107. **Beatty, P. G., Harlan, J. M., Rosen, H., Hansen, J. A., Ochs, H. D., Price, T. D., Taylor, R. F., and Klebanoff, S. J.,** Absence of monoclonal-antibody-defined protein complex in boy with abnormal leucocyte function, *Lancet,* 1, 535, 984.

108. **Beatty, P. G., Ledbetter, J. A., Martin, P. J., Price, T. H., and Hansen, J. A.,** Definition of a common leukocyte cell-surface antigen (Gp95-150) associated with diverse cell-mediated immune functions, *J. Immunol.,* 131, 2913, 1983.

109. **Kohl, S., Springer, T. A., Schmalstieg, F. C., Loo, L. S., and Anderson, D. C.,** Defective natural killer cytotoxicity and polymorphonuclear leukocyte antibody-dependent cellular cytotoxicity in patients with LFA-1/OKM-1 deficiency, *J. Immunol.,* 133, 2972, 1984.

110. **Krensky, A. M., Mentzer, S. J., Claryberger, C., Schmalstieg, F. C., Anderson, D. C., Burakoff, S. J., and Springer, T. A.,** Heritable lymphocyte function-associated antigen-1 deficiency: Abnormalities of cytotoxicity and proliferation associated with abnormal expression of LFA-1, *J. Immunol.,* 135, 3102, 1985.

111. **Mentzer, S. J., Bierer, B., Anderson, D. C., Schmalstieg, F. C., Springer, T. A., and Burakoff, S. J.,** Abnormal cytolytic activity of LFA-1 deficient CTL clones, *J. Clin. Invest.,* 78, 1387, 1986.

112. **Collins, T., Krensky, A. M., Clayberger, C., Fiers, W., Gimbrone, M. A., Burakoff, S. J., and Pober, J. S.,** Human cytolytic T lymphocyte interactions with vascular endothelium and fibroblasts: Role of effector and target cell molecules, *J. Immunol.,* 133, 1878, 1984.

113. **Barbosa, J. A., Mentzer, S. J., Kamarick, M. E., Hart, J., Strominger, J. L., Bino, P. A., and Burakoff, S. J.,** Somatic cell hybrid approach of human lymphocyte function associated antigen (LFA-3). Gene mapping and role in CTL-target cell interactions, *J. Immunol.,* 136, 305, 1986.

114. **Gromkowski, S. H., Krensky, A., Martz, E., and Burakoff, S. J.,** Functional distinctions between LFA-1, LFA-2 and LFA-3 membrane proteins on human CTL are revealed with trypsin pretreated target cells, *J. Immunol.,* 134, 244, 1985.

Chapter 8

# TOWARD UNDERSTANDING TARGET BINDING AND LYSIS BY NATURAL KILLER CELLS

**Gunther Dennert**

## TABLE OF CONTENTS*

*　This work was supported by USPHS grants CA 37706, CA 39501, and CA 39623.

# I. INTRODUCTION

Natural killer cells (NK) are a class of lymphocytes able to lyse in vitro a variety of tumor targets as well as certain normal cells without prior antigen exposure.[1] They acquired notoriety because of their unique properties, resulting in the hypothesis that they may be the prime effectors in immunosurveillance of tumors and may be a first line of defense against microbial infections.[2] Moreover, they are thought to play a role in the regulation of hemopoiesis. The first evidence for this latter role of NK cells was the finding by Cudkowicz and colleagues that there is a correlation between the ability of F1 hybrid mice to acutely reject parental bone marrow grafts and their NK activity.[3] Further experiments then showed that NK cells may lyse syngeneic bone marrow cells in vitro.[4] More recently, it was reported that mice that are genetically deficient in NK activity[5] when injected with either enriched populations of NK cells or cloned NK cell lines, regain the ability to reject bone marrow grafts.[6] Taken together, these experiments suggest that NK cells likely play an important role in the acute rejection of bone marrow grafts. Another interesting correlation between in vivo NK activity and resistance was uncovered in certain viral infections[7] leading to the suggestion that NK cells may also play a role in resistance to certain microbial infections. Strong support for this hypothesis has recently been obtained in NK deficient mice infected with murine cytomegalo virus.[8] In these experiments, a small number of cloned NK cells injected into NK deficient newborn mice was able to confer complete resistance to the lethal effect of the virus. There is also increasing support for the participation of NK cells in the resistance to certain tumors.[9] Direct evidence for this was obtained by injecting NK deficient mice with enriched populations of NK cells or cloned cell lines with NK activity. Such NK reconstituted mice express resistance to the transplantable melanoma tumor B16 and the occurrence of radiation induced leukemia.[9] Because of the important role NK cells appear to play in immunosurveillance against neoplasia and resistance to microbial infections, it is important to understand how NK cells perform these functions. It is the aim of this chapter to summarize our knowledge in this area, primarily in the context of the recently cloned cell lines with natural killer activity.

# II. TARGET RECOGNITION AND BINDING AS A PREREQUISITE OF TARGET CELL DESTRUCTION

Several different mechanisms of target lysis have been proposed for NK cells, some of which involve secretion of lymphotoxins which can be assayed in cell supernatants,[10] while others involve intimate contact between effector and target cell.[11,12] The NK clones isolated in our laboratory require target contact for cytolysis, and supernants of these cells do not contain demonstrable cytolytic activity. Assay of NK clones on a panel of tumor targets (Figure 1) reveals that certain targets are lysed by NK effectors cells, while others are not. The failure of certain cells to serve as lysable targets could be due to either a lack of antigenic determinants enabling binding by NK cells or resistance to the lytic mechanism. A way to distinguish between these two possibilities is to test targets in cold target *inhibition* assays. In these assays, effector cells are mixed with $^{51}$Cr labeled targets like YAC-1, and unlabeled targets are added to the reaction mixture in various ratios. Inhibition of isotope release indicates that the effector cells bind to the unlabeled targets, resulting in lower lysis of the labeled targets. Targets inhibiting in a cold target inhibition assay are considered to express antigens recognizable by the effector cells. The results illustrated in Figure 1 show that, in general, cells that are lysable in a direct cytolytic assay are able to act as cold target inhibitors. The reverse, however, is not necessarily the case. Target cell B/C-N, for instance, is a good cold target inhibitor, but is not lysable in a direct cytolytic assay. It therefore appears that B/C-N expresses target antigens which enable the effector to bind, but no lysis occurs. The

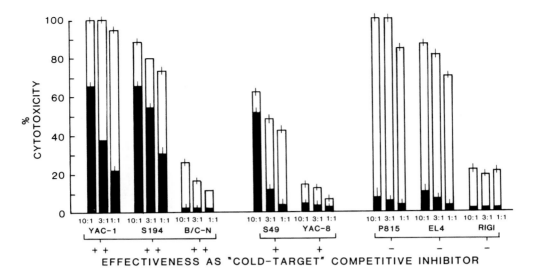

FIGURE 1. Ability of NK11.6.D6 to lyse YAC-1, Chang, S49, Raji, R1G1, EL4, P815 and B/C-N in the absence (black bars) or presence of 4 μg/mℓ Con A (white bars). Spontaneous $^{51}$Cr release from targets was determined in the presence of 4 μg/mℓ Con A, although Con A did not increase spontaneous $^{51}$Cr release. The 5-hr time-point is given at the E/T ratios of 1:1, 3:1, and 10:1.

targets P815, EL4, and R1G1 are not lysed by NK cells and could have either one of two defects: lack of target antigens, or both lack of antigens and resistance to the lytic mechanism. To distinguish between the two possibilities, NK cells were incubated with their targets in the absence or presence of the lectin Concanavalin A (Con A) which enables effector cells to bind to targets in the absence of appropriate target antigen. Results in Figure 1 indeed demonstrate that two of the targets, P815 and EL4, that do not show lysis by NK cells in the absence of Con A, show high lysis in the presence of the lectin. This suggests that both targets lack NK target structures yet are susceptible to the lytic mechanism. In contrast, R1G1 shows only poor lysis in the presence of Con A and, therefore, does not only lack NK target structures but is also resistant to cytolysis. Taken together, these results show that NK mediated lysis requires killer target cell binding and that binding does not necessarily result in target lysis. In the following, we will discuss experiments aimed at elucidating which cell surface components on the target cell are involved in binding of the effector cell and able to trigger the lytic process.

## III. WHAT TARGET STRUCTURES ARE RECOGNIZED BY NK EFFECTOR CELLS?

The poorly defined cytolytic specificity of NK cells has resulted in much speculation on the target structure of the NK cell receptor. Early on, it was observed that NK cells may express some species specificity since mouse NK cells appear to primarily lyse mouse targets while human NK cells preferentially lyse human targets.[13] Cloning of murine NK cells[14] then showed that individual NK clones express indistinguishable target specificity, suggesting that they have identical receptors.[15] Many suggestions were made in regard to what this receptor specificity may be. One of the more recent ones was based on the observation that the susceptibility of targets to NK mediated lysis positively correlates with the expression of the cell surface transferrin receptor. Transformed neoplastic cells express many more transferrin receptor molecules on their cell surface than normal cells to a finding which could explain the preferential sensitivity of transformed cells to NK mediated lysis. In support of this hypothesis, Vodinelich et al.[16] reported that purified transferrin receptor molecules may inhibit competitively NK mediated lysis. The hypothesis, however, was not supported by further critical experiments. For instance, in the murine system[17] the expression of transferrin receptors on targets does not correlate with the susceptibility of these targets to NK lysis. Moreover, in the human NK system mouse L cells transfected with the human transferrin receptor gene, and expressing this molecule on its cell surface, were able to absorb human NK cells but did not undergo cell lysis.[17] The expression of the human transferrin receptor on L cells, therefore, was sufficient to mediate NK binding but not lysis. It is, therefore, clear that other molecules besides the tranferrin receptor have to be present for target lysis to occur.[17]

## IV. WHAT IS THE NK TARGET RECEPTOR?

The question of what antigenic determinants on target cells are recognized by NK cells has been complicated by the fact that NK cells may interact with their targets via two entirely different mechanisms. One mechanism involves the native NK receptor, assayed by in vitro cytotoxicity, while the other involves the participation of Fc receptors for IgG. The latter mechanism is called antibody dependent cell mediated cytotoxicity (ADCC) and can be assayed in vitro by incubating NK effector cells with targets in the presence of antitarget cell antibody. Previous experiments had suggested that NK cells and K cells that are responsible for ADCC of nucleated targets are one and the same cell type. For instance it was reported that patients with the Chediak-Higashi syndrome are both NK deficient and lack ADCC activity.[18] Moreover, it was known from single-cell cytolytic assays that one effector cell may simultaneously lyse a target in an ADCC reaction and lyse another target in the absence of target cell specific antibody.[19] It is, therefore, not surprising that our cloned NK cells express ADCC activity.[20] Target cells that lyse poorly in the presence of NK cells may lyse much better in the presence of target cell specific antibody of IgG but not of IgM isotype. It is, therefore, clear that antibody bound via the Fc receptor to the NK effector may serve as an antigen receptor in the lytic reaction. In recent studies we have shown that the mechanism of acute bone marrow allograft rejection involves NK cells[6] and that the specificity of this rejection depends on the presence of target cell specific immunoglobulin in the graft recipient.[20] This suggests that NK mediated ADCC indeed plays a physiological role in vivo.

A more difficult problem is to explore the nature of the native NK receptor. A recent approach to this quesiton was made possible by the cloning of the β-gene of the thymus-derived lymphocyte (T cell) receptor in mouse and man.[21,22] A β-gene probe was used to examine whether murine NK clones express and rearrange the β-gene in their DNA. Several independently derived lines with NK activity were analyzed, three of which were cloned from normal splenocytes, i.e., NK3, NK B61A2, and NK B61B10. All five cell lines tested express rearranged β-genes.[23] Very similar results were obtained with NK cells enriched from spleen, as well as from uncloned cell lines with NK activity.[23] Since β-gene rearrangement is seen in both DNA and mRNA of NK cells, it was likely that respective receptor polypeptides are expressed on their cell surface. Using radioiodination, it was indeed found that a 90 kDalton heterodimer is present on NK cells, and studies are in progress to analyze the function of this molecule (unpublished results). Taken together, these results suggest two conclusions: (1) NK and T cells may be related ontogenetically because they express common cell surface antigens, and (2) they may acquire like specificity in culture.[23] Another conclusion is that NK cell and T cell receptors are closely related because both cell types express a rearranged β-gene. The question then arises as to why the specificity of T cells and NK cells is so different. There is no reasonable explanation for this at present, but as pointed out above, NK cells may be able to distinguish between targets of different species which may be a reflection of specificity for histocompatibility antigens.

## V. THE TRIGGERING STEP: TARGET CELLS EMIT SIGNALS RESULTING IN MOVEMENTS OF THE GOLGI APPARATUS

Experiments employing various lysosomal inhibitors had pointed to the importance of an intact secretory system in NK cells required for the expression of cytoxicity.[24,25] It had also been observed that the Golgi apparatus (GA), which plays an important role in secretion,[26] occupies a position close to the target binding site during cytolysis.[27,28] The localization of the GA in killer target conjugates could be due to either a close association of the antigen receptor to the GA, or due to reorientation of the GA towards the target binding site after the initial binding. In order to distinguish between these two possibilities, the localization of the GA in effector target conjugates was assessed at early times after target binding. To do this, advantage was taken of the availability of antibody specific for either the GA or the microtubules. In the interphase cell, the GA and microtubule organizing center (MTOC) are closely associated. The latter structure is that part of the interphase cell that contains the two centrioles from which the microtubules emanate. The co-localization of MTOC and GA in interphase cells was verified for NK cells by using double labeling immunofluorescence microscopy and specific antibody for both structures. Thus, staining of the MTOC is indicative of the localization of the GA and vice versa.[29] Cloned NK cells were conjugated with the NK targets YAC-1 or S194 and conjugates fixed various times after conjugation followed by staining with antibody reagents specific for the MTOC. Experiments showed that at early times, i.e., up to 20 min after conjugation, less than 70% of the effector cells have their GA oriented toward the target binding site (Figure 2). This result suggests that the NK antigen receptor does not have a polar orientation close to the GA. Interestingly, at later times, i.e., 30 min or later after conjugation, essentially all effector cells had their GA oriented toward the target contact area. Taken together, these observations suggest that GA orientation in the effector cell is initially random but is followed by a rapid reorientation of this organelle towards the target binding site.[29] It was suspected that GA reorientation could be an important and perhaps obligatory step in the initial phase of target lysis. In order to collect evidence for this speculation, the cellular requirements for GA reorientation were examined. Results showed that there was an absolute correlation between cell lysis and GA reorientation.[30,31] For instance, when NK cells are conjugated with the lysable targets YAC-1 and S194, the GA was always observed to be oriented toward the target binding site (Table 1). In contrast, when lysis resistant targets like YAC-8 and B/C-N (Fig. 1, Table 1) are conjugated to NK cells, no GA reorientation is observed. These results suggest that the mere binding of NK effector cells to their targets is not sufficient to initiate GA reorientation. One could therefore hypothesize that lysis resistant NK targets lack a specific cell surface component and therefore are unable to emit the signal that triggers GA reorientation in the effector. Next, one could ask whether NK clones that have lost their lytic activity but bind to lysable targets are able to reorient their GA. A derivative of NK cell line, NK3, had lost its cytolytic activity after prolonged culture but was still able to bind to YAC-1. Results with NK3 showed that no GA reorientation takes place in this cell after binding to YAC-1.[31]

Taken together, these results suggest that targets emit a signal to the NK effector resulting in GA reorientation. This reorientation does not take place in certain NK effector cells which have lost their cytolytic activity. To collect further support for the hypothesis that GA reorientation is an obligatory prerequisite for target lysis, conditions known to inhibit cytolysis by NK cells were employed. Since NK mediated lysis requires the presence of $Ca^{++}$, the absence of this divalent cation on GA reorientation was studied. Results showed that in the absence of $Ca^{++}$, target binding does occur but no GA reorientation takes place (Table 1). In order to assess whether functional microtubules are important for GA reorientation, the drug nocodazole, which depolymerizes microtubules[32] was tested for its effect on GA

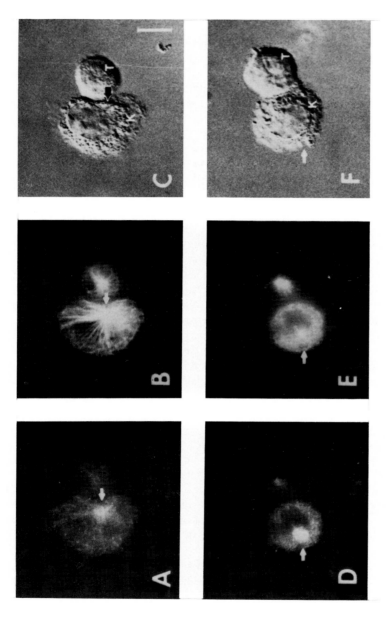

FIGURE 2. Close association of MTOC and GA in NK target conjugates. Couples of NK cells and YAC-1 observed 15 min after mixing. Nomarski optics images of two different couples are shown (C, F). The corresponding cells were double immunofluorescently labeled to reveal their GA (A, D) and their MTOC (B, E). The example in A to C is representative of the majority (65%) of the population of couples, that in D to F of the minority (35%). The GA (arrow in A) and the MTOC (arrow in B) in the NK cell are coordinately positioned facing towards the TC, whereas in example D to F, the two organelles are coordinately positioned facing away from the target cell. The bar in C indicates 10 μm. (From Kupfer, A., Dennert, G., and Singer, S. J., Proc. Nat'l. Acad. Sci. USA, 80, 722, 1983. With permission.)

### Table 1
## CORRELATION BETWEEN TARGET CELL LYSIS AND GA/
## MTOC REORIENTATION IN NK TARGET CONJUGATES

| Effector cells | Target cells | Cytolysis | GA/MTOC reorientation | Ref. |
|---|---|---|---|---|
| NKB61A2 | YAC-1 | + | + | 30 |
|  | S194 | + | + | 30 |
|  | YAC-8 | − | − | 29 |
| NK3 | YAC-1 | − | − | 30 |
| NKB61A2 | YAC-1 + EGTA | − | − | 30 |
|  | B/C-N | − | − | 31 |
|  | YAC-1 + Nocodazole | − | − | 33 |
|  | YAC-1 + Nocodazole + Con A | + | + | 33 |

reorientation. It is important to note that depolymerization of microtubules by nocodazole causes dispersion of the elements of the GA into the cell periphery without, however, significantly impairing cellular secretion.[33] Incubation of NK cells with nocodazole depolymerizes the microtubules and thereby eliminates them, but when the drug is given together with the microtubule stabilizing agent, taxole, an abortive MTOC is formed that can be visualized with anti-tubulin antibody.[34] NK cells that were treated in this way and subsequently conjugated to YAC-1 targets[29] do not show GA reorientation (Table 1). Moreover, assay of cytolytic activity of NK cells treated with nocodazole/taxol[29] reveals that these conjugates do not progress to target lysis. The drug-induced effects appear to be fully reversible since removal of the drug leads to a rapid reappearance of microtubules, reorientation of the GA, and onset of target lysis.[29] Since it had previously been shown that nocodazole-induced GA dispersion does not interfere with cellular secretion *per se*[33] one would assume that microtubule depolymerization in NK cells should still allow for secretion of cytolytic molecules. Due to the dispersion of the GA, however, this secretion would not be focused and therefore presumably the cytolytic components less effective. If this interpretation is correct, then increasing the overall binding area between the effector cell and target should lead to an increase in target lysis. The lectin Con A is known to increase the binding area between NK effector cells and target cells. Con A therefore should be able to at least partially overcome the nocodazole induced inhibition of target cell lysis[34] which was indeed observed (Table 1). These results suggest that neither a compact GA nor an intact MTOC are absolutely necessary for target lysis but, rather, both enhance the cytolytic effectivity of the effector cell.

The events preceding target cell lysis therefore require an initial binding of the effector to the target, followed by GA reorientation, which requires signalling from the target (Figure 3). Whenever conditions are chosen that interfere with either GA reorientation or cytolysis one or the other of the effects are invariably inhibited (Figure 3, Table 1). On the other hand, inhibition of GA reorientation by microtubule depolymerization can be compensated for by the addition of Con A (Table 1). Therefore, GA orientation is not an obligatory step, but appears to make the cytolytic reaction more effective. NK to target conjugation is followed by specific recognition events, since non-lysable targets do not trigger GA reorientation. GA reorientation is, therefore, not merely a fortuitous event resulting from cell-cell binding. This is also supported by the observation that target cells never reorient their own GA towards the effector binding site.[29]

## VI. NK GRANULES CONTAIN CYTOLYTIC COMPONENTS ABLE TO LYSE TARGET CELLS

Ultrastructural analysis of NK target cell conjugates revealed that the presumably GA-

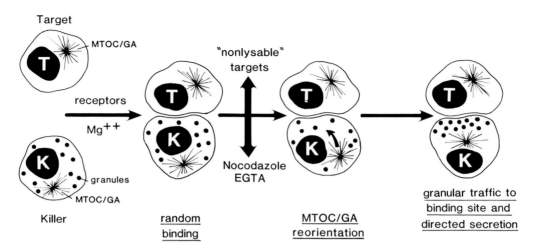

FIGURE 3.    Schematic outline of the events leading to target cell lysis.

derived dense granules tend to collect close to the target binding site.[11] This observation led to the hypothesis that NK granules may contain the cytolytic components responsible for cell lysis. In support of this, Henkart et al.[35] demonstrated that granules from a rat leukemia that expresses NK activity are able to lyse target cells in a $CA^{++}$ dependent reaction. It was therefore important to examine whether our cloned NK cell lines similarly contain granules able to lyse target cells. Results showed that NK granules isolated by Percoll gradient centrifugation lyse targets like YAC-1 and sheep erythrocytes.[36] Granules were found not to be target-specific, which suggests that they do not express antigen-specific receptors.[36] An interesting observation was that the granules isolated from cloned NK cells lyse nucleated targets more efficiently than erythrocyte targets,[36] which is in contrast to previous results with a rat leukemia tumor with NK activity which showed preferential granule mediated lysis on erythrocyte as compared to nucleated targets.[35] It is, therefore, possible that the lysis observed with granules from our NK clones has a different molecular basis than that previously described for granules from a rat leukemia.

## VII. NK GRANULES CONTAIN TUBULAR STRUCTURES THAT APPEAR TO BE RESPONSIBLE FOR TARGET LYSIS

Cell lysis by the membrane attack complex of complement has been extensively studied in the past and inspired experiments aimed at proving that cell mediated cytolysis follows similar pathways.[37] Since complement lesions can be visualized by negative staining electronmicroscopy,[38] a direct approach to the question whether cell mediated lysis procedes via similar mechanisms was feasible. Using this approach, Dourmashkin et al.[39] were the first to report the presence of tubular or ring-like structures on target cells incubated with cytolytic effector cells from human peripheral blood. In subsequent experiments, we employed cloned NK cells incubated with YAC-1 targets to demonstrate that similar tubular structures as the ones described before can be found on target membranes.[11] Essentially, two types of tubular structures were observed and called polyperforin 1 (P1) and polyperforin 2 (P2), respectively.[11] P1 has an outer and inner diameter of 26 and 16 nm, respectively, while the equivalent dimensions of P2 are 11 and 5 nm. Putative side views of these structures suggest that they are tubular complexes with a length of 16 (P1) and 12 nm (P2), respectively.[11] Morphologically, there is some similarity of these structures to mouse complement lesions, but the overall dimensions of P1 and P2 are different from those of complement lesions. It is not known presently whether there are similarities in the subunit structure between mouse complement and P1 and P2. On the basis of electron microscopic and biochemical studies, it was suggested that NK effector cells secrete granule-derived cytolytic molecules of tubular structure that insert into target membranes, leading to membrane perforation and target death.[11] A critical test of this hypothesis was to show that NK granules give rise to P1 and P2 which insert into target membranes. To find out, erythrocyte ghosts were loaded with labeled marker proteins and incubated with isolated granules in the presence of $Ca^{++}$. Proteins with a molecular weight below 250,000 Daltons were released, while β-galacto-sidase with a molecular weight of 500,000 Daltons was not released (Figure 3). A similar result was obtained with complement-mediated lysis of similarly loaded erythrocyte targets (Figure 4). These results suggest that the overall dimension of lesions induced by granules and complement are similar, supporting the view that the tubular structures observed previously by electron microscopy may indeed be the cytolytic molecules responsible for NK-mediated target cell lysis.[36]

## VIII. CONCLUSIONS

One of the least understood events in NK cytolysis is the initial recognition of the target by the effector. We know that this recognition may proceed via target adsorbed antibody that binds to NK Fc receptors, resulting in triggering of cytolytic events. An unresolved question, however, is what the nature and specificity of the native NK receptor may be. Expression of the rearranged β-gene in the DNA of NK cells[22] raises the question of whether NK cell receptors may be a form of T cell receptor. It is possible, however, that the T cell receptor on NK cells is not functional and merely a reflection of the ontogenic relationship between NK cells and T cells. The finding that there are targets like P815 and EL4 that do not adhere to NK cells could provide an approach to find out what the NK receptor recognizes, but this approach has not been successful, so far. Experiments with the nonlysable targets YAC-8 and BCN suggest that for successful target lysis to occur, two kinds of cell surface antigens on the target have to be present. One is required for binding of the effector to the target and the other for triggering of GA reorientation. It is not known presently whether one antigen epitope may fulfill both functions or whether the two functions are always due to two different determinants. One of the target antigens which is involved in NK effector target binding has been identified as the human transferrin receptor. Target cells expressing this antigen, however, are not always lysed, and it is an open question as to whether the transferrin receptor by itself induces GA reorientation in the effector cell. An interesting question is whether NK receptors occupy a specific polar region close to the GA or whether receptors are randomly distributed. Our experiments are not conclusive either way. They do show, however, that if such restricted localization of receptors exists, then it is not defined with regard to the position of the MTOC/GA complex (Figure 3). The intriguing observation was made that although target binding occurs randomly with regard to the position of the GA, progression of cytolysis is always accompanied by reorientation of the GA to the target binding site (Figure 3). The various conditions examined that inhibit either cytolysis or GA reorientation invariably inhibit the other (Figure 3). It is therefore suggested that the reorientation of the GA is an important early event in cytolysis. This event, however, does not appear to be obligatory, rather it makes the lytic mechanism more effective in that it focuses the secretion of cytolytic molecules toward the target (Figure 5). At the present time we can only speculate about the next steps following GA reorientation. It appears that NK granules collect at the target binding site (Figures 3 and 5), which may be facilated by the MTOC/GA complex providing cytoskeletal tracks for the movement of granules to the target binding site. Isolated granules from NK cells can be shown to be nonspecifically cytolytic to target cells (Figure 4). Therefore, one would speculate that the specificity of NK lysis is dictated

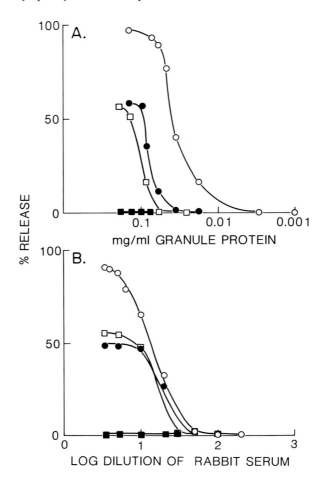

FIGURE 4.    Release of macromolecules from human erythrocyte ghosts by the action of granules (A) and complement (B). Ghosts were loaded with labeled α-bungarotoxin (closed circles), Fab fragments (open circles), immunoglobulin G (closed squares), or β-galactosidase (open squares), and their release by the action of granules (A) or complement (B) was monitored. In a typical experiment 140 μℓ erythrocyte ghosts, loaded as described in Reference 36, were incubated with granules or with rabbit serum plus rabbit antihuman erythrocyte antibody. CaCl$_2$ (5m*M* final concentration) was added to start the reaction with granules, and MgSO$_4$ (50 mg/ℓ plus Ca(NO$_3$)$_2$·4H$_2$O (100 mg/ℓ) was added to initiate the complement-mediated reaction. Incubation was carried out at 37°C for 30 min, followed by centrifugation of the ghosts, washing, and counting of radioactivity. Radioactivity remaining inside the ghosts was compared to controls in which granules or complement were replaced with buffer. Results are expressed as percentage of radioactivity released from erythrocyte ghosts as compared to untreated controls.

on the level of the NK antigen receptor rather than on the level of the granule or cytolytic effector molecules. Cytolytic granules insert lesions of defined size into target membranes which appear to be similar in size to those of complement lesions (Figure 5). This suggests that the P1 and P2 structures previously seen by electron microscopy on cell membranes of targets incubated with NK cells very likely originate from the granules. This mechanism of target cell lysis would pose an interesting question, i.e., what the protective mechanism in the effector cell may be that suppresses autolysis by granule-derived cytolytic molecules. These and many other questions pertaining to the final stages of cell mediated lysis are now an area of intensive experimentation, and the next few years will, we hope, provide many of the missing parts of this interesting problem.

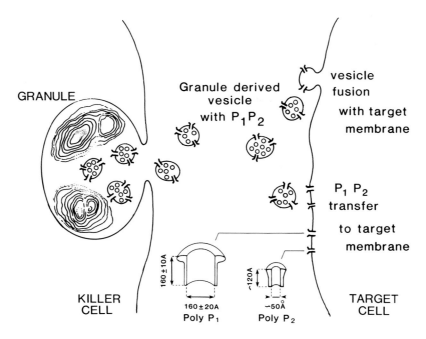

FIGURE 5. Schematic outline of the events leading to deposition of lytic $P_1$ and $P_2$ into the target membrane. Vesicles either fuse with the target membrane, or $P_1$ or $P_2$ are transferred from the vesicle to the membrane.

# REFERENCES

1. **Herberman, R. B. and Holden, H. T.,** Natural cell-mediated immunity, *Adv. Cancer Res.,* 27, 305, 1978.
2. **Koide, Y. and Takasugi, M.,** Specificities in natural cell-mediated cytotoxicity against lymphoblastoid cell lines. I. Selective inhibition by cross competition, *Eur. J. Immunol.,* 8, 818, 1978.
3. **Kiessling, R., Hocman, P. S., Haller, O., Shearer, G. M., Wigzell, H., and Cudkowicz, G.,** Evidence for a similar or common mechanism for natural killer cell activity and resistance to hemopoietic grafts, *Eur. J. Immunol.,* 7, 655, 1977.
4. **Holmberg, L. A., Miller, B. A., and Ault, K. A.,** The effect of natural killer cells on the development of syngeneic hematopoietic progenitors, *J. Immol.,* 133, 2933, 1984.
5. **Roder, J. C. and Duwe, A. K.,** The beige mutation in the mouse selectively impairs natural killer cell function, *Nature,* 278, 451, 1979.
6. **Warner J. F. and Dennert, G.,** Effects of a cloned cell line with NK activity on bone marrow transplants, tumour development and metastasis *in vivo, Nature,* 300, 31, 1982.
7. **Welsh, R. M.,** Mouse natural killer cells: Induction, specificity, and function, *J. Immunol.,* 121, 1631, 1978.
8. **Bukowski, J. F., Warner, J. F., Dennert, G., and Welsh, R. M.,** Adoptive transfer studies demonstrating the anti-viral effect of natural killer cells *in vivo, J. Exp. Med.,* 161, 40, 1985.
9. **Haller, O., Hansson, M., Kiessling, R., and Wigzell, H.,** Non-conventional NK cells may play a decisive role in providing resistance against syngeneic tumor cells *in vivo, Nature,* 270, 609, 1977.
10. **Wright, S. C. and Bonavida, B.,** Selective lysis of NK resistant target cells by a soluble mediator released from murine spleen cells and human peripheral blood lymphocytes, *J. Immunol.,* 126, 1516, 1981.
11. **Podack, E. R. and Dennert, G.,** Cell-mediated cytolysis: assembly of two types of tubules with putative cytolytic function by cloned natural killer cells, *Nature (London),* 302, 442, 1983.
12. **Kupfer, A., Dennert, G., and Singer, S. J.,** Polarization of the Golgi apparatus and the microtubule organizing center within cloned natural killer cells bound to their targets, *Proc. Natl. Acad. Sci. USA,* 80, 722, 1983.
13. **Roder, J. C., Richter, L. A., and Jondal, M.,** Target-effector interaction in the human and murine natural killer system, *J. Exp. Med.,* 150, 471, 1979.

14. **Dennert, G.**, Cloned lines of natural killer cells, *Nature,* 287, 47, 1980.

15. **Dennert, G., Yogeeswaran, G., and Yamagata, S.**, Cloned cell lines with natural killer activity. Specificity function and cell surface markers, *J. Exp. Med.,* 153, 545, 1983.

16. **Vodinelich, L., Sutherland, R., Schneider, C., Newman, R., and Greaves, M.**, Receptor for transferrin may be a "target" structure for natural killer cells, *Proc. Natl. Acad. Sci. USA,* 80, 835, 1983.

17. **Newman, R. A., Warner, J. F., and Dennert, G.**, NK recognition of target structures: Is the transformation receptor the NK target structure? *J. Immunol.,* 133, 1841, 1984.

18. **Klein, M., Roder, J., Haliotis, T., Kores, S., Jett, J. S., Herberman, R. B., Katz, P., and Fauci, A. S.**, Chediak-Higashi gene in humans. II. The selectivity of the defect in natural killer and antibody-dependent and cell mediated cytotoxicity function, *J. Exp. Med.,* 151, 1049, 1980.

19. **Bradley, T. P. and Bonavida, B.**, Mechanism of cell mediated cytotoxicity at the single cell level. Natural killing and antibody-dependent cellular cytotoxicity can be mediated by the same human effector cell as determined by the two-target conjugate assay, *J. Immunol.,* 129, 2260, 1979.

20. **Warner, J. J. and Dennert, G.**, Bone marrow graft rejection as a function of antibody directed natural killer cells, *J. Exp. Med.,* 161, 563, 1985.

21. **Yanagi, Y. et al.**, A human T cell specific cDNA clone encodes a protein having extensive homology to immunoglobulin, *Nature,* 308, 145, 1984.

22. **Hedrick, S. M., Cohen, D. I., Nielsen, E. A., and Davis, M. A.**, Isolation of cDNA clones encoding T cell specific membrane associated proteins, *Nature,* 308, 149, 1984.

23. **Yanagi, Y., Cacue, M., Kronenberg, M., Orin, B., Rohel, D., Kiyoliari, T., Carson, R., Toyouaga, B., Rosenthal, K., Dennert, G., Hengartner, H., Hood, L., and Hiak, T. W.**, Natural killer cell rearrange and express the β chain of the T cell antigen receptor, *Nature (London),* 314, 631, 1985.

24. **Carpen, O., Virtanen, I., and Saksela, E.**, Ultrastructure of human natural killer cells: Nature of the cytolytic contacts in relation to cellular secretion, *J. Immunol.,* 128, 2691, 1982.

25. **Carpen, O., Virtanen, I., and Saksela, E.**, The cytotoxic activity of human natural killer cells requires the intact secretory apparatus, *Cell Immunol.,* 58, 97, 1981.

26. **Farquhar, M. G. and Palade, G. E.**, The Golgi apparatus (complex) — (1954—1981) — from artifact to center stage, *J. Cell. Biol.,* 91, 77a, 1981.

27. **Bykovskaja, S. N., Rytenko, A. N., Rauschenbach, M. O., and Bykovsky, A. F.**, Ultrastructural alteration of cytolytic T-lymphocytes following their interaction with target cells. I. Hypertrophy and change of orientation of the Golgi apparatus, *Cell Immunol.,* 40, 164, 1978.

28. **Geiger, G., Rajen, D., and Berke, G.**, Spatial relationships of microtubule-organizing centers and the contact area of cytotoxic T lymphocytes and target cells, *J. Cell. Biol.,* 95, 137, 1982.

29. **Kupfer, A., Dennert, G., and Singer, S. J.**, Polarization of the Golgi apparatus and the microtubule organizing center within cloned natural killer cells bound to their targets, *Proc. Natl. Acad. Sci. USA,* 80, 7224, 1983.

30. **Kupfer, A. and Dennert, G.**, Reorientation of the microtubule organizing center and the Golgi apparatus in cloned cytotoxic lymphocytes triggered by binding to lysable target cells, *J. Immunol.,* 133, 2762, 1984.

31. **Kupfer, A., Dennert, G., and Singer, S. J.**, The reorientation of the Golgi apparatus and the microtubule organizing center in the cytotoxic effector cell is an obligatory early event in the lysis of bound target cells, *J. Mol. Cell. Immunol.,* 2, 37, 1985.

32. **Robbins, E. and Gonata, N. K.**, Histochemical and ultrastructural studies on HeLa cell cultures exposed to spindle inhibitors with special reference to the interphase cell, *J. Histochem. Cytochem.,* 12, 704, 1964.

33. **Rogalski, A. A., Bergmann, J. E., and Singer, S. J.**, The effect of microtubule assembly status on the intracellular processing and surface expression of an integral protein of the plasma membrane, *J. Cell. Biol.,* in press.

34. **Dennert, G., Kupfer, A., Anderson, C. G., and Singer, S. J.**, Reorientation of the Golgi apparatus and the microtubule organizing center: Is it a means to polarize cell mediated cytotoxicity? *International Workshop on the Mechanism of All Mediated Cytotoxicity Analysis,* Henkart, P., Ed., Academic Press, in press.

35. **Henkart, P. A., Millard, P. J., Reynolds, C. W., and Henkart, M. P.**, Cytolytic activity of purified cytoplasmic granules from cytotoxic rat granular lymphocyte tumors, *J. Exp. Med.,* 160, 75, 1984.

36. **Criado, M., Lindstrom, J. M., Anderson, C. G., and Dennert, G.**, Cytotoxic granules from killer cells: Specificity of granules and insertion of channels of defined size into target membranes, *J. Immunol.,* in press.

37. **Sundsmo, J. S. and Muller-Eberhard, H. J.**, Neoantigen of the complement attack complex on cytotoxic human peripheral blood lymphocytes, *J. Immunol.,* 122, 2371, 2378, 1979.

38. **Henney, C. S. and Mayer, M. M.**, Specific cytolytic activity of lymphocytes: Effect of antibodies against complement components C2, C3, and C5, *Cell. Immunol.* 2, 702, 1971.

39. **Dourmashkin, R. R., Deteix, P., Simone, B., and Henkart, P. A.**, Electron microscopic demonstration of lesions in target membranes associated with antibody-dependent cellular cytotoxicity, *Clin. Exp. Immunol.,* 42, 554, 1980.

40. **Dennert, G.**, unpublished.

Chapter 9

# THE HOMOLOGY BETWEEN SPECIFIC AND NONSPECIFIC LECTIN- OR OXIDATION-DEPENDENT CTL/TARGET INTERACTIONS

**Gideon Berke and Zvi Keren**

## TABLE OF CONTENTS

# I. INTRODUCTION

## A. Specific CTL-Mediated Lysis

The mechanism whereby cytolytic T lymphocytes (CTL) induce specific, irreversible, damage to target cells (TC) has been a subject of two decades of intensive research (recent reviews[1-6]). CTL/TC interaction resulting in lysis is initiated by a receptor-mediated, $Mg^{2+}$-dependent recognition and adhesion step (conjugation)[7-11] followed by a temperature- and $Ca^{2+}$-dependent irreversible step, whereupon the lethal hit is delivered,[12-14] culminating in TC disintegration and recycling of the effector to start a new lytic interaction.[15,16] A basically similar sequence of events has been proposed in recent years in natural-killer (NK) induced lysis (for review see References 17 to 19). Yet the exact nature of the lethal hit in both CTL or NK is enigmatic. Recently, perforation of the TC membrane by ring-shaped structures (i.d. 10 to 15 nm) of effector cells (CTL/NK) origin, structurally and functionally analogous to lesions produced by the membrane-attack complex of complement, has been suggested to be the mechanism by which CTL and NK inflict irreversible damage to the TC membrane.[5,6,20-22] Berke and Rosen,[23] however, have not been able to detect such ring structures following lysis induced by in vivo primed, specifically sensitized peritoneal exudate CTL (see note added in proof).

## B. Nonspecific Lectin- and Oxidation-Dependent Cytotoxicity (LDCC and ODCC) and CTL Targeting by Antibody

In contrast to the exquisite specificity of CTL-medited lysis,[4,24,25] under certain conditions CTL can lyse virtually any TC — both allogeneic, syngeneic and even autologous, nonspecifically. These conditions include:

1.  Presence of certain mitogenic lectins, notably Concanavalin A (Con A) and phytohemagglutinin (PHA)[26-31]
2.  The cells are subjected mild oxidation by periodate ($NaIO_4$) or by neuraminidase followed by galactose oxidase (NAGO)[32,33]
3.  Cross-linking CTL and TC through antibodies against the CTL-receptor or receptor-associated determinants such as T3 or T11[34-39]

In a recent report,[40] however, a pepsin $F(ab')_2$ fragment of T3 antibody has been shown to be an effective mediator of (nonspecific) CTL-induced lysis, suggesting that physical, antibody-mediated bridging of effector and TC may, in fact, not be necessary at all to induce lysis. Confirmation and extension of the latter report is required, as it appears to contradict an earlier study stressing cell-cell contact for lysis to occur,[34] as well as to indicate involvement of a soluble cytocidal mediator that can lyse bystander cells.

## C. Mechanism of TC Recognition in LDCC and ODCC

Although generally considered as excellent cell agglutinating agents, the manner by which lectins and oxidants mediate CTL/TC interactions resulting in nonspecific lysis is not at all clear. Because only T cell mitogenic lectins are effective inducers of LDCC, (Table 1), the mere agglutination (bridging) between CTL and TC clearly is not sufficient to initiate lysis. Therefore a (putative) lectin-induced "activation" step following initial "bridging", has been proposed as the second signal delivered by the lectin in LDCC.[30,31,41-42] Lectin and oxidation-dependent, nonspecific killing resulting from "passive" CTL/TC binding, also seems to be in conflict with killer/anti-killer experiments which show selective inactivation of only B anti-C CTL interacting with A anti-B CTL[43,44] and a lack of simultaneous, mutual lysis when A anti-B CTL react with B anti-A CTL.[45] The above killer/anti-killer, as well as other experiments,[34,37] have indicated that TC binding through the CTL receptor, or

**Table 1**
**LYSIS AND CONJUGATE FORMATION MEDIATED BY MITOGENIC**
**AND NONMITOGENIC LECTINS**

| Lectin | Lysis[a] (% ± S.D.) | No. conjugates per 0.5 μℓ[b] |
|---|---|---|
| Mitogenic | | |
| Con A | 46.0 ± 25.0 | 64 ± 11 |
| PHA | 77.0 ± 15.0 | 68 |
| LCA | 87.0 ± 16.0 | 57 ± 19 |
| Non-mitogenic | | |
| PNA | 4.3 ± 0.9 | 1.5 |
| WGA | 15.3 ± 7.5 | 2 |
| SBA | 14.0 ± 3.8 | — |
| PWM | 6.2 ± 1.9 | 7.5 |

[a] Triplicate cultures of ConA-stimulated (CTL) splenocytes of DBA/2 origin were reacted with $^{51}$Cr-labeled EL4 target cells. Mitogenic lectins were used at 2 to 10 μg/mℓ; nonmitogenic lectins at 20 to 50 μg/mℓ. CTL/TC ratio was 10:1. Incubation time was 90 min at 37°C.

[b] Con A-induced splenocytes of DBA/2 origin, or BALB/c anti-EL4, or C57BL/6 anti-P815 alloimmune peritoneal exudate CTL were mixed with EL4 or P815 (1 × 10⁶ cells each), centrifuged at 170 × g for 10 min at room temperature, resuspended vigorously with a Pasteur pipette (10 strokes) and examined microscopically. The number of conjugates per 0.5 μℓ shown was determined in 1 to 3 experiments.

Modified from Berke, G., Rosen, D., and Moscovitch, M., *Immunology,* 49, 585, 1983.

receptor-associated molecules such as T3 or T11, is a prerequisite for lysis.[1,44] Involvement of CTL (antigen) receptor(s) even in nonspecific LDCC and ODCC, has been proposed[46-49] and will be discussed below.

In this article we review experiments carried out in our laboratory to uncover the mechanisms by which lectins and oxidants nonspecifically mediate CTL/TC interactions resulting in lysis. We consider two models to explain LDCC (and ODCC). In the first, proposed originally by Green et al.,[41] and Parker and Martz,[50] the lectin (Con A) plays a dual role: (1) "gluing" CTL and immunologically irrelevant TC simply through lectin-binding receptors, and (2) "activating" the TC-bound CTL to kill. In the second,[2,46,47] we proposed that Con A (in LDCC) and oxidation products (in ODCC) "modify" TC surface components including MHC determinants, inducing the appearance of a multitude of new cell surface determinants which thus render the TC nonspecifically recognizable by the authentic CTL antigen receptor(s), rather than only through lectin-binding receptors. Another major difference beween the two models is that no lectin specific "activation" signal is attributed to the lectin in the second.

## II. THE DUAL ROLE OF LECTINS AND OXIDANTS IN LDCC AND ODCC: A REEXAMINATION

The observation that only mitogenic lectins effectively mediate LDCC (although deviations from this rule following neuraminidase treatment of the TC have been reported[51]) has been interpreted to indicate a two-stage mechanism: (1) lectin-mediated intercellular (CTL/TC) "bridging" or "gluing", followed by (2) lectin-induced "activation" of the TC-bound CTL by the lectin.[29,41,50] In ODCC, CTL/TC interaction has been thought to result from intercellular Schiff-base formed between free aldehydes (-CHO), generated at the cell surface by mild chemical (NaIO₄) or enzymatic (galactose oxidase) oxidation, and cell surface amino groups on the opposing cell. Next we shall consider the role(s) of Con A in "gluing" CTL and TC and in activating the TC-bound CTL.

**Table 2**
### THE FUNCTIONS OF CON A IN LDCC

| Cell mixtures tested | CTL/TC conjugation or lysis of TC | |
|---|---|---|
| | Expected | Observed |
| CTL + TC (nonspecific) | − | − |
| (Con A-CTL) + TC | + + + + | + |
| CTL + (Con A-TC) | + + + + | + + + + |
| (Con A-CTL) + (ConA-TC) | + + + + | + + + |
| (Con A-CTL) + Con A | + + + + | + + + |

*Note:* CTL, cytotoxic T lymphocyte; TC, target cell; Con A-TC and Con A-CTL denotes pretreated target and killer cells, respectively.

## A. Lectin as a "Glue" of Killer and Target Cells

Arguments have been presented in support of the idea that in LDCC the lectin functions to "glue" CTL and TC simply through lectin-binding receptors. These have been discussed before in detail (for review, see Berke,[2] Bonavida et al.,[42] and Sitkovsky et al.[49]) and will be dealt with here in brief. Against the trivial "gluing" role of Con A in mediating CTL/TC interactions, experiments have been carried out which show that Con A-pretreatment of the TC but not of the CTL result in effective TC lysis[46,47] (Table 2). This TC preference in Con A pretreatment has been previously observed by others,[28] but only received scant attention.[31,41,50] We argued[46] that if Con A simply "glued" effector and target cells, comparable killing would be expected when either effector or target were pretreated with Con A. A similar, though not as clear-cut, preference for the TC was observed with phytohemagglutinin (PHA). A comparable degree of lysis resulted when either effector or target cells were pretreated with *Lens culinaris* lectin (LcA).[52] Therefore, lectins must be considered individually, and we limit our discussions to Con A only.

Failure of Con A-pretreated CTL to lyse TC may be due to their inactivation or inability to establish cell-to-cell contact (conjugate formation) with the TC. Lectin-induced inactivation of the CTL has been excluded,[46] although it is clear that Con A-treated CTL can be lysed by either other CTL or autologous CTL (Con A-pretreated or not).[2,49,53] We next evaluated the influence of lectin pretreatment on CTL/TC conjugation.[52] Although the general agglutinating properties of lectins, which produce cell clumping, somewhat impaired the precise enumeration of CTL/TC conjugate formation,[3,10] conjugation, like cytolysis, occurred preferentially when lectin-treated TC were reacted with untreated effectors; lectin-treated CTL conjugated with untreated TC less effectively (Table 2). Preferential binding of lectins (Con A or LcA) to TC was excluded by showing effective binding to both target and effector cells (Figure 1).[52]

Why nonmitogenic lectins are poor mediators of LDCC has not been clear.[51] Effective binding to either target or effector cells was observed with LDCC-nonsupporting (nonmitogenic) lectins (Figure 1c). For example, wheat germ agglutinin (WGA) — an LDCC nonsupporting lectin, binds to both CTL or TC even more effectively than the LDCC-active lectin, Con A. Interestingly, nonmitogenic lectins, unlike Con A, PHA, or LcA, do not mediate CTL/TC conjugation and hence lysis (Table 1). Taken together, the data suggests that the mitogenic lectins (and certainly nonmitogenic lectins) do not simply "glue" CTL and TC to form conjugates, as passive "gluing" would not explain preferential CTL/TC conjugation and lysis when TC is pretreated.

A striking observation, made originally by Gately and Martz[30] is that the number of

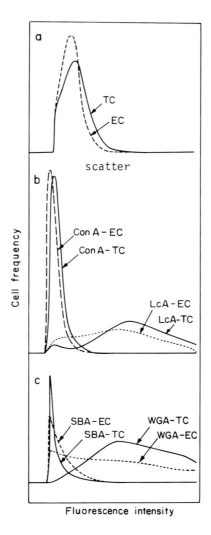

FIGURE 1. FACS analysis of lectin binding to effector and target cells. Scatter distribution of effector and target cells (a). FI-Con A or FI-LCA (b) (LDCC supporting lectins) and FI-SBA or FI-WGA (c) (nonsupporting lectins), were used at 10 μg/mℓ. Con A-stimulated blasts of DBA/2 origin were used as effectors (EC) and EL4 as TC. (Modified from Berke, G., Rosen D., and Moskovitch, M., *Immunology,* 49, 585, 1983.)

conjugates formed between specifically sensitized CTL and TC is not increased in the presence of Con A. When examining the binding of in vivo primed BALB/c anti-EL4 peritoneal exudates (at a lymphocyte/target ratio of 1:1), we scored 35% conjugate formation with and without Con A. If Con A merely bridged lymphocytes and TC, both CTL and nonCTL in the population would be expected to form conjugates, giving rise to high conjugation in the presence of the lectin. However, if as has been proposed,[46,47] Con A mediates conjugate formation only of CTL, then nonCTL would only be aggregated by Con A, a process clearly distinguishable from established firm CTL/TC conjugates. We noticed that in certain "weak" CTL systems, giving rise to small conjugation/lysis, the inclusion of Con A during effector/target interaction could produce a considerable increase in the CTL/TC conjugation and lysis, possibly due to increasing avidity of CTL/TC interaction.

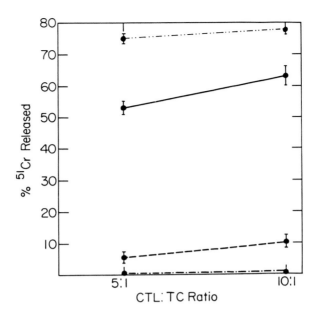

FIGURE 2.   Inhibition of lysis by reduction of pre-formed CTL/O-TC conjugates. $^{51}$Cr-labeled EL4 cells were oxidized by NaIO$_4$. 2mM 10 min at room temperature. After washing, they were mixed with CTL (T lymphoblasts) at different effector/target ratios, centrifuged, and resuspended in NaBH$_4$, 2 mM 10 min at room temperature. Following a second centrifugation, NaBH$_4$ was removed and fresh RPMI-medium was added. For specific lysis, BALB/c anti-EL4 were reacted with intact EL4 as TC. ( — ). IO$_4$ —treated EL4: ( - - -), reduced conjugates; (-·-·-), reduced, IO$_4$-treated EL4; (-···-···-), reduced conjugates in specific lysis. Results are the mean of 5 experiments ± standard error.

## B. Testing for Intercellular Schiff-Base Mediation of CTL/TC Interaction Through ODCC

We exploited the strategy of killer and target pre-oxidation (see Table 2), to study if CTL/TC bridging in ODCC occurs through formation of intercellular Schiff-bases. As in LDCC, oxidation of the TC resulted in effective ODCC; oxidized CTL exposed to nonoxidized TC produced a low level of lysis only. These results are incompatible with the idea that in ODCC, CTL/TC interaction occurs simply through the formation of intercellular Schiff-bases. An additional objection to such a mechanism stems from the finding that the NaBH$_4$, a strong reducing agent, dissociates preformed conjugates and inhibits ODCC (Figure 2).[54] If effector and target were held together chemically via the Schiff-bases, reduction would be expected to stabilize, rather than dissociate CTL/O-TC conjugates, (oxidized target cells).

## C. Lectins as "Activators" of Cytolytic Lymphocytes — Activation of What?

Because only T-cell mitogenic lectins effectively mediate LDCC, a lectin-dependent "activation" step has been proposed.[31,42,50] Although logical, it seems that the state of CTL activation (lectin-mediated or otherwise) specifically relevant to killing, has not been clearly demonstrated or even well-defined. Nor is it even known which specific CTL-function must be "activated" for CTL to lyse, as effectors may be fully lytic, and the role of lectin may be only to establish effective binding. Kinetic analyses[1,12] have not revealed a considerable lag period in CTL-mediated lysis that is compatible with a lengthy step of lectin or antigen-mediated gene-activation in killing, though a short (1 to 10 min) lag is consistently observed.[12] Furthermore, we recently observed a potent T cell mitogen — staphylococcal enterotoxin B (SEB) — capable of generating cytocidal cells in vitro as effectively as Con A, but which is unable to mediate CTL/TC interaction resulting in lysis.[55] Interestingly, Bradley and

## Table 3
## LACK OF RECIPROCAL LYSIS OF CON-A TREATED CTL AND UNTREATED CTL

| Group | %[51]Cr released |
|---|---|
| (Con A-[51]Cr-CTL) + CTL | 66.6 ± 2.0 |
| (Con A-CTL) + ([51]Cr-CTL) | 0.9 ± 0.3 |
| (Con A-[51]Cr CTL) | 19.7 ± 1.2 |

*Note:* Unlabeled and [51]Cr-labeled CTL (Con A-stimulated lymphoblasts of DBA/2 origin) were pretreated with Con A at 10 μg/mℓ at 37°C and diluted 10-fold with medium. Untreated CTL were added to the Con A-treated CTL, spun, and resuspended in medium. Following cocentrifugation, the cells were incubated for 2 hr at 37°C, then assayed for released radioactivity. The number of Con A-treated effectors in each assay was 5 × 10⁵. (Modified from Berke, G. et al., *J. Immunol.*, 127, 782, 1981.)

Bonavida[51] have demonstrated an opposite example; namely, that nonmitogenic lectins such as SBA or PNA induce LDCC if the TC (but not CTL) are pretreated with neuraminidase. Therefore the ability of mitogenic lectins to transform lymphocytes from an inactive or "memory" state to effectors capable of lysis cannot be equated simply with their function in mediating CTL/TC interaction in LDCC. Evidence against the putative "activating" role of lectin in the cytolytic mechanism of CTL comes from experiments using CTL as both effectors and targets.[46] In these experiments, conjugation between Con A-CTL and an identical target (also a CTL) was assured, since untreated CTL could bind to and lyse Con A-treated TC. Although it was predicted that CTL could lyse Con A-CTL, we questioned whether Con A-CTL, now conjugated to CTL, would lyse the CTL. The results of these experiments (Table 3) indicate that lysis is not symmetrical between Con A-CTL and CTL. That is, lysis occurred only in the direction of the Con A-coated (CTL) cell. These CTL anti-CTL experiments demonstrate that Con A per se, does not act as a CTL activator, since if it did, conjugation of two CTL (Con A-CTL and CTL) via Con A linkage would lead to activation of both CTL and result in mutual lysis; but this did not occur. The observation that lysis proceeds only in the direction of the Con A-treated partner (Table 3) and not bidirectionally, as predicted by the "bridging" and "activation" model, suggests that lectin facilitates antigenically irrelevant TC lysis by affecting some structure(s) of the TC that is involved in LDCC. It further indicates that the lectin does not directly affect cytolysis-related structures on the CTL.[49,50]

### D. Induction of LDCC by Con A-Sepharose is Due to Con A Eluted from the Beads
In an attempt to characterize the putative "activation signal" of Con A in LDCC and to exclude (cellular) internalization of the lectin during that presumed process, Ballas et al.[56] employed Con A coupled to Sepharose beads (Con A-Seph). Because Con A-Seph effectively supported LDCC in a 3 hr assay, it was concluded that the presumed "activation" signal (Con A dependent) could be delivered solely at the membrane of the effector cell. Since this experiment is important to our understanding of the mechanism of lectin-dependent lymphocytotoxicity, we decided to check if some of the Con A, believed to be covalently and irreversibly bound to the beads, in fact dissociated and reacted with the target rather than the effector cells. Testing several preparations of Con A-Sepharose, we found that enough Con A can dissociate from the beads during the 3 hr incubation to account for considerable LDCC[57] suggesting that LDCC induced by Con A-Seph was probably mediated by free Con A dissociating from the beads rather than by Con A bound to the beads. Further, direct evidence that the dissociated Con A, like free Con A, exerted its effect on the TC and not the CTL has been presented.[57]

## Table 4
## LYSIS OF TM-TREATED AND UNTREATED TARGET CELLS

| | | | % lysis ± S.E. | | | |
|---|---|---|---|---|---|---|
| | | | +TM | | −TM | |
| CTL | TC | CTL:TC | TC + ConA | TC − ConA | TC + ConA | TC − ConA |
| T lymphoblasts (poly-clonally) activated | EL4 | 10:1 | 5.6 ± 0.6 | 0.8 ± 0.8 | 73.0 ± 3.9 | 1.0 ± 1.1 |
| | | 5:1 | 3.0 ± 1.5 | 0 | 61.3 ± 4.7 | 0.3 ± 0.5 |
| | | 2:1 | 2.1 ± 0.2 | 0.3 ± 0.3 | 49.3 ± 1.9 | 0 |
| | L1210 | 10:1 | 2.5 ± 1.5 | 0 | 29.0 ± 1.5 | 0 |
| | | 5:1 | 1.1 ± 1.1 | 0 | 13.0 ± 2.8 | 0 |
| | | 2:1 | 1.3 ± 1.1 | 0 | 6.1 ± 2.4 | 0 |
| | RDM-4 | 10:1 | 0.7 ± 0.6 | 0 | 26.7 ± 1.9 | 0.4 ± 0.4 |
| | | 5:1 | 0.4 ± 0.4 | 0 | 20.2 ± 1.9 | 0 |
| | | 2:1 | 0 | 0 | 12.2 ± 0.6 | 1.2 ± 1.2 |

*Note:*  EL4, L1210, and RDM-4 cells were treated with papain and then cultured with tunicamycin (TM), 2, 1, and 0.2 μg/mℓ, respectively. After 12 hr of incubation, the cells were washed, labeled with $^{51}$Cr, treated with Con A, 10 μg/mℓ for 30 min at 37°C, washed, and resuspended in PBS-FCS 10%. The TC were then mixed with polyclonally activated T-lymphoblasts and the mixtures were centrifuged for 10 min at room temperature. The cytotoxic assay proceeded for 1.5 to 2 hr. The results are the mean percent $^{51}$Cr released of 3 experiments ± S.E. (Modified from Keren, Z. and Berke, G., *Cell. Immunol.*, 89, 458, 1984.)

## E. Target Cell Surface Molecules That May be Involved in LDCC and ODCC

The foregoing data indicated that some TC structures affected by lectins and oxidants play a role in both LDCC and ODCC, respectively. Experiments have been presented[46] which suggest that at least some of the TC structures affected by Con A in LDCC or by oxidants in ODCC are products of the MHC. These included

1.    Demonstration that the lytic susceptibility of papain-treated TC in LDCC, ODCC, and in specific CTL-mediated or H-2 antibody plus complement-induced lysis, paralleled MHC expression on the cell surface
2.    The finding that genetically H-2 deficient TC are relatively less susceptible to lysis as compared with their H-2 positive counterparts (see below)
3.    The observation that lysis could be blocked effectively by antibodies against MHC-Ag of the TC type and not by antibodies against non-MHC cell surface determinants.[47]

Papain-treated TC become refractory to lysis induced by specific CTL or in LDCC/ODCC; they regain susceptibility following a 3 hr incubation without the enzyme. Resistance/susceptibility to lysis correlates well with surface expression of MHC antigens.[47] Interestingly, papain-treated TC, allowed to recover in the presence of tunicamycin (TM) — a potent inhibitor of N-linked glycosylation — are completely refractory to lysis (Table 4).[58] Additional experiments have shown that the ability of TM-treated TC to bind CTL nonspecifically (in LDCC) and form conjugates was seriously impaired; hence, lack of LDCC against TM-treated TC maybe wholly attributed to their failure to form conjugates. Inhibition of Con A-dependent lysis and conjugation could be explained easily if TM-treated TC bound no Con A, particularly since the TC have previously been shown to be important in Con A binding[46] (Table 2). Testing the Con A-binding capacity of TM-TC using $^{125}$I-Con A with and without α-methyl mannoside (αMM) and by FACS analysis of FITC-Con A binding, revealed comparable Con A-binding to TM-treated and untreated cells.[58] Hence, failure of TM-TC to undergo LDCC was probably due to failure of the lectin to bind to a *unique* (glycosylated) component(s) important for LDCC.

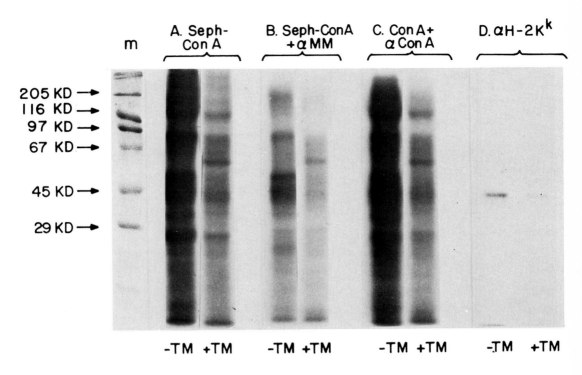

FIGURE 3. SDS-PAGE of [125]I-labeled RDM-4 cell lysates after affinity absorption on Sepharose-Con A. Lysates from untreated and TM-treated cells were incubated with (A) Sepharose-Con A; (B) Sepharose-Con A in the presence of α MM 100 mM. After 30 min the beads were washed and then boiled in sample buffer for 3 min, and the supernatant was taken to SDS-PAGE. (C) and (D) are immunoprecipitates of RDM-4 lysates reacted with Con A (C) and anti-H-2K[k] (D). Immunoprecipitation was carried out at 4°C for 12 hr. Precipitates were absorbed on SAC-I bacterial protein A, washed, and the pellets were boiled for 3 min before SDS-PAGE. (Modified from Keren, Z. and Berke, G., *Cell. Immunol.*, 85, 556, 1984.)

The specific Con A-binding, TC component(s) involved in LDCC were further investigated by analyzing [125]I-labeled cellular components derived from control and TM-treated cells, exploiting the ability of the latter to bind Con A (probably through O-linked residues), while exhibiting refractoriness to lysis. Figure 3 shows two major components, of 30 and 45 kDaltons, detectable in untreated cells but not in TM-treated cells. αMM, 100 mM, retarded absorption and therefore elution of both components from Sepharose-Con A beads (Figure 3B). Immunoprecipitates of Con A + anti-Con A (Figure 3c) confirmed the presence of the 30- and 45-kDalton products in untreated cells. Anti-H-2K[k] (mAb) precipitated a distinct 45-kDalton product from untreated cells, but only a minimal amount from TM-treated cells (Figure 3d); the latter observation was expected in view of considerable reduction in H-2 surface expression following TM treatment.[58] These results indicated a possible role for a 45-kDalton component (possible K and D end products of H-2), as well as of a 30-kDalton, in Con A interactions with the TC which are relevant to LDCC. As shown before,[47,58] anti-EL4 as well as H-2[b] antibodies from congenic strains inhibited LDCC. The binding of [125]I-labeled Con A to antibody-treated cells, however, was not significantly affected. Hence LDCC blocking by MHC-antibodies was not due to an overall reduction in Con A-binding to the TC; alteration of Con A binding to a specific (MHC?) component seemed a more likely possibility.

Papain (but not trypsin) can remove most, if not all, MHC Class I (and some rare Class II) determinants from the cell surface. Papain treated TC were refractory to LDCC or ODCC (although their capacity for Con A binding and oxidation were not significantly affected).

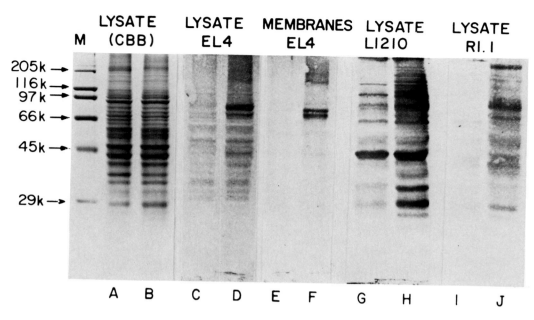

FIGURE 4. Blot analysis of lysates and membrane fractions of oxidized cells. Aliquots from untreated (lane A,C,E,G, and I) and $IO_4^-$-treated (lanes B,D,F,H, and J) EL4, L1210, and R1.1 cells were subjected to SDS-PAGE (10% slab gel). Lanes A-B show Coomassie brilliant blue (CBB) staining of the lysates, lanes C-D and G-L are blots on nitrocellulose filter of all cell lysates, and lanes E-F are blots of membrane fractions prepared from EL4. After blotting the filters were probed with alkaline-phosphatase hydrazide (APHz) (1/750). (Modified from Keren, Z. and Berke, G., *Eur. J. Immunol.*, 16, 1049, 1986.)

However, although trypsinized cells lost about half their susceptiblity in ODCC, they retained full susceptibility to LDCC, indicating that, in addition to papain-sensitive determinants, certain trypsin-sensitive non-MHC molecules contribute to ODCC. Based on the lysis of papain-treated cells which had been allowed a short recovery period prior to testing, involvement of a non-MHC determinant(s) in LDCC has been recently proposed.[59,60] The authors suggested that in LDCC the lectin perturbs the TC membrane, inducing expression of a papain-sensitive, non-class I determinant, important for lysis in LDCC (see relevant discussions in References 61 and 62).

Oxidized determinants on the cell surface in cell lysates and on membranes have been analyzed using a new method for identifying cell surface aldehydes generated by oxidation.[54] Aldehyde bound to major bands corresponding to 125-, 87-, and 82 kDalton have been detected in oxidized-EL4, and at 115- and 40-kDalton in oxidized-L1210 and 300-, 95-, and 83-kDalton in oxidized-R1.1 (Figure 4). That the free aldehydes were bound to cell surface glycoproteins was verified by the observation that similar molecular species appeared in oxidized membranes (Figure 4). Importantly, papain-treated TC (refractory to LDCC) did not express the oxidized determinants and trypsin-treated TC expressed aldehydes bound to different cell surface molecules.[54]

## F. LDCC and ODCC Against MHC "Deficient or Negative" Cells

Our data indicate that at least some of the cell surface determinants involved in LDCC and ODCC are MHC products.[2,47,58] However, the contribution of MHC proteins to lysis in LDCC and ODCC deserves further discussion, for a number of reports utilizing MHC deficient or negative target cells have been published indicating that these determinants have no role in lysis. In an earlier study, Bevan and Hyman[63] reported that the H-2-negative lymphoma cells R1.3 (R1$^-$) underwent LDCC and concluded that MHC antigens do not

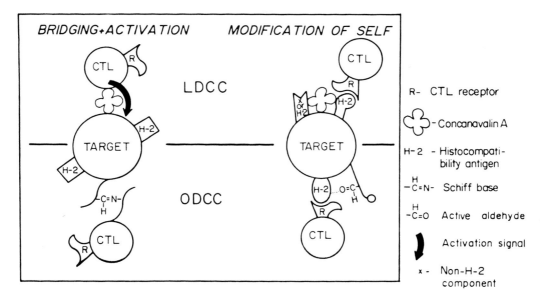

FIGURE 5.    Alternative models for LDCC and ODCC. (Left) bridging and activation: CTL/TC interaction occurs solely through lectin-binding receptors (LDCC) or intercellular Schiff-bases (ODCC). MHC-H-2 determinants of the target are not involved. The CTL is triggered to lyse by the lectin. (Right) modification of self (our proposal): The CTL recognize lectin or aldehyde-induced polyspecific modifications in MHC antigens of the target. Non-MHC determinants may be involved as well.

play a role in CTL-mediated lysis beyond recognition. However, as pointed out in their own study, the susceptibility of the R1$^-$ cells to LDCC was in fact considerably lower than that of the H-2 positive controls R1.1 (R1$^+$). A similar differential susceptibility (R1$^+$ vs. R1$^-$) has been observed by us[47] as well as by others[64] (see, for example, Table 1 in Reference 64). In another system Golstein et al.[65] have shown that mouse embryonal carcinoma cells F9, devoid of serologically detectable H-2 components (Qa-T1a products have not been tested, see below), were lysed in LDCC but not in specific CTL-mediated lysis. In that study, however, whether lysis was due to natural killers (NK) or not, was not rigorously determined. (Unpublished experiments by M. Moscovitch in our lab, showed considerable inhibition of NK-induced F9 killing by asialo-GM$_1$ antibody, indicating the possible contribution of NK activity). It is noteworthy that some F9 cells can be induced to differentiate in vitro to endodermal cells expressing MHC-Ag and can be lysed directly by CTL.[66] When transplanted in vivo, certain embryonal carcinoma cells express MHC-Ag and are then rejected immunologically.[67] Furthermore, monoclonal H-2$^b$ antibody detected a small percentage of F9 embryonal carcinoma cells expressing MHC-Ag and evidence has recently been presented, suggesting a role for Qa T1a MHC Class I products in the lysis of those cells.[68,69] The total refractoriness either to antigen-specific CTL-mediated conjugation and lysis or to LDCC, of mouse, human and chicken red blood cells, known to display either extremely low or undetectable quantities of MHC-determinants is noteworthy.[47,58]

## G. How Lectins and Oxidants Mediate CTL/TC Interactions: A Theory

A key element in our theory on LDCC and ODCC is that the lectin itself or intercellular Schiff-bases, respectively, play an indirect role only in mediating CTL/TC intercellular recognition. Further, lectin- or oxidant-induced "activation" of the effector cell is not an integral or necessary component in our interpretation of LDCC and ODCC although it cannot be formally excluded at the present time. We propose (Figure 5) that the fundamental mechanism whereby CTL recognize TC in LDCC and ODCC is analogous to that employed in specific CTL/TC interaction, i.e., through the interaction of the CTL antigen receptor(s) with the TC MHC antigens, and perhaps other cell surface determinants[62] modified by the lectin or oxidants. This analogy between specific and lectin-dependent, T-cell killing is further supported by the finding that both types of killing processes are multiphasic, proceeding through $Mg^{2+}$-dependent conjugation, $Ca^{2+}$-dependent programming for lysis, then killer-cell independent lysis.[30] Also, both processes are similarly influenced by metabolic, cytoskeletal and pharmacological inhibitors as well as by the effects of antibodies against various CTL and TC surface components involved in CTL/TC interaction.[42,49]

Our data furthers the analogy between specific CTL-induced lysis and nonspecific LDCC and ODCC, by suggesting that the same CTL receptors and lytic machinery are involved. CTL probably react (nonspecifically) with TC-MHC gene products "modified" by lectin or by oxidation (see Figure 5). In the original version of our hypothesis,[47] the term "modification" implied mainly lectin/oxidant-induced redistribution (clustering) of TC-MHC antigens which increased the avidity of CTL/TC interactions. A similar situation may be found in a report by Bradley and Bonavida[51] showing LDCC by nonmitogenic lectins after removing sialic acid residues from the cell's surface. While there is considerable evidence to indicate *direct* Con A binding to MHC-Ag (as well as to non-MHC-Ag) which could induce clustering/modification of MHC-Ag and account for TC recognition in LDCC, the results in ODCC appear to be somewhat different.[54] In ODCC, MHC-H-2 antigens of the TC appear to be involved in recognition, as deduced from blocking by H-2 antibodies and the refractoriness to lysis of H-2 negative cells such as R1[-] and red blood cells and of papain-treated cells. Yet, we have recently found[54] distinct trypsin-sensitive, non-MHC components that may play a role in ODCC. This is reminiscent of the proposed involvement of non-MHC determinants in specific CTL/TC interactions.[61,62] We have observed that O-TC possess free, stable aldehydes bound to some of the above trypsin-sensitive non-MHC molecules which, possibly in concert with H-2 determinants, but not through formation of covalent complexes, that play a role in recognition and lysis in ODCC. We propose that in ODCC active aldehyde groups located on non-MHC determinants, react with adjacent H-2 (and perhaps other cell surface molecules) to create a *multitude* of new (H-2) antigenic conformations recognizable by the CTL.[24,25] In LDCC direct lectin/MHC-Ag interaction and probably additional cell surface determinants, appear to play a role in processing of the TC so that it becomes recognizable (nonspecifically) by the CTL-receptor. The proposed mechanism(s) for ODCC and LDCC now becomes an extension of the now "classical" MHC-restriction to polyclonal MHC-recognition. The mechanism of TC recognition in specific CTL-mediated lysis, LDCC, and ODCC is basically similar, i.e., recognition of modified MHC determinants. Lectin and oxidants, unlike specific Ag, induce a multitude of MHC modifications on the cell surface, giving rise to polyclonal (nonspecific recognition and lysis). Recent experiments on the serological activities of oxidized TC indicate considerable alteration in the binding of MHC antibodies, possibly due to MHC conformational alterations induced by oxidation (Figure 6).

## NOTE ADDED IN PROOF REGARDING THE MECHANISM OF CTL-MEDIATED CYTOTOXICITY IN SPECIFIC AND LECTIN-DEPENDENT CYTOLYSIS

Once CTL-target cell binding is achieved (conjugate formation)[10] the provision of $Ca^{2+}$ and heat (37°C) sets off violent lytic machinery, and some lymphocyte-bound target cells become lysed within several minutes.[1-3] The notion that a Complement- (C) like lytic mechanism is involved in lymphocytotoxicity was suggested by Dourmashkin et al.,[70] who observed C-like lesions (I.D. 10 to 20 nm) following lysis induced in antibody-dependent cellular cytotoxicity (LDCC) and after NK attack, using negative staining electron micros-

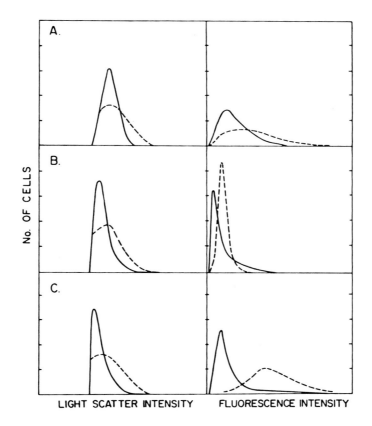

FIGURE 6. FACS analysis of antibody-binding to untreated and oxidized cells. Oxidized (dashed line) and untreated (solid line) EL4 cells ($2 \times 10^6$) were treated for 30 min at 4° with (A) monoclonal anti-H-2K$^k$ (16-3-1); (B) polyvalent BALB/c anti-EL4, 1/500; (C) monoclonal anti-H-2K$^b$ (2-08-4), 1/500. As second antibody, FITC-conjugated rabbit anti-mouse IgG was used (1/20). 20,000 Cells were counted at 450 volts using FACS II, Becton, and Dickinson.

copy. Secretory lytic granules of the effector cell origin, which contain the lytic protein(s) perforin 1 (and 2) and/or cytolysin, were suggested to be the origin of the above C-like lesions.[20-22] On the other hand, close examination of commonly used in vivo primed cytolytic T lymphocytes (CTL) directly derived from the site of graft rejection (PEL)[1] revealed neither formation of the above C-like lesions during lysis of the target, nor the presence of cytocidal granules, perforin 1 and/or cytolysin in these highly potent cells.[23,71] However, cultivation of the in vivo primed PEL-CTL in IL-2 led to the acquisition of cytocidal granules as well as BLT-esterase activity.[72] These results suggested two distinct pathways in lymphocytotoxicity.[72,73] While not discounting the proposed role of secretory lytic granules in lysis induced by at least cells which possess them, particularly IL-2 dependent CTL and NK cells growing in vitro under the influence of massive quantities of IL-2, an alternative lytic mechanism not involving secretory lytic granules and the formation of C-like "rings" has been proposed[3,73] for in vivo primed CTL. Further evidence in support of the latter mechanism comes from experiments showing lysis in the absence of granule exocytosis even with granule-containing cytolytic lymphocytes.[74-76]

# REFERENCES

1. **Berke, G.,** Interaction of CTL and target cells, *Prog. Allerg.,* 27, 69, 1980.
2. **Berke, G.,** Cytotoxic T lymphocytes. How do they function? *Immunol. Rev.,* 72, 5, 1983.
3. **Berke, G.,** How lymphocytes kill infected cells, *Microbiol. Sci.,* 2, 44, 1985.
4. **Nabholtz, M. and MacDonald, H. R.,** Cytolytic T lymphocytes, *Ann. Rev. Immunol.,* 1, 273, 306.
5. **Henkart, P.,** Mechanism of lymphocyte-mediated cytotoxicity, *Ann. Rev. Immunol.,* 3, 31, 1985.
6. **Podack, E.,** The molecular mechanism of lymphocyte-mediated tumor cell lysis, *Immunol. Today,* 6, 21, 1985.
7. **Brondz, B. D., Egorov, I. K., and Drizlikh, G. I.,** Private specificities of H-2K and H-2D loci as possible selective targets for effector lymphocytes in cell-mediated immunity, *J. Exp. Med.,* 141, 11, 1975.
8. **Golstein, P., Svedmyr, E. A. J., and Wigzell, H.,** Cells mediating specific *in vitro* cytotoxicity. I. Detection of receptor-bearing lymphocytes. *J. Exp. Med.,* 134, 1385, 1971.
9. **Stulting, R. D. and Berke, G.,** Nature of lymphocyte-tumor interaction. A general method for cellular immunoabsorption, *J. Exp. Med.,* 137, 932, 1973.
10. **Berke, G., Gabison, D., and Feldman, M.,** The frequency of effector cells in populations containing CTL, *Eur. J. Immunol.,* 5, 813, 1975.
11. **Martz, E.,** Early steps in specific tumor cell lysis by sensitized mouse T-lymphocytes. I. Resolution and characterization, *J. Immunol.,* 115, 261, 1975.
12. **Berke, G. and Amos, D. B.,** Mechanism of lymphocyte-mediated cytolysis. The LMC cycle and its role in transplantation immunity, *Transplant. Rev.,* 17, 71, 1973.
13. **Golstein, P. and Smith, E. T.,** Mechanism of T-cell-mediated cytolysis: The lethal hit stage, in *Contemporary Topics in Immunobiology,* Vol. 7, Stutman, O., Ed., Plenum, New York, 1977, 273.
14. **Martz, E.,** Mechanism of specific tumor-cell lysis by alloimmune T lymphocytes: Resolution and characterization of discrete steps in the cellular interaction, in *Contemporary Topics in Immunobiology,* Vol. 7, Stutman, O., Ed., Plenum, New York, 1977, 301.
15. **Berke, G., Ax, W., Ginsburg, H., and Feldman, M.,** Graft reaction in tissue culture. II. Quantification of the lytic action on mouse fibroblasts by rat lymphocytes sensitized on mouse embryo monolayers, *Immunology,* 16, 643, 1969.
16. **Berke, G., Sullivan, K. A., and Amos, D. B.,** Tumor immunity *in vitro:* destruction of a mouse ascites tumor through a cycling pathway, *Science* (Washington), 177, 433, 1972.
17. **Clark, W. R. and Golstein, P., Eds.,** *Mechanisms of Cell Mediated Cytotoxicity: Advances in Experimental Medicine and Biology,* Vol. 146, Plenum, New York, 1982.
18. **Henkart, P. and Martz, E., Eds.** *Mechanisms of Cell Mediated Cytotoxicity: Advances in Experimental Medicine and Biology,* Vol. 184, Plenum, New York, 1985.
19. **Herberman, R. B., Reynolds, C. W., and Ortaldo, J.,** Mechanism of cytotoxicity by natural killer cells, *Ann. Rev. Immunol.,* 4, 651, 1986.
20. **Henkart, M. P. and Henkart, P. A.,** Lymphocyte mediated cytolysis as a secretory phenomenon, in *Mechanisms of Cell Mediated Cytotoxicity,* 146, Clark, W. R. and Golstein, P. Eds., Plenum, New York, 1982, 227.
21. **Millard, P. J., Henkart, M P., Reynolds, C. W., and Henkart, P. A.,** Purification and properties of cytoplasmic granules from cytotoxic rat LGL tumors, *J. Immunol.,* 132, 1, 1984.
22. **Podack, E. R. and Konigsberg, P.J.,** Cytolytic T cell granules: Isolation, structure, biochemical and functional characterization, *J. Exp. Med.,* 160, 695, 1985.
23. **Berke, G. and Rosen, D.,** Circular lesions detected on membranes of target cells lysed by antibody and complement or natural killer (spleen) cells but not by in vivo primed CTL, in *Membrane Mediated Cytotoxicity, UCLA Symposia, Park City, 1986,* Bonavida, B. and Collier, R. J., Eds., Alan R. Liss, New York, 1987, 367.
24. **De Waal, L. P., Nathenson, S. G., and Melief, C. J. M.,** Direct demonstration that CTL recognize conformational determinants and not primary amino acid sequences, *J. Exp. Med.,* 158, 1720, 1983.
25. **Sherman, L. A.,** Recognition of conformational determinants on H-2 by CTL, *Nature,* 297, 511, 1982.
26. **Forman, J.,** The specificity of thymus derived T-cells in cell-mediated cytotoxic reactions, *Transplant. Rev.,* 29, 146, 1976.
27. **Bevan, M. J. and Cohen, M.,** Cytotoxic effects of antigen- and mitogen-induced T cells on various targets, *J. Immunol.,* 114, 559, 1975.
28. **Bonavida, B. and Bradley, T. P.,** Studies on the induction and expression of T cell mediated immunity. V. Lectin-induced non-specific cell-mediated cytotoxicity by alloimmune lymphocytes, *Transplantation,* 21, 94, 1976.
29. **Bradley, T. P. and Bonavida, B.,** Mechanism of cell-mediated cytotoxicity at the single cell level. III. Evidence that cytotoxic T lymphocytes lyse both antigen-specific and -nonspecific targets pretreated with lectins or periodate, *J. Immunol.,* 127, 208, 1980.

30. **Gatley, M. K. and Martz, E.,** Comparative studies on the mechanism of nonspecific, Con A-dependent cytolysis and specific T cell-mediated cytolysis, *J. Immunol.,* 119, 1711, 1977.
31. **Green, W. R.,** Studies on the mechanism of lectin-dependent T cell-mediated cytolysis: Use of *Lens culinaris* hemagglutinin A to define the role of lectin, in *Mechanisms of Cell Mediated Cytotoxicity,* 146, Clark, W. R. and Golstein, P., Eds., Plenum, New York, 1982, 81.
32. **Novogrodsky, A.,** Induction of lymphocyte cytotoxicity by modification of the effector or target cells with periodate or with neuraminidase and galactose oxidase, *J. Immunol.,* 114, 1089, 1975.
33. **Schmitt-Verhulst, A.-M. and Shearer, G. M.,** Effects of sodium periodate modification of lymphocytes on the sensitization and lytic phases of T cell-mediated lympholysis, *J. Immunol.,* 116, 947, 1976.
34. **Spitz, H., Yssel, H., Leeuwenberg, J., and De Vries, J. E.,** Antigen-specific cytotoxic T cell and antigen-specific proliferating T cell clones can be induced to cytolytic activity by monoclonal antibodies against T3, *Eur. J. Immunol.,* 15, 88, 1985.
35. **Leeuwenberg, J. F. M., Spitz, H., Tax, W. J. M., and Capel, P. J. A.,** Induction of nonspecific cytotoxicity by monoclonal anti-T3 antibodies, *J. Immunol.,* 134, 3770, 1985.
36. **Hoffman, R. W., Bluestone, J. A., Leo, O., and Shaw, S.,** Lysis of anti-T3-bearing murine hybridoma cells by human allospecific CTL clones and inhibition of lysis by anti-T3 and anti-LFA-1 antibodies, *J. Immunol.,* 135, 5, 1985.
37. **Kranz, D. M., Tonegawa, S., and Eisen, H. N.,** Attachment of an anti-receptor antibody to non-target cells renders them susceptible to lysis by a clone of cytotoxic T lymphocytes, *Immunology,* 81, 7922, 1984.
38. **Perez, P., Hoffman, R. W., Shaw, S., Bluestone, J. A., and Segal, D. M.,** Specific targeting of CTL by anti-T3 linked to anti-target cell antibody, *Nature,* 316, 354, 1985.
39. **Siliciano, R. E., Pratt, J.C., Schmidt, R. E., Ritz, J., and Reinherz, E. L.,** Activation of cytolytic T lymphocyte and natural killer cell function through the T11 sheep erythrocyte binding protein, *Nature,* 317, 428, 1985.
40. **Schrezenmeier, H., Kurrle, R., Wagne, H., and Fleischer, B.,** Activation of human T lymphocytes. III. Triggering of bystander cytoxocity in CTL clones by antibodies against T3 or by a calcium ionophore, *Eur. J. Immunol.,* in press.
41. **Green, W. R., Ballas, Z. K., and Henney, C. S.,** Studies on the mechanism of lymphocyte-mediated cytolysis. XI. The role of lectin in lectin-dependent cell-mediated cytotoxicity, *J. Immunol.,* 121, 1566.
42. **Bonavida, B., Bradley, T., Fan, J., Hiserodt, J., Effros, R., and Wexler, H.,** Molecular interactions in T cell mediated cytotoxicity, *Immunol. Rev.,* 72, 119, 1983.
43. **Golstein, P.,** Sensitivity of CTL to T cell-mediated cytotoxicity, *Nature,* 255, 81, 1974.
44. **Kuppers, R. C. and Henney, C. S.,** Evidence for direct linkage between antigen recognition and lytic expression in effector T cells, *J. Exp. Med.,* 143, 684, 1976.
45. **Fishelson, Z. and Berke, G.,** T lymphocyte-mediated cytolysis: Dissociation of the binding from the lytic mechanism of the effector cells, *J. Immunol.,* 120, 1121, 1978.
46. **Berke, G., Hu, V., McVey, E., and Clark, W. R.,** T lymphocyte-mediated cytolysis. I. A common mechanism for target recognition in specific and lectin-dependent cytolysis, *J. Immunol.,* 127,776, 1981.
47. **Berke, G., McVey, E., Hu, V., and Clark, W. R.,** T lymphocyte mediated cytolysis. II. Role of target cell histocompatibility antigens in recognition and lysis, *J. Immunol.,* 127, 782, 1981.
48. **Sitkovsky, M. V., Pasternack, M. S., and Eisen, H. N.,** Inhibition of CTL activity by Concanavalin A, *J. Immunol.,* 129, 1372, 1982.
49. **Sitkovsky, M. V., Schwartz, M. A., and Eisen, H. N.,** Cell-cell contact proteins in antigen-specific and antigen-nonspecific cellular cytotoxicity, in *Mechanisms of Cell Mediated Cytotoxicity,* Vol. 2., Henkart, P. and Martz, E., Eds., Plenum, New York, 1984, 429.
50. **Parker, W. L. and Martz, E.,** Lectin-induced nonlethal adhesions between cytolytic T lymphocytes and antigenically unrecognizable tumor cells and nonspecific "triggering" of cytolysis, *J. Immunol.,* 124 25, 1980.
51. **Bradley, T. P. and Bonavida, B.,** Mechanism of cell-mediated cytotoxicity at the single cell level. V. The importance of target cell structures in cytotoxic T lymphocyte-mediated antigen in nonspecific lectin-dependent cellular cytotoxicity, *J. Immunol.,* 129, 2352, 1982.
52. **Berke, G., Rosen, D., and Moscovitch, M.,** T lymphocyte-mediated cytolysis. III. Delineation of mechanisms whereby lectins and oxidants mediate lymphocyte-target recognition, *Immunology,* 49, 585, 1983.
53. **Bradley, T. P. and Bonavida, B.,** Studies on the induction and expression of T cell mediated immunity. VII. Inactivation of autologous cytotoxic T lymphocytes when used as both effectors and targets in a lectin-dependent cellular cytotoxic reaction, *Transplantation,* 26, 212, 1978.
54. **Keren, Z. and Berke, G.,** Interaction of periodate-oxidized target cells and cytolytic T lymphocytes: A model system of polyclonal MHC restriction, *Eur. J. Immunol.,* 16, 1049, 1986.
55. **Zehavi-Willner, T. and Berke, G.,** The mitogenic activity of staphylococcal enterotoxin B (SEB): A monovalent T cell mitogen that stimulates cytolytic T lymphocytes but cannot mediate their lytic interaction, *J. Immunol.,* 137, 2682, 1986.

56. **Ballas, Z. K., Green, W. R., and Henney, C. S.,** Studies on the mechanism of T-cell mediated lysis. XIII. Lectin-dependent T cell-mediated cytotoxicity is supported by Con A-coupled Sepharose Beads, *Cellul. Immunol.*, 59, 411, 1981.

57. **Keren, Z. and Berke, G.,** The pathway of lectin-mediated lymphocytotoxicity using Con A coupled Sepharose beads, *Cellul. Immunol.*, 85, 556, 1984.

58. **Keren, Z. and Berke, G.,** Selective binding of Concanavalin A to target cell MHC antigens is required to induce conjugation and lysis by cytolytic T lymphocytes in lectin-dependent cytotoxicity, *Cellul. Immunol.*, 89, 458, 1984.

59. **Bonavida, B. and Katz, J.** Studies on the induction and expression of T cell-mediated immunity. XV. Role of non-MHC papain-sensitive target structures and Lyt-2 antigens in allogeneic and xenogeneic lectin-dependent cellular cytotoxicity (LDCC), *J. Immunol.*, 135, 1616, 1985.

60. **Bonavida, B., Ostergaard H., and Katz, J.,** Mechanism of T-dependent cytotoxicity: Role of papain-sensitive non-Class I target molecules and expression of target antigen for cytotoxicity, in *Mechanisms of Cell Mediated Cytotoxicity*, Vol. 2, Henkart, P., and Martz, E., Eds., Plenum, New York, 1984, 415.

61. **Gromkowski, S. H., Heagy, W., and Martz, E.,** Blocking of CTL-mediated killing by monoclonal antibodies to LFA-1 and Lyt-2,3, *J. Immunol.*, 134, 70, 1985.

62. **Martz, E., Heagy, W., and Gromkowski, S. H.,** The mechanism of CTL-mediated killing: Monoclonal antibody analysis of the role of killer and target-cell mediated proteins, *Immunol. Rev.*, 72, 73, 1983.

63. **Bevan, M. J. and Hyman, R.,** The ability of H-2$^+$ and H-2$^-$ cell lines to induce or be lysed by cytotoxic T cells, *Immunogenetics*, 4, 7, 1977.

64. **Hünig, T.,** Monoclonal anti-Lyt-2.2 antibody blocks lectin-dependent cellular cytotoxicity of H-2 negative target cells, *J. Exp. Med.*, 159, 551, 1984.

65. **Golstein, P., Kelley, F., Avner, P., and Gachelin, G.,** Sensitivity of H-2-less target cells and role of H-2 in T cell-mediated cytolysis, *Nature*, 262, 693, 1976.

66. **Knowles, B. B., Pan, S., Solter, D., Linnenbach, A., Croce, C., and Huebner, K.,** Expression of H-2, laminin and SV-40T and TASA on differentiation of transformed murine teratocarcinoma cells, *Nature*, 288, 615, 1980.

67. **Ostrand-Rosenberg, S.,** H-2 negative teratocarcinoma cells become H-2 positive when passaged in genetically resistant host cells, *J. Immunol.*, 126, 6, 1984.

68. **Bell, S. M. and Stern, P. L.,** Rat natural killer cell and cytotoxic T cell lysis of H-2-negative murine embryonal carcinoma cells, *Eur. J. Immunol.*, 15, 59, 1985.

69. **Aspinall, R. and Stern, P. L.,** Analysis of the xenogeneic T-cell response to Murine H-2 Negative Embryonal Carcinoma Cells, *Immunology*, 54, 549, 1985.

70. **Dourmashkin, R. R., Deteix, P., Simone, C. B., and Henkart, P.,** Electron microscopic demonstration of lesions on target cells membranes associated with antibody-dependent cytotoxicity, *Clin. Exp. Immunol.*, 43, 554, 1980.

71. **Berke, G. and Rosen, D.,** Are lytic granules and perforin 1 thereof, involved in lysis induced by in vivo primed, peritoneal exudate CTL? *Transpl. Proc.*, 19, 412, 1987.

72. **Berke, G. Rosen, D.,** IL-2 mediated induction of lytic granules, perforin, and BLT-esterase in potent, granule-free CTL indicates an alternative function of lytic granules, in *Proc. 18th Leuc. Cult. Conf. 19-24 June, 1987, La Grande Motte.* (Reference incomplete).

73. **Berke, G.,** Lymphocyte-mediated cytolysis. The mechanism whereby early membrane derangements result in target cell death, in Cytotoxic T Cells: Biology and Relevance to Disease, *Proc. N.Y. Acad. Sci. U.S.A.* in press.

74. **Treen, G. and Sitkovsky, M. V.,** *Nature,* (1987) in press.

75. **Ostergaard, H. and Clark, W.,** *J. Immunol.*, (1987) in press.

76. **Ostergaard, H., Kane, K., Mescher, M. and Clark, W.,** *Nature,* (1987) in press.

*Section II.A: Cytolytic Mechanism — Complement*

Chapter 10

# ASSEMBLY AND STRUCTURE OF THE MEMBRANE ATTACK COMPLEX (MAC) OF COMPLEMENT

**Eckhard R. Podack**

## TABLE OF CONTENTS

# I. HISTORICAL PERSPECTIVES

In 1964 Borsos et al.[1] discovered the ultrastructural complement lesions on membranes attacked by complement and presented evidence that these lesions were associated with the cytolytic activity of complement. Studies in 1970 by Lachman and collaborators [2,3] clearly demonstrated that the five terminal complement proteins C5, C6, C7, C8, and C9 were necessary *and* sufficient to form lesions on membranes.

Mayer, in 1972,[4] formulated the "doughnut hypothesis" of complement lysis bringing together, for erythrocyte lysis, the concept of the one hit theory with the ultrastructural observation of membrane lesions. He postulated that the "hit" is achieved by the structure forming the lesion and described it as a "doughnut" that forms a stable pore in the membrane. Lysis of the cell then proceeds by colloid osmotic differences between cell interior and external milieu following ionic equlibration across the transmembrane pore.

The molecular nature of the membrane lesion remained uncertain except that it was known that the five terminal proteins were required for its formation.[2,3] In 1976 Tranum-Jensen and Bhakdi[5] and Podack et al.[6] independently showed that the structure responsible for the membrane lesions is a protein complex of C5b to C9. Yet, it still was controversial how these five proteins could form a tubular complex. Biesecker et al.[8] proposed a dimeric structure $(C5b-9)_2$, whereas Bhakdi maintained the concept of a monomeric complex having essentially the same structure as SC5b-9 complex in solution or when bound to membranes without S-protein.[7]

These controversies were resolved with the discovery that C9 alone, in its polymerized form (Chapter 11), forms complexes akin to the MAC.[9] It became clear that the circular ultrastructural membrane lesion is formed by C9 polymerizing with C5b-8 to form the MAC.[10,11] This molecular concept for the first time allowed the explanation of all previous observations, including complex heterogeneity, differing functional pore sizes and membrane disruption independent of osmotic forces. In 1984 the relationship of C6, C7, C8α-γ, and C9 as transmembrane channel formers in the MAC emerged from studies by Podack,[12] suggesting a common ancestry for these four proteins. Most recent evidence from Podack,[13] Tschopp et al.,[14] and Rao et al.[15] is in support of the molecular model for the MAC shown in Figure 1. Thus from the first observation of membrane lesions to the elucidation of their molecular nature, 20 years of active research were necessary.

# II. STRUCTURE OF THE MAC

Figure 1 shows the current molecular model of the MAC.[12] C9 is polymerized around the C5b-8 complex. The tubular transmembrane part of the MAC is formed by one chain of C6, C7, C8α-γ and 10-16 molecules C9. The precise arrangement of C6, C7, C8α-γ is not known except that they are contained in the rod-like structure of C5b-8 adjacent to and embedded in the membrane, and form part of the MAC tubule. The subunits of C5 (C5bα and C5β) and C8β are apparently not part of the MAC tubule. The tubule is resistant to dissociation by SDS, and those peptide chains not forming it are dissociated upon boiling the MAC in SDS. C6, C7, C8α-γ and poly C9 remain together in an SDS resistant tubular complex with a molecular weight of ~1300 kDalton. In this molecular model the *pore-formers proper* are C6, C7, C8α-γ, and C9, presumably in a heteropolymeric tubular assembly. As will be discussed below, evidence is accumulating to suggest that these four proteins and C8β have arisen together with Perforin 1 (P1) of cytolytic lymphocytes, from an ancestral gene by duplication. The gene products may therefore be considered as members of the perforin family.[13] The subunits of C5b and C8β may, in this context, be defined as helper molecules of complement for the membrane perforating protein family C6, C7, C8α-γ, and C9.

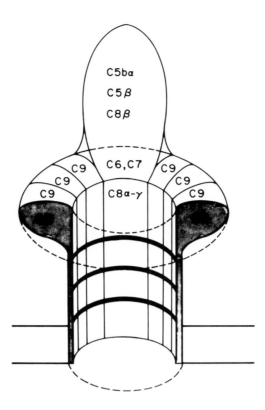

FIGURE 1. Hypothetical model of the structure of the membrane attack complex of complement. The transmembrane tubule is formed by 10 to 16 C9 molecules, one chain of C6, C7, and C8α-γ. The precise arrangement of the latter three peptides is not known. The C8β chain and the chains of C5b are not integrated into the channel but form an attachment to the transmembrane tubule.

## A. Assembly of the MAC: Formation of C5b-8 as the C9 Receptor Complex

MAC assembly is initiated by proteolytic cleavage of C5. C5b remains associated with the membrane through C3b and acts as receptor for C6. The forming C5b-6 complex still is associated with the activating membrane through C3b. Only after binding of C7 to C5b-6 and formation of the amphiphilic C5b-7 complex from the two hydrophilic precursors, is the direct contact of C5b-7 with the membrane established. For the first time in the complement sequence are the complement proteins, i.e., those of C5b-7, anchored via a hydrophobic membrane binding site in the *hydrocarbon core* of the bilayer.

### 1. Formation of Hydrophobic Membrane Binding Domains

The hydrophilic amphiphilic transition through protein-protein interactions and the formation of a hydrophobic membrane combining site are the characteristic and unique biochemical feature of the membrane perforating terminal complement proteins and other proteins of the perforin family. The ability to exist in a hydrophilic environment and to form amphiphilic complexes is the essential functional hallmark of perforins. The amphiphilic transition has been analyzed in detail for C9 (Chapter 11) and clearly is due to a major conformational change of the inserting or perforating proteins upon protein-protein association (Figure 2). The analysis of the insertional complex formation of C5b-7 suggests a similar reaction sequence (Figure 2). Here the reacting poreformers are, in all probability, C6 and C7, thus forming the hydrophobic membrane binding site upon unfolding.[16] The function of C5b is to bind C6 and C7, thus bringing them into close contact and sterically

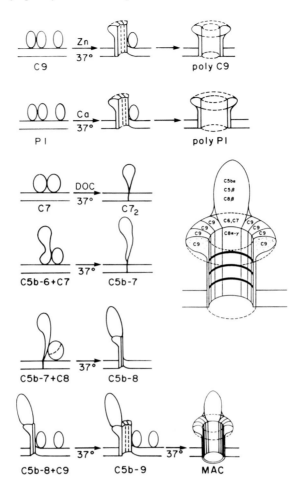

FIGURE 2. Formation of hydrophobic membrane binding sites through protein-protein association and conformational rearrangement (unfolding). The same basic principle is observed (from top to bottom) in: C9 polymerization (C9 unfolding); P1 polymerization (P1 unfolding); C7 dimerization (C7 unfolding); C5b-7 complex formation (C6, C7 unfolding); C5b-8 complex formation (C8α-γ unfolding); and MAC formation (C9 unfolding).

orienting the complex in such a way that the nascent membrane binding site can immediately insert into the bilayer.

### 2. The Binding Site of C5b-7

This hydrophobic site is functionally different from the ones created upon binding of C8 or C9 in that the C5b-7 complex does not, on natural membranes, mediate pore formation. C5b-7 thus is not cytolytically active. This observation would suggest that the hydrophobic tail of C7 is hydrophobic on its entire surface and thus does not cause any significant disturbance in the lipid packing of the membrane. The tendency of C5b-7 to aggregate within the plane of the membrane supports this hypothesis

The complete hydrophobicity of C5b-7's tail is an important functional feature developed late in evolution (see below) that appears to improve the insertional efficiency of the complex.

### 3. The Binding Site of C5b-8

Of the two noncovalently linked subunits of C8, the C8α-γ chain is inserted into the lipid bilayer.[17] The function of C8β is to mediate contact of C8 with C5b-7 (presumably through C5b) and to allow close contact of C8α-γ with C5b-7.[18] The insertion of C8α-γ, in all probability, involves conformational rearrangement and unfolding as described for C7 and C9, mediating close contact between the hydrophobic tail of C5b-7 and C8α-γ and creating a new membrane inserted domain of C5b-8. This domain is different in its functional properties from that formed by C5b-7 in two aspects.

1.  C5b-8 mediates formation of small membrane pores (~12Å diameter) and causes cytolysis in the absence of C9.[19,20] This observation suggests that the hydrophobic domain of C5b-8 is not hydrophobic in its entirety. Similar to unfolded C9, it is probable that one surface of this domain (to be located on the convex side of the MAC-poly C9 tubule) is hydrophobic, whereas the opposite surface (to be located towards the tubule lumen) is hydrophilic. The hydrophilic, but membrane-embedded surface, by repelling lipid molecules may create a functional defect, a pore, in the membrane.
2.  C5b-8 cannot spontaneously insert into membranes like C5b-7. C8 in fact is an inhibitor of C5b-7 mediated lysis, presumably by binding to C5b-7 prior to its insertion and preventing this reaction.[21] This finding is in support of the idea discussed above that C8α-γ forms, at least in part, a hydrophilic surface on the membrane-associated domain of C5b-8 and that this surface prevents membrane insertion. Thus, unfolding and insertion of C8α-γ have to be simultaneous events proceeding in the membrane as is also true for C9.

## B. C9 Polymerization

C5b-8 is the receptor for and accelerator of C9 polymerization. Under similar conditions (normal ionic strength and pH at 37°), spontaneous C9 polymerization requires 2 to 3 days.[9] Zn-mediated polymerization requires 2 to 3 hr,[22] and C5b-8-mediated polymerization requires 2 to 3 min.[23] In addition to accelerating tubular C9 polymerization, C5b-8 directs the site of poly C9 insertion to its own binding site and facilitates C9's insertions into natural membranes, into which C9 alone cannot insert even during polymerization. The mechanism by which C5b-8 induces C9 polymerization is not known. Free C8 has affinity for free C9,[10] and the two proteins form a stoichiometric, reversible complex at low ionic strength. It is probable that C5b-8 also has a single C9 binding site of higher affinity for C9 than monomeric C8. Interaction of C9 with this site may induce the unfolding of C9 and set into motion the chain reaction leading to a tubular poly C9 complex. How C9 unfolding by C5b-8 is achieved is a matter of speculation. Since C5b-8 has hydrophobic sites, it may in some way resemble detergent-mediated C9 polymerization; alternatively, C9 binding to C5b-8 may perturb its tertiary structure sufficiently to cause its unfolding; the possibility has not been excluded that C5b-8 has enzymatic activity and causes cleavage of the one, initially interacting, C9 molecule, thus facilitating its unfolding. The authors's working hypothesis is that C5b-8 imitates an activated (unfolded) C9 molecule and provides a nucleation site for tubule formation just like an unfolded C9 molecule does. This model implies polymerization by physical association without covalent modification of C9. It also implies homologies between C5b-8 peptides and C9.

C5b-8 mediated C9 polymerization gives rise to complexes with various C5b-8 to C9 ratios. The final structure depends on the density of C5b-8, its state of clustering, and on the availability of C9. In addition, local membrane factors may influence the propensity of C9 polymerization by C5b-8. Thus the complex shown in Figure 1 is only one of the possible structures of the MAC that would assemble under idealized conditions of a single C5b-8 bound to a permissive membrane in the presence of excess C9. For detailed discussions of the MAC heterogeneity see chapters 12 and 13 and Reference 40.

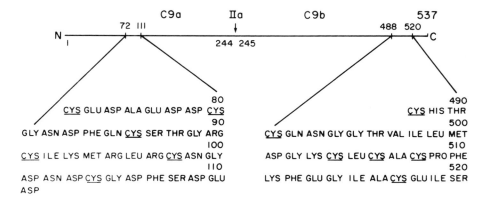

FIGURE 3. Schematic representation of the two cysteine-rich domains of C9.[25] The N-terminal domain (AA #73-111) is homologous to the LDL-receptor, the C-terminal domain (AA #488-520) is homologous to the EGF-receptor-precursor. Evidence is accumulating that these domains are present in C6, C7, C8α, C8β, C9, and Perforin 1.

## Table 1
## PROPERTIES OF MEMBERS OF THE PERFORIN FAMILY

| Name | Mol wt (kDalton) | Cross-reaction with anti C9 | EGFP domain | LDL-R domain | Function |
|---|---|---|---|---|---|
| Perforin 1 (murine) | 70 — 75 | Yes | Yes | ? | Poreformation CTL, NK |
| C9 | 73 | Yes | Yes | Yes | Poreformation complement |
| C8α | 68 | Yes | Yes | Yes | Poreformation, C9-binding |
| C8β | 68 | No | Yes | Yes | C5b-7binding |
| C7 | 110 | Yes | ? | ? | Membrane insertion |
| C6 | 120 | Yes | ? | ? | Membrane insertion |

## III. THE PERFORIN FAMILY OF COMPLEMENT AND CYTOLYTIC LYMPHOCYTES

It is apparent from the discussion above that C6, C7, C8α-γ, and C9, as well as the cytolytic lymphocyte protein perforin 1, have many structural functional features in common. Based on this recognition, Podack[12] first postulated similar structural domains in these proteins. Subsequent analyses by Podack[13] and Tschopp et al.[14] revealed immunological cross-reactivity between C6, C7, C8α-γ, C9 and perforin when the molecules were reduced. Since antiserum raised against reduced C9 reacted also with the reduced LDL-receptor, it was concluded that the cystein-rich domain of C9, which is homologous to similar domains in the LDL-receptor, occurs also in C6, C7, C8α-γ, and perforin 1. Similarly, antigenic evidence suggests that the EGFP type cystein-rich domain (AA #488-520) is present at least in C7 as well as in C9 (Figure 3). Table 1 lists the properties of the individual members of the perforin family known to date.

Recent sequence determination of C8α and perforin 1 directly confirmed these predictions. C8α contains regions that are homologous to C9 AA #75-101, corresponding to the cysteine rich LDL-receptor-like domain, and to AA #488-520, corresponding to the EGFP-domains of C9.[15] C8α, in addition, has a 59% homology region to C9 AA #313-345 which represents a very hydrophobic region. The sequence of C8β was recently obtained. C8β also contains the cysteine-rich domains found in C9 and thus also is a member of the perforin family. Mouse perforin 1 is 27% homologous to human C9, including the cysteine-rich EGFP type domain of C9.[41] Whether P1 also contains the LDL-receptor-like domain has not yet been determined.

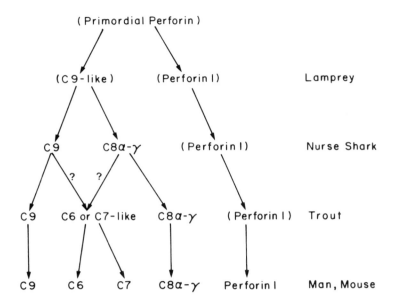

FIGURE 4. Hypothetical evolution of complement and lymphocyte perforins. Proteins in parentheses are inferred. For details see text.

## A. Evolution of the Perforin Family

No studies are available on the presence of P1 in species other than mouse and humans. Thus the discussion on P1 evolution below is conjectural. In contrast, studies on the MAC of complement have been carried out in several species including trout, shark, and lamprey. The picture that is emerging from these studies is summarized in Figure 4. It is postulated that a primordial perforin gene initially duplicated to give rise to a secreted C9-like protein and a cellular perforin. In the lamprey, the C9 like soluble protein is not yet associated with the C3-like opsonin.[25] This association, i.e., the acquisition of cytolytic and pore-forming functions of complement, is achieved in the shark.[26] The MAC in this species is comprised apparently of C8 and poly C9, with C8 presumably directly interacting with C3b. We postulate that the C8α and C8β gene arose from the C9 gene. The association of C8α-γ and C8β provided the basis for the linkage of polymerizing C9 to C3b in the shark.

In the trout,[27] C5b and a C6- or C7-like protein have evolved. C5 clearly came from C3, whereas the C6- or C7-like protein are derived either by duplication of the C9 or the C8α-γ gene. In the mammal, finally, all terminal proteins have evolved. It is obvious from this species comparison that the evolution focused mainly on the insertional reaction of C5b-7. The reason for this may have been to adapt to the increased sophistication of bacterial targets to evade MAC attack at the insertional step. In addition, the stepwise assembly allowed the fine control by S-protein of C9 polymerization and of C5b-7 insertion. It is becoming apparent that control of C9 polymerization may be important for protection of the host from host complement.

## IV. CONTROL OF C9 POLYMERIZATION AND MAC ASSEMBLY

MAC assembly is under the control of soluble and membrane-bound inhibitors. Soluble inhibitors prevent lysis of innocent bystander cells at the site of complement activation and inhibit the futile consumption of C9 in fluid phase. Host-membrane proteins interfere with the action of C9 and protect host cells from accidental complement lysis.

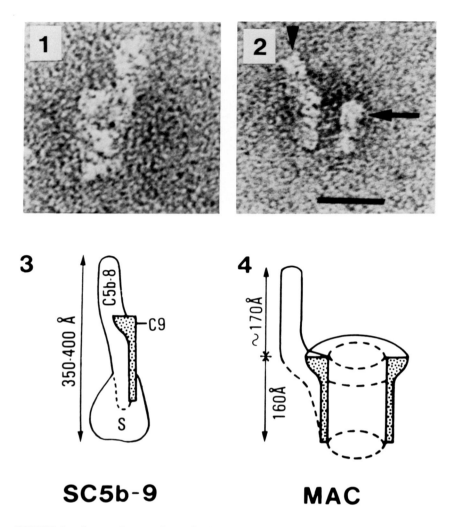

FIGURE 5. Structural comparison of soluble and membrane-associated C5b-9 complexes. (Panel 1 and 3) SC5b-9, lacking the poly C9 tubule; hydrophilic soluble complex. (Panel 2 and 4) MAC, amphiphilic with tubular structure; membrane-associated complex.

## A. Soluble Inhibitors: The S-Protein

Complement activation often occurs on nonmembranous particles, such as immune complexes and carbohydrate-containing cell walls. C5, activated on solid particles, will allow the formation of C5b-7. However, since this complex on these particles lacks a substrate for hydrophobic insertion, the complex is released from the activating particle and may attach to innocent bystander cells.[28] In the presence of C8 and C9, the bystander cells will then be lysed unless insertion of C5b-7 is prevented.

S-protein is a plasma protein with 200 to 300 μg/mℓ concentration, inhibiting bystander lysis. Upon release from activating particles, C5b-7 binds with high affinity to S-protein.[29] Two or three S-protein molecules associate with the hydrophobic combining site of C5b-7, rendering the SC5b-7 complex soluble. SC5b-7 allows the binding of C8 and of two or three molecules C9. C9 polymerization, however, is blocked in the presence of S-protein in the complex.[30,31] Figure 5 shows the structural comparison of SC5b-9 (soluble) with the MAC (amphiphilic). The most obvious difference is the lack of a tubular structure in SC5b-9 owing to the inhibition of C9 polymerization.

## 1. Multiple Functions of S-Protein

In complement, S-protein subserves two functions, as described above. First, inhibition of bystanders lysis by inhibition of C5b-7 insertion, and second, inhibition of C9 polymerization.

In addition, S-protein participates in coagulation by association with thrombin. In the presence of heparin, S-protein protects thrombin from inactivation by antithrombin III.[32] Another function of S-protein is its role as cell adhesion protein. Jenne et al.[33] found that S-protein is identical with vitronectin, a protein that had been isolated, based on its function as cell adhesion factor of plasma.[34,35] S-protein in cell adhesion is functionally similar to fibronectin; however, because of its smaller size (80 kDalton), it is present and can also function in the extravascular space.

The domain structure of S-protein reveals several interesting features. The N-terminal part of the molecule is identical with somatomedin C. This region is followed by the tripeptide Arg-Gly-Asp, which is the ligand for cellular S-protein receptors. Further toward the C-terminus S-protein contains a glycosaminoglycan (heparin) binding site and sites that are potential cleavage sites for thrombin and tryspin. S-protein contains a free sulfhydryl group and can form soluble S-S-linked dimers.[31]

Several observations suggest that S-protein can undergo comformational changes that might expose one or several of the above-mentioned functional domains.

1. Upon binding to C5b-7, S-protein covers up the hydrophobic binding site of this complex. S-protein itself thus must have a hydrophobic domain that becomes available on binding to C5b-7.
2. The heparin-binding site of S-protein is not available in native S-protein, and hence S-protein does not bind to heparin-Sepharose. Upon denaturation of S-protein with urea or upon binding of S-protein to the SC5b-9 complex. S-protein or SC5b-7, respectively, will bind to heparin-Sepharose, suggesting that a conformational change in S-protein exposed the heparin binding site.[36]
3. Numerous cells express S-protein receptors that are different from the fibronectin receptor.[37] It would seem probable that the tripeptide-ligand in S-protein becomes available to receptor interaction only after conformational reorganization of S-protein subsequent to surface adherence or C5b-9 or thrombin-ATIII binding.

The postulated conformational change of S-protein upon complex formation could provide a mechanism for clearance and participation in inflammatory reactions of SC5b-9 and S,IIa, ATIII-complexes, the end-products of complement activation and coagulation.

## B. Membrane Inhibitors: the C8 Binding Protein

Following the initial observation by Hansch et al.,[38] Schoenermark et al.[39] recently described the isolation of a 68-kDalton protein from human erythrocytes named C8 binding protein (C8bp) based on its affinity for C8. This protein seems to protect host cells from the action of complement by interfering with the action of C9. Although the precise details have not been elucidated, C8bp seems to mediate its action in the following way. When C5b-7 becomes bound to human erythrocytes and binds C8 to form the C5b-8 complex, the membrane-bound C8bp interferes with the subsequent action of C9 by blocking C9's polymerization or insertion. The action of C8bp is species-specific: for instance, human C8bp will block human C9 but not guinea pig C9.

C8bp is deficient in paroxysmal nocturnal homoglobinuria type III. This may suggest that C8bp is related to DAF, the decay accelerating factor responsible for the control of the C3-convertase (see chapter 4).

## V. PERSPECTIVES

It is now quite evident that complement and cytolytic lymphocytes use related proteins (C9 and P1) for pore formation and induction of cytolysis. However, despite this similarity, it is also evident that subsequent events leading to bacterial lysis by complement or to nuclear damage by lymphocytes may be quite different. An important helper factor for complement mediated bactericidal activity is lysozyme, which gains access through complement pores to the peptidoglycan layer that then is enzymatically degraded. It is probable that the poly P1 pores are also utilized as an entry mechanism for additional cytolytic lymphocyte factors. These factors may then be responsible for the nuclear damage observed in lymphocyte-mediated nucleated cell lysis. It is thus evident that the formation of a pore in both systems is not in itself the end-point of the cytolytic mechanism, but rather is the initial event leading to the ultimate target death.

## REFERENCES

1. **Borsos, T., Dourmashkin, R. R., and Humphrey, J. H.,** Lesions in erythrocyte membranes caused by immune hemolysis, Nature, 202, 251, 1964.
2. **Lachman, P. J., Bowyer, D. E., Nicol, P. A. E., Dawson, R. M. C., and Munn, E. A.,** Studies on the terminal stages of complement lysis, *Immunology,* 24, 135, 1973.
3. **Hesketh, R. R., Dourmashkin, R. R., Payne, S. N., Humphrey, J. H., and Lachman, P. J.,** Lesions due to complement in lipid membranes, *Nature (London),* 233, 620, 1971.
4. **Mayer, M. M.,** Mechanism of cytolysis by complement, *Proc. Natl. Acad. Sci. USA,* 69, 2954, 1972.
5. **Tranum-Jensen, J., Bhakdi, S., Bhakdi-Lehnen, B., Bjerrum, O. J., and Speth, V.,** Complement lysis; the ultrastructure and orientation of the C5b-9 complex on target sheep erythrocyte membranes, *Scand. J. Immunol.,* 7, 45, 1978.
6. **Podack, E. R. Halverson, C., Esser, A. F., Kolb, W. P., and Muller-Eberhard, H. J.,** SC5b-9: regeneration of the ability to interact with lipid by the selective removal of S-protein, *J. Immunol.,* 120, 492, 1977.
7. **Bhakdi, S., Bhakdi-Lehnen, B., and Tranum-Jensen, J.,** Proteolytic transformation of SC5b-9 into an amphilic macromolecule resembling the C5b-9 membrane attack complex of complement, *Immunology,* 37, 901, 1979.
8. **Biesecker, G., Podack, E. R., Halverson, C. A., and Muller-Eberhard, P. J.,** C5b-9 dimer: isolation from complement lysed cells and ultrastructural identification with complement dependent membrane lesions, *J. Exp. Med.,* 149, 448, 1979.
9. **Podack, E. R. and Tschopp, J.,** Polymerization of the ninth component of complement (C9): formation of poly (C9) with a tubular structure resembling the membrane attack complex of complement, *Proc. Natl. Acad. Sci. USA,* 79, 574, 1982.
10. **Podack, E. R., Tschopp, J., and Muller-Eberhard, P. J.,** Molecular organization of C9 within the membrane attack complex of complement: Induction of circular C9-polymerization by the C5b-8 assembly, *J. Exp. Med.,* 156, 268, 1982.
11. **Tschopp, J., Podack, E. R., and Muller-Eberhard, P. J.,** Ultrastructure of the membrane attack complex of complement: detection of the tetramolecular C9-polymerizing complex C5b-8, *Proc. Natl. Acad. Sci. USA,* 79, 7474, 1982.
12. **Podack, E. R.,** Molecular composition of the tubular structure of the membrane attack complex, *J. Biol. Chem,,* 259, 8641, 1984.
13. **Podack, E. R.,** Perforins: A family of pore forming proteins in immune cytolysis, in *UCLA-Symposium Proceedings: Membrane Mediated Cytotoxicity,* Collier, Bonavida, Eds., Alan R. Liss, New York, 1986.
14. **Tschopp, J., Masson, D., and Stanley, K. K.,** Structural/functional similarity between proteins involved in complement and cytotoxic T-lymphocyte-mediated cytolysis, *Nature (London),* 322, 831, 1986.
15. **Rao, A. G., Howard, O. M. Z., Ng., S. N., Snider, J. V., Whitehead, A. S., Colten, M. R., and Sodetz, J. M.,** Characterization of a cDNA clone encoding the α-subunit the eighth component of human complement (C8), *Abstracts, 6th International Conference of Immunology,* Toronto, 197, 1986.
16. **Preissner, K. T., Podack, E. R., and Muller-Eberhard, H. J.,** The membrane attack complex of complement: relation of C7 to the metastable membrane binding site of the intermediate complex C5b-7, *J. Immunol.,* 135, 445, 1985.

17. **Podack, E. R., Stoffel, W., Esser, A. F., and Muller-Eberhard, H. J.,** Membrane attack complex of complement: Distribution of subunits between the hydrocarbon phase of membranes and water, *Proc. Natl. Acad. Sci. USA,* 78, 4544, 1981.
18. **Monahan, J. B. and Sodetz, J. M.,** Role of the β-subunit in interaction of the eighth component of human complement with the membrane bound cytolytic complex, *J. Biol. Chem.,* 356, 3258, 1981.
19. **Ramm, L. E., Withlow, M. B., and Mayer, M. M.,** Size of the transmembrane channel produced by complement proteins C5b-8, *J. Immuunol.,* 129, 1143, 1982.
20. **Stolfi, R. L.,** Immune lytic transformation: a state of irreversible damage generated as a result of the reaction of the eighth component in the guinea pig complement system, *J. Immunol.,* 100, 46, 1968.
21. **Nemerow, G. R., Yamamoto, K. I., Lint, T. F.,** Restriction of complement mediated membrane damage by the eighth component of complement: a dual role for C8 in the complement attack sequence, *J. Immunol.,* 123, 1245, 1979.
22. **Tschopp, J.,** Circular Polymerization of the membranolytic ninth component of complement: dependence on metal ions, *J. Biol. Chem.,* 259, 10569, 1984.
23. **Tschopp, J., Podack, E.E. and Muller-Eberhard, H. J.,** The membrane attack complex of complement: C5b-8 complex as accelerator of C9 polymerization, *J. Immunol.,* 134, 495, 1985.
24. **DiScipio, R. G., Gehring, M. R., Podack, E. R., Kan, C. C., Hugli, T. E., and Fey, G. H.,** Nucleotide sequence of cDNA and derived amino acid sequence of human complement component C9, *Proc. Natl. Acad. Sci. U.S.A,* 81, 7298, 1984.
25. **Nonaka, M. Fujii, T., Kaidoh, T., Nonaka, M., Sakai, S., and Takahashi, M.,** Purification and characterization of a primordial complement protein (C3) of lamprey, *Immunobiology,* 163, 304, 1983.
26. **Jensen, J. H., Festa, E., Smith, D. S., and Cayer, M.,** The complement system of the nurse shark: hemolytic and comparative characteristics, *Science,* 213, 566, 1981.
27. **Nonaka, M., Yamagudi, N., Natsiumi-Sakai, S., and Takahashi, M.,** The complement system of rainbow trout, *J. Immunol.,* 126, 1487, 1981.
28. **Lint, T. F., Behrends, C. C., Baker, P. J., and Gewurz, H.,** Activation of the complement attack mechanism in the fluid phase and its control by C5b-7 INH: lysis of normal erythrocytes initiated by zymosan, entotoxin and immune complexes, *J. Immunol.,* 117, 1440, 1976.
29. **Podack, E. R., and Muller-Eberhard, H. J.,** Binding of desoxycholate, phosphatidyl choline vesicles, lipo-protein and of the S-protein to complexes of terminal complement proteins, *J. Immunol.,* 121, 1025, 1978.
30. **Podack, E. R., Preissner, K. T., and Muller-Eberhard, H. J.,** Inhibition of C9-polymerization within the SC5b-9 complex of complement by S-protein, *Acta. Path. Microbiol. Immunol. Scand.,* Sect. C, (Suppl. 284), 92, 89, 1984.
31. **Dahlback, B. and Podack, E. R.,** Characterization of human S-protein an inhibitor of the membrane attack complex of complement. Demonstration of a free, reactive thiol group, *Biochemistry,* 24, 2368, 1984.
32. **Podack, E. R., Dahlback, B., and Griffin, J. H.,** Interaction of S-protein of complement with thrombin and antithrombin III during coagulation. Protection of thrombin by S-protein from antithrombin inactivation, *J. Biol. Chem.,* 261, 7387, 1986.
33. **Jenne, D. and Stanley, K. K.,** Molecular cloning of S-protein, a link between complement, coagulation and cell substrate adhesion, *EMBO J.,* 4, 3153, 1986.
34. **Barnes, D. W., and Silnutzer, J.,** Isolation of human serum spreading factor, *J. Biol. Chem.,* 258, 12548, 1983.
35. **Suzuki, S., Oldberg, Å., Hayman, E. G., Pierschbader, M. D., and Ruoslahti, E.,** Complete amino acid sequence of human vitronectin deduced from cDNA. Similarity of cell attachment sites in vitronectin and fibronectin, *EMBO J.,* 4, 2519, 1985.
36. **Barnes, D. W., Reing, J. E., and Amos, B.,** Heparin binding properties of human serum spreading factor, *J. Biol. Chem.,* 260, 9117, 1985.
37. **Pytela, R., Pierschbacher, M. D., and Ruoslahti, E.,** A 125/115 kDa cell surface receptor specific for vitronectin interacts with arginine-glycine-aspartic acid adhesion sequence derived from fibronectin, *Proc. Natl. Acad. Sci. U.S.A,* 82, 5766, 1985.
38. **Hansch, G. M., Hammer, C. H., Vanguri, P., and Shin, M. L.,** Homologous species restriction in lysis of erythrocytes by terminal complement proteins, *Proc. Natl. Acad. Sci. U.S.A,* 78, 5118, 1981.
39. **Schonermark, S., Rauterberg, E. W., Shin, M. L., Loke, S., Roelcke, D., and Hansch, G. M.,** Homologous species restriction in lysis of human erythrocytes: a membrane derived protein with C8 binding capacity functions as an inhibitor, *J. Immunol.,* 136, 1772, 1986.
40. **Podack, E. R.,** The molecular mechanism of cytolysis by complement and cytolytic lymphocytes, *J. Cell Biochem.,* 30, 133, 1986.
41. **Podack, E. R., and Lowrey, D. M.,** Properties and function of cytolytic lymphocyte granules: homology of C9 (complement) and perforin 1. in: Proceedings of the 14th International Cancer Congress, Eckhardt, S., Ed., Elseviers Science, Amsterdam, in press.

Chapter 11

# STRUCTURE AND FUNCTION OF C9 AND POLY C9

## Jürg Tschopp and Eckhard R. Podack

### TABLE OF CONTENTS

## I. INTRODUCTION

Sixty years after the discovery of the complement system,[1] Green et al.[2] showed that complement-mediated cytolysis most likely involved the formation of discrete pores on cell membranes. This conclusion was based on the observation that large molecules, e.g., albumin, could prevent target cell lysis when it was present in high concentration in the medium, while small molecules failed to block lysis. It was concluded that colloid-osmotic swelling and rupture of the membrane was responsible for the lysis of target cells. In 1964, the putative pores were visualized for the first time [3] by electron microscopy of complement-lysed membranes of erythrocytes. Since the concept of the bilayer membrane was to be proposed only eight years later by Singer and Nicholson,[4] the exact molecular nature of these complement "holes" or "lesions" remained unexplained. In 1970, Lachmann and co-workers demonstrated that only the five terminal complement proteins C5-C9[5,6] were required for lesion formation and membrane impairment.

Haxby et al. and Kinsky et al.[7,8] first demonstrated that the lipid bilayer is the target of the five terminal components of complement. Their studies revealed that C5-C9 could directly impair the integrity of pure lipid bilayers independent of enzymatic activity. Since bilayer membranes composed of phospholipid analogues resistant to lipase attack were lysed by C5-C9, a physical rather than chemical destruction of membranes by complement was postulated by these authors.[8,9]

Mayer's foresighted theoretical contribution to the mechanism of complement lysis represents one of the breakthroughs in complement research.[10] Mayer proposed the hypothesis (the "doughnut" hypothesis, as it became to be known) that the complement lesion seen in the electron microscope is formed by a stable, protein-walled pore inserted in the bilayer membrane. This doughnut, stably associated with the lipid bilayer through hydrophobic forces, was postulated to form a transmembrane channel allowing ionic equilibration across the target membrane and resulting in colloid osmotic lysis of the target cell. It was not clear at that time how the five terminal complement proteins might assemble to form this putative pore structure.

Another 10 years of active research were required before C9 was identified as the protein directly responsible for the formation of the ultrastructurally defined membrane lesion.[11] It was shown that C9 alone could polymerize to form complexes structurally similar to those described for the complete C5b-C9 complex. Monomeric precursor C9, upon circular polymerization, undergoes a hydrophilic-amphiphilic transition, allowing it to insert into the lipid bilayer membrane to form the cylindrical transmembrane complex proposed by Mayer's doughnut hypothesis.[10]

The mechanism of channel formation on target cells by polymerizing proteins is not unique for the complement system. Other cytolytic proteins using the same principle are the perforins isolated from cytotoxic T- or NK-cells (see chapter 15, this issue) and bacterial toxins such as *Staphylococcus aureus* α-toxin,[12] aerolysin,[13] and Streptolysin O.[14] More recently, it was reported that the amoeba *N. fowleri* contains a channel-forming cytotoxic protein with properties similar to C9 and perforin.[15]

This review will be limited to a discussion of the molecular action of C9, in particular to the molecular mechanism of pore formation and membrane impairment by this protein. The aspects of C9 as part of the membrane attack complex are the subject of another section of this book.

## II. POLYMERIZATION OF C9

### A. Conditions Favoring C9 Polymerization

C9 is a plasma protein with a concentration of 60 to 70 μg/mℓ.[16,17] It can be isolated in

**Table 1**
**PROPERTIES OF C9 AND POLY C9**

| | C9 | Poly C9 |
|---|---|---|
| Subunits | 1 | 2—19 |
| pI | 4.95[18] | |
| Carbohydrate | 7.8[16]—15%[23,26] | |
| Sulfhydryl groups | 0 | 0.2—0.3[32] |
| Disulfide bonds | 12[23](11)[26] | |
| Molecular weight | (A)77,000 ± 4,000[19] | (C) 1.1 × 10$^6$ ± 150,000[19] |
| | (B)70,000 ± 5,000[19] | (A)1.09 × 10$^6$ ± 118,000[19] |
| | (C)71,000[16] | (E)1.078 × 10$^6$ ± 194,000[19] |
| | (D)79,000[47] | |
| Secondary structure | 24% α-helix | 22% α-helix |
| | 32% β-structure | 38% β-structure |
| Tertiary structure | Sphere-like molecule | Tubular polymer |
| | 4 × 8 nm | Height: 16 nm |
| | | Outer diameter: 21 nm |
| | | Inner diameter: 10 nm |

(A) Sedimentation equilibrium; (B) light scattering; (C) SDS-PAGE; (D) s-rate / diffusion coefficient; (E) electron scattering.

good yield according to procedures published by Biesecker et al.[16] and Luzio et al.[18] C9 is a single-chain, glycosylated protein with an average apparent mol wt of approximately 71,000 (Table 1). The mol wt of monomeric C9 determined by sedimentation equilibrium is slightly higher, i.e., 74,000[19] (Table 1). Monomeric C9 exhibits a high propensity to polymerize circularly into tubular complexes with an inner diameter of 10 mn and a height of 16 mn (Figure 1). The following conditions promote C9 polymerization:

1. **Metal ions and low ionic strength** — In the presence of low concentrations of $Zn^{2+}$ or, less efficiently, $Cu^{2+}$ or $Cd^{2+}$ ions, C9 starts to polymerize at 37°C into circular complexes (Table 2). Lowering the ionic strength in the presence of $Ca^{2+}$ ions also induces circular polymerization, whereas EDTA completely blocks the reaction.[20] The initial observation that C9 polymerization takes place upon prolonged incubation (3 days) at 37°C was probably due to the presence of traces of metal ions in water. Using ultrapure water,[20,21] C9 polymerization was absolutely dependent on the addition of metal ions.

2. **Chaotropic agents** — In the presence of 0.6 *M* guanidine-HCl or 1 *M* urea,[22] C9 forms long linear aggregates with a mean width of approximately 8 nm. These complexes are soluble in buffers without added detergent, indicating that no hydrophobic domains are exposed. By increasing the guanidine-HCl concentration to 4 *M*, the aggregates are dissociated into monomeric C9.[22] Upon rapid removal of the chaotrope, C9's hemolytic activity is completely restored. The complete refolding of C9 is probably due to the structural stability of the cysteine-rich domains present in C9 (see paragraph 4).

3. **Detergents** — The exposure of C9 to various detergents such as deoxycholate, octylglucoside, or NP-40 above their critical micellar concentrations leads to noncircular polymerization of C9.[22] These C9 polymers have exposed hydrophobic domains, since upon detergent removal, they are able to insert into lipid bilayers.

4. **Enzymatic digestion** — Limited digestion of C9 by trypsin cleaves C9 after position 390 [23] (see paragraph 4). Two noncovalently linked fragments with an apparent molecular mass of 53 kDalton and 20 kDalton are generated (Figure 2).[24] C9 nicked by

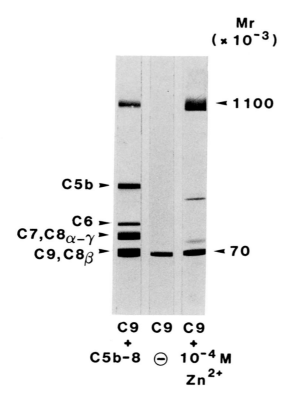
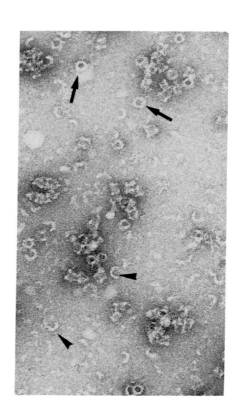

FIGURE 1.    Ultrastructure of C9 (right panel) polymerized in the presence of $10^{-4}$ $M$ ZnCl$_2$.[20] Ot-poly C9 (arrowheads) and ct-poly C9 (arrows) can be distinguished. SDS-polyacrylamide gel analysis of C9, C5b-8, and Zn$^{2+}$ induced C9 polymers. Note the appearance of a high molecular weight band (1.1 MDalton) upon C9 polymerization corresponding to ct- poly C9 (see text). The inner diameter of ct-poly C9 corresponds to 10 nm.

trypsin polymerizes within 8 hr.[24] Tubular complexes are formed with a similar ultrastructure as observed in Zn$^{2+}$ induced C9 polymers (Figure 2). However, the tubular complexes often are not symmetrical in a side view and seem to lack a domain close to C9's lipid interacting site. These complexes still recombine with lipid vesicles using the detergent-dialysis procedure. *Staphylococcus aureus* V8 protease splits C9 close to the N-terminus,[23] and the rate of C9 polymerization of V8-treated C9 is also accelerated.[25] In contrast, C9 cleaved by thrombin after position 244 [23,26] exhibits no increased tendency to polymerize.[24,27] Trypsin- and V8-nicked C9 are also lytically more active. In the case of trypsinized C9, the hemolytic activity increases almost 2.5 times.[24]

5.    **C5b-8 complex** — C5b-8 is the natural inducer of C9 polymerization[28] (see chapter 10). C5b-8 binds one copy of C9 and the consequent restricted unfolding of C9 (see below) induces C9 polymerization.[28,29] Poly C9 and C5b-8 thereby form a tight complex, the membrane attack complex.

The physical environments leading to C9 polymerization are summarized in Table 3. It appears that monomeric C9 has a meta-stable conformation. Agents which destabilize this labile conformation lead to restricted unfolding of C9. Chaotropic agents at low concentration can cause a perturbation of C9's tertiary structure. Detergents may have a similar effect. They may act in addition by shifting the equilibrium of monomeric to unfolded, amphiphilic form of C9, since they can interact with the hydrophobic domain(s) of the latter structure. Enzymes may destabilize C9 by increasing the flexibility of monomeric C9, thereby facil-

## Table 2
### INFLUENCE OF METAL IONS ON C9 POLYMERIZATION

| Metal ion | Residual C9 activity (metal ion conc 13 $\mu M$)[a] (%) | Residual monomeric C9 (metal ion conc 13 $\mu M$)[b] (%) | ct-poly C9[c] | |
|---|---|---|---|---|
| | | | 13 $\mu M$[d] (%) | 65 $\mu M$[d] (%) |
| Mg$^{2+}$ | >85 | ND[e] | <5 | ND |
| Ca$^{2+}$ | >85 | ND | <5 | ND |
| Cu$^{2+}$ | 72 | 75 | 8 | 18 |
| Zn$^{2+}$ | <5 | <5 | 38 | 46 |
| Cd$^{2+}$ | 76 | 78 | <5 | 6 |
| Hg$^{2+}$ | >85 | 82 | <5 | <5 |
| TBS[f] | >85 | >85 | <5 | |
| TBS[g] | 37 | 35 | 35 | |
| EDTA (1 m$M$)[f] | >85 | >95 | <5 | |
| EDTA (1 m$M$)[g] | 58 | 45 | <5 | |
| NaCl (1.15 $M$)[g] | 37 | ND | <5 | |
| NaCl (50 m$M$)[g] | <5 | ND | 70 | |

[a]  13 $\mu M$ corresponds to 1 metal ion per C9 molecule. C9 loses its hemolytic activity upon polymerization.
[b]  Measured by sedimentation velocity analysis.
[c]  Measured by SDS-PAGE; tubular poly C9 is resistant to dissociation by SDS.
[d]  Metal ion concentration.
[e]  ND, not determined.
[f]  Sample incubated 2 hr at 37°C.
[g]  Sample incubated 3 days at 37°C.

itating the unfolding. The decrease in ionic strength favors the amphiphilic form of C9 due to the lowering of the dielectric constant and facilitating C9-C9 contact. In contrast, high ionic strength conditions stabilize the monomeric nature of C9. It is proposed that the *unfolded* C9 exhibits a high affinity for monomeric C9 and can serve as nucleus for further C9 polymerization (see detailed discussion of mechanism in paragraph 4).

## B. Structural Changes Accompanying C9 Polymerization

Monomeric C9 can be seen by electron microscopy as a globular protein with approximate dimensions of 5 × 8 nm.[22] The monomeric molecule often contains a crevice filled with negative stain (Figure 3). Upon polymerization, C9 doubles its length, and tubules with a mean inner diameter of 10 nm and a length of 16 nm are formed. Poly C9 tubules bear a 21 nm wide torus and have a height of 16 nm (Figure 3). In solution the poly C9 tubule form staggered aggregates due to the association of the hydrophobic domains exposed on the end of the poly C9 tubule opposite to the torus. The overlapping site in these aggregates indicates that the hydrophobic part of poly C9 is 4 nm long. Polymeric C9 (poly C9) consists of heterogenous complexes that contain various numbers of protomers in closed or open tubular form, as discussed below.

### 1. Closed Tubular Poly C9 (ct-poly C9)

In ct-poly C9, each C9 has two neighboring C9 molecules, hence ct-poly C9 is extremely stable.[30] It is resistant to dissociation by boiling in 2% SDS even under reducing conditions (Figure 4). Chaotropes at high concentration are also ineffective. The only agent that dissociates ct-poly C9 is guanidine-thio-cyanate (Figure 4). The closed complex is resistant to enzymatic digestion by trypsin. Based on this extreme physical and chemical stability, ct-poly C9 can be isolated in the presence of SDS (Figure 5) in a sucrose gradient.[30] On SDS-PAGE, ct-poly C9 migrates with an apparent mol wt of 1.1 × 10$^6$ (Figure 4 and Figure 5),

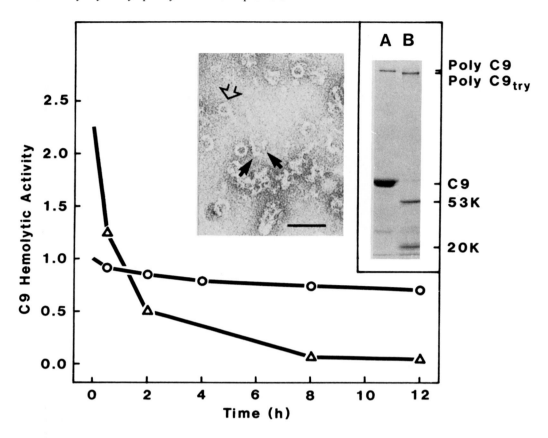

FIGURE 2.   Polymerization of trypsin-nicked C9 (C9try).[24] Native monomeric C9 (○ — ○) and trypsin-treated C9 (△ — △) were incubated at 37°C, and the residual hemolytic activity determined. The ultrastructure of poly C9$_{try}$ is shown in the inset. The two arrows point to poly C9 having different tubular lengths within the same complex. A top view of a poly C9 is shown by an open arrow. The SDS-polyacrylamide gel analysis of C9$_{try}$ (B) and C9 (A) exposed to 37°C for 8 hr, is shown in the other inset. The scale bar corresponds to 50 nm.

## Table 3
### AGENTS MEDIATING C9 POLYMERIZATION

| Agent | Presumed mechanism | Type of C9 polymer[a] | Remark |
|---|---|---|---|
| Detergents | Effect on tertiary structure, binding to hydrophobic crevices | Mostly ot-poly C9 | |
| Chaotropes | Effect on tertiary structure | Linear poly C9 | Polymers hydrophilic, not unfolded ? |
| Metal ions | Increased C9-C9 contact | ct-poly C9 and ot-poly C9 | |
| Decreased ionic strength | Increased C9-C9 contact | ot- and ct-poly C9 | Polymerization at room temperature in presence of Zn$^{++}$ |
| Proteolytic enzymes | Increased peptide backbone flexibility | ot- and ct-poly C9 | |
| C5b-8 | Restricted unfolding of C9 | ot- and ct-poly C9 | Physiological C9-polymerase |

[a]   C9 polymers are categorized as ct- and ot-poly C9 (see text). In ct-poly C9 the tubules are not closed. Linear poly C9 shows little curvature and little tendency to form ring structures.

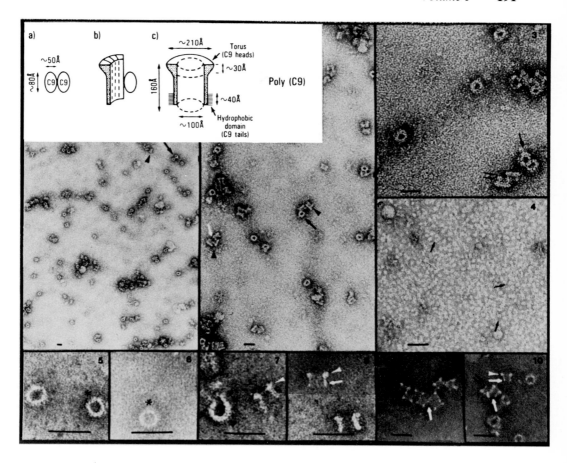

FIGURE 3. Ultrastructure of monomeric C9 (panel 4) and of poly (C9) (other panels). Panels 1 and 2 are low-magnification field views. Panels 3 to 10 are high-mangification views of smaller areas. The scale bars represent 40 nm in each panel. Note the globular structure of monomeric C9 (panel 4) and the presence of stain inside the molecule (black arrows). Poly (C9) (panels 1 to 3 and 5 to 10) appears as ring structure (top view, black arrows) or as rectangular structures (side views, black arrowheads). In side views the torus (C9 heads, panel c, white arrowheads, panels 7, 8, and 10), the hydrophobic segment (C9 tails, panel C, white arrows, panels 2 and 8 to 10), and an intervening segment may be distinguished. Note the overlapping area (parallel black arrows, panels 2, 3, 9, and 10), corresponding to the length of the hydrophobic segment. The inset (a to c) shows a schematic view of polymerizing C9.

and analysis by analytical ultracentrifugation indicates a sedimentation coefficient of $s_{20,w}$ = 27 S. Ct-poly C9 is not a uniform complex. The mol wt of this complex varies from 1.1 × 10⁶ ± 194,000 (SD) as determined by sedimentation equilibrium and electron scattering in the scanning transmission electron microscope.[19] 75% of the complexes contain between 14 to 16 protomers according to the latter methods, but C9 complexes with 11 (lower limit) or 19 (upper limit) are also found. This difference of protomer-number is also reflected in the inner diameter of ct-poly C9, which varies from 9 to 12 nm. Figure 6 shows the image of ct-poly C9 containing different numbers of protomers as revealed by image enhancement using rotational autocorrelation analysis (courtesy Dr. R. Guckenberger, Max-Planck-Institute for Biochemistry, Martinsried, FRG). The observed heterogeneity of ct-poly C9 indicates that the C9-C9 contact is not a completely rigid interaction, but allows a certain degree of flexibility.

## 2. Open Tubular Poly C9 (ot-poly C9)

Using $Zn^{2+}$ to polymerize C9, at most 50% (w/w) of C9 are in the ct-form. The rest are

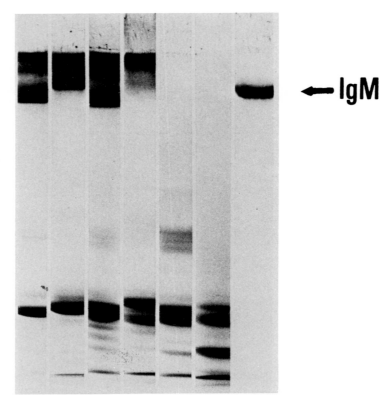

FIGURE 4.    Stability of ct-poly C9 to denaturing agents. SDS-polyacrylamide analysis of poly C9 is shown after the following treatments. Track 1, 2% SDS, 20 m*M*
iodoacetamide for 5 min at 100°C; track 2, 2% SDS, 2% mercaptoethanol for 5 min
at 100%; track 3, 8 *M* guanidine-HCl, 20 m*M* iodoacetamide for 3 hr at 60°C; track
4, 8 *M* guanidine-HCl, 20 m*M* dithiothreitol for 3 hr at 60°C; track 5, 8 *M* guanidine-
thiocyanate, 20 m*M* iodoacetamide, 3 hr at 60°C; track 6, 8 *M* guanidine-thiocyanate,
20 m*M* dithiothreitol for 3 hr at 60°C; track 7, IgM, 2% SDS, 20 m*M* iodoacetamide.
(From Podack, E. R. and Tschopp, J., *J. Biol. Chem.*, 257, 15204, 1982. With
permission.)

circular polymers forming an open or incomplete tubule. These intermediates contain 2 to
approximately 12 C9, and have failed to form a closed tubule, either due to steric circumstances or due to exhaustion of the C9 pool. Ultrastructurally, they have the form of half-
rings or three-quarter rings when analyzed in a top view (Figure 1). Ot-poly C9, in contrast
to the ct-form, is dissociated by SDS (Figure 4) and is sensitive to trypsin digestion.[30]

The unusual stability of poly C9 may be functionally important, since it confers protection
to the physical or chemical degradation of poly C9 by target defence mechanisms after
insertion as cytolytic transmembrane channel. The stability of the tubules is, at least in part,
due to the cysteine-rich domains (see paragraph 4). Poly C9 may further be stabilized by
spontaneous disulfide exchange between adjacent C9 protomers.[31] This process is greatly
accelerated in the presence of low concentrations of glutathione.[32,33] Presumably, glutathione
catalyzes the formation of disulfide bonds through thiol-disulfide exchange.[32]

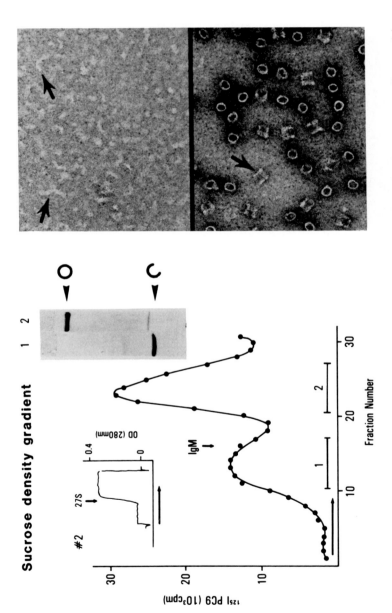

FIGURE 5.    Stability and isolation of ct-poly C9. Poly C9 was solubilized in 2% SDS and then centrifuged on a sucrose gradient containing 1% DOC. Pool 1 corresponds to ot-poly C9, pool 2 to ct poly-C9. SDS-PAGE analysis of the two pools is shown in the inset; the right panel shows the ultrastructure of ot- (top) and ct-poly C9 (bottom) treated with SDS. Ct-poly C9 sediments as a 27S complex in the presence of DOC (inset).

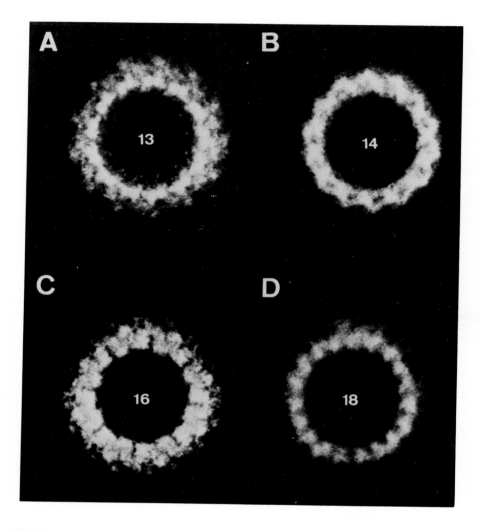

FIGURE 6.    Image enhancement by rotational autocorrelation analysis of ct-poly C9 containing different protomer numbers (In collaboration with Dr. R. Guckenberger, Max-Planck-Institute for Biochemistry, Martinsried, Germany). Complexes with 13, 14, 16, and 18 C9 protomers are shown.

## III. LIPID INSERTION OF C9

### A. Hydrophilic-Amphiphilic Transition

During polymerization, monomeric C9 undergoes a considerable conformational change. It doubles its length from 8 nm to 16 nm and increases the content of β structure from 32 to 38%.[34] The amount of α-helix remains constant. New antigenic sites are exposed during this transition. Several monoclonal antibodies have been described which react only with poly C9 but not with the monomeric form.[35,36] The restricted unfolding of C9 during polymerization exposes hydrophobic domains: poly C9 thus behaves like an integral membrane protein. If polymerization is induced in the presence of single bilayer phospholipid vesicles, lipid insertion of polmerizing C9 occurs.[34] Polymerizing C9 penetrates 4 nm into and across the lipid bilayer. The remaining part of the tubule projects 12 nm above the surface of the lipid bilayer (Figure 7). Poly C9 is stably inserted in the membrane and forms transmembrane channels as evidenced by the following observations:

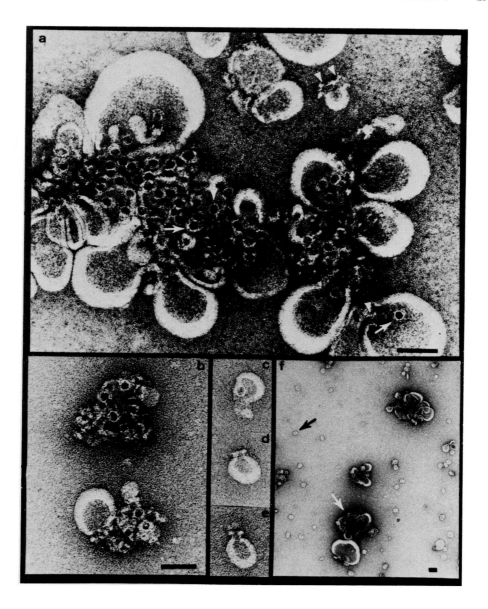

FIGURE 7. Ultrastructure of poly C9-vesicle complexes. Poly C9 was formed in the presence of small unilamellar vesicles at a C9 (monomer) to vesicle ratio of (a) 6:1; (b) 50:1; and (c,d,f) 12:1. For comparison, a MAC-vesicle complex is shown in panel (e). (From Tschopp, J. et al., *Nature*, 298, 534, 1982. Copyright 1982 Macmillan Journals. With permission.)

1. Poly-C9 vesicle complexes float in a sucrose gradient even in the presence of 2 M NaCl.[34]
2. Vesicles carrying poly C9-complexes allow negative stain to enter into the lipid membrane, suggesting a channel size of 10 nm for ct-poly C9 pore. Poly C9-vesicle conjugates release carboxyfluorescein entrapped in the vesicles.[34]
3. C9 inserted into planar lipid bilayers leads to discrete step conductance increases.[37,38] From the conductance an average channel size of 7 nm can be estimated.
4. Using membrane-restricted photoactivatable probes incorporated in the lipid vesicles, polymerizing C9 becomes labeled. Monomeric C9 is only faintly labeled, whereas both ct- and ot-poly C9 interact with the probe[39,40] (Figure 8).

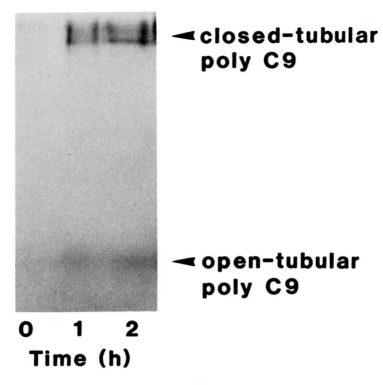

**◄closed-tubular poly C9**

**◄ open-tubular poly C9**

**0     1     2**

**Time (h)**

FIGURE 8.    Lipid insertion of polymerizing C9. C9 was polymerized in the presence of small unilamellar vesicles containing the radioactive, photoactivatable probe TID. Both ct- and ot-poly C9 are labeled after lipid insertion, i.e., after 1 or 2 hr of incubation in the presence of $Zn^{2+}$. Note the absence of labeling of monomeric C9 at time 0.

Figure 9 summarizes these results in schematic form. C9 weakly interacts in its monomeric form with the artificial lipid bilayer. Polymerization can be induced, for instance with $Zn^{2+}$ (see above). C9 starts to polymerize and to insert into the lipid bilayer. Heterogeneous poly C9-complexes are formed, having a protomer number varying from 2 to 19 C9. The two types of tubules, i.e., ct-poly C9 or ot-poly C9 form different types of transmembrane channels. As shown by the membrane-restricted probe [3-(trifluoromethyl)-3-($^{125}$I-iodo-phenyl)]diazirine (TID), both forms are in contact with the hydrocarbon core of the membrane.[39] In the case of ct-poly C9, the inside of the tubule is completely separated from the surrounding lipid bilayer. Hydrophilic surfaces are aligned inside the pore, excluding the lipid molecules from the channel. The hydrophobic domains are aligned at the outside of the tubule, i.e., at the interface of C9 and the lipid bilayer. On the other hand, channels created by ot-poly C9 are delimited by a combination of protein and lipids.[41] Whereas the hydrophobic domains of ot-poly C9 interact with the lipid bilayer, the hydrophilic sites at the inside of the tubule are now exposed to lipids. Lipids will be repelled, allowing membrane channels to form. This mechanism requires that the lipid-protein interaction is extremely strong in order to avoid the ejection of poly C9 due to the energetically unfavorable exposure of hydrophilic sites to the lipids. Different channel sizes will be caused by ot-poly C9 depending on the degree of polymerization.[39,41] This model accounts therefore, at least in part, for the observed functional channel size heterogeneity of the MAC (see Chapter 10).

Although C9 inserts into lipid vesicles, it does not enter into natural membranes such as erythrocyte membranes. Even at very high C9 concentrations, no hemolysis occurs.[34] The presence of C5b-8 on the red blood cell membrane is absolutely required for successful lipid entry of C9. Stanley et al. propose that C5b-8 causes a local fluidization of the membrane,

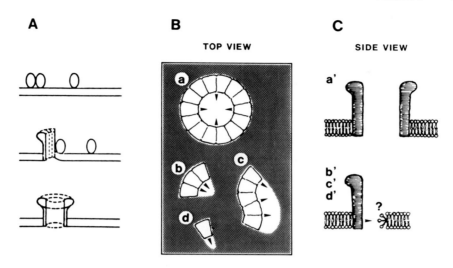

FIGURE 9. Schematic model of C9-lipid insertion and channel formation. (A) Hydrophilic-amphiphilic transition of C9. Monomeric C9 interacts weakly with the bilayer membrane of phospholipid vesicle (a). It then unfolds and polymerizes, thereby exposing hydrophobic domains that insert into the hydrocarbon core (b,c) of the membrane. (B,C) Hypothetical model of transmembrane channel formation by poly C9. (a, a') The inside of tubular poly C9 is devoid of any lipid due to the hydrophilic domains of C9 facing the inside of the protein channel, thus allowing passage of macromolecules of up to 10 nm (protein channel). (b, b') Nontubular poly C9 is bound to the membrane by hydrophobic domains, as shown in (a). The hydrophilic sites aligned on one side are now facing the hydrocarbon core of the lipid bilayer. Lipids are repelled (arrows) and a mixed protein-lipid channel is formed. The structure of the lipid bilayer facing the hydrophilic areas of C9 remains to be determined. It is possible that these mixed protein-lipid channels could form transmembrane channels even with one C9 (d) or with noncircular aggregates (b, c).

forming a small and unstable pore.[42] C9 is allowed to enter into this pore and then rapidly interact with C5b-8. C9 consequently unfolds and polymerizes to form a membrane channel. This hypothesis is supported by Esser et al.,[43] showing that monomeric C9 inserts only into artificial bilayers with low surface pressure. Presumably, C9 inserted in the pore and bound to C5b-8 at 4°C is still in a conformation sensitive to trypsin, suggesting that it has not yet undergone the conformational rearrangement.[44,45]

## IV. AMINO ACID SEQUENCE AND STRUCTURE OF C9

### A. Sequence of C9

cDNA molecules coding for C9 have been recently cloned either by using an expression system in *E. coli*[23] or by means of oligonucleotide probes synthesized according to known parts of the amino acid sequence of C9.[26] The nucleotide-deduced peptide chain is 537 amino acids long (Figure 10), corresponding to a mol wt of 60,700. Since the mol wt of C9 is approximately 71,000, C9 contains presumably 15% carbohydrates, which is considerably higher than the 7.8% oligosaccharide content determined by Biesecker.[16] The majority of carbohydrate is present in the carboxyterminal fragment after limited proteolysis of C9 by thrombin[46] (residues 245 to 837). Two asparagine-linked carbohydrate moieties have been identified at residues 256 and 393.[23] Carbohydrates present in the aminoterminal part of thrombin split C9 (residues 1 to 244) presumably are O-linked and account for 25% of the total content.[46] C9 is synthesized as a pro-C9 including a 21 amino-acid long leader sequence. This leader sequence is typically found in secreted molecules and is cleaved off by the signal peptidase, giving rise to the mature C9 molecule.

Limited digestion of C9 by thrombin[46] or trypsin[24] leads to the formation of two fragments. The amino acid sequences of the carboxyterminal fragment have been partly determined,

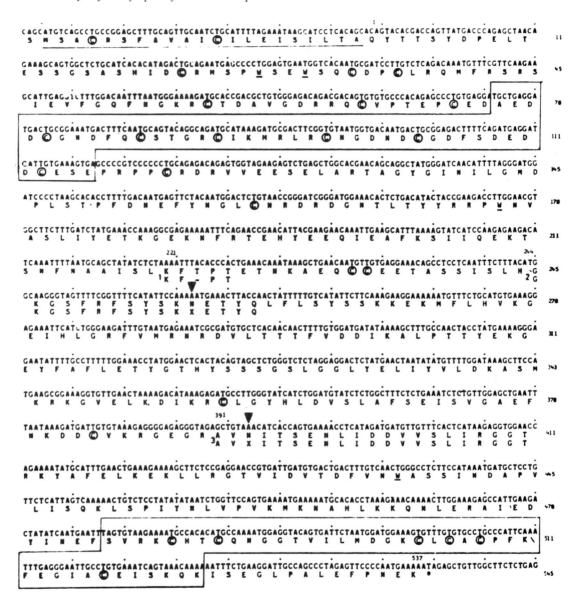

FIGURE 10.    Nucleotide and amino acid sequence of C9. The aminoterminal sequences of fragments generated by chymotrypsin,[1] thrombin,[2] and trypsin[3] are indicated. N-linked carbohydrates are marked by an arrowhead. The sequence most likely corresponding to the leader peptide is underlined. The two cysteine-rich domains are boxed. Cysteine residues are encircled. (From Stanley, K. K. et al., *EMBO J.,* 4, 375, 1985. With permission.)

allowing the localization of the cleavage sites within C9's sequence. Thrombin cleaves between residues 244 and 245. The segment comprising amino acids 1 to 244 is designated C9a, and the segment comprising amino acid 245 to 537 is C9b. Trypsin cleaves after residue 390.

## B. Lipid Binding Site

Although C9 interacts with the lipid bilayer, there exists no long hydrophobic stretch which could account for this interaction as found in other membrane proteins. Thus, C9 interacts with the lipid bilayer with an hydrophobic element present only in the secondary

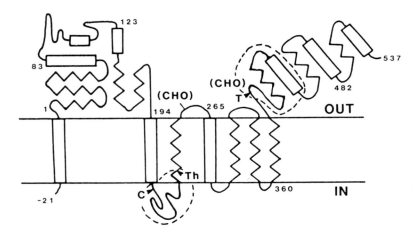

FIGURE 11.  Predicted structural model of C9 as proposed by Stanley et al.[42] The regions predicted to be α-helix are shown as open boxes, whereas β-structures are shown as zigzag lines. Turns, coils or structure without clear prediction are indicated by a simple wavy line. Proteolytic cleavage sites are shown for chymotrypsin (C), α-thrombin (Th), and trypsin (T). N-linked carbohydrate attachment sites are marked with CHO. The regions predicted to be associated with the membrane lie between the horizontal lines.

or tertiary structure. A prediction of the secondary structure of C9 by Stanley[42] and co-workers (Figure 11), suggests that C9 contains an α-helix corresponding to the leader sequence which is highly hydrophobic. According to the algorithm[55] used, there exist at least six other elements of α- or β-structure which presumably are inserted in the lipid bilayer. They are all located in the central part of C9, between residues 197 and 398. Some of these theoretically possible lipid-interacting structures are, however, not in contact with the lipid bilayer:[39,40] the thrombin fragment C9a (residues 1 to 244) is not labeled using the membrane-restricted probe TID. Thus, residues 197 to 244, including one amphiphatic α-helix and one β-structure, can be excluded as possible candidates for membrane-spanning segments. Moreover, the 20 kDalton fragment of trypsin-cleaved C9 (residues 392 to 537) is labeled by the probe, suggesting that other membrane-interacting segments exist in addition to those shown in Figure 11.

## C. Cysteine-Rich Domains

One of the salient features of the C9 sequence is the presence of clustered cysteines. 12 cysteines occur close to the N-terminus, another cluster of 6 cysteines close to the C-terminus, with the remaining 6 cysteines scattered throughout the amino acid sequence. The sequence published by DiScipio[26] places at position 22 an Arg instead of a Cys, as found by Stanley.[23] This reduces the 24 cysteines to an odd number. Since no free sulfhydryl-groups are found[32,47] in native C9, this result indicates that one free sulfhydryl-group has to be blocked. The two published sequences also differ at position 395, where a threonine[26] was found instead of a proline.[23] C9 thus may be synthesized as polymorphic protein.

The cysteine cluster in C9a shows high structural and sequence homology to the cysteine-rich repeat unit of the LDL-receptor (Figures 12, 13). It comprises amino acids 76 to 116 of C9 and is highly negatively charged. This cluster of negative charges is particularly strong in the sequence

Asp-Cys-Gly-Asp-Phe-Ser-Asp-Glu-Asp-Glu-Glu-Cys

which is also the sequence exhibiting the highest homology with the LDL-receptor.[23,48] This

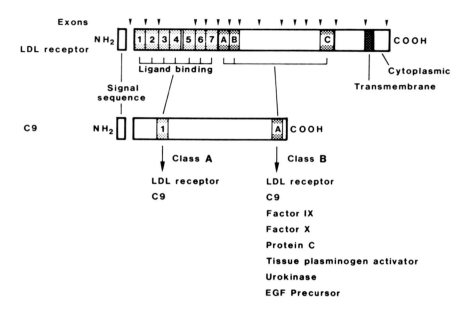

FIGURE 12.   The location of cysteine-rich domains in the LDL-receptor and C9. The exon organization of the LDL-receptor is shown by arrowheads.

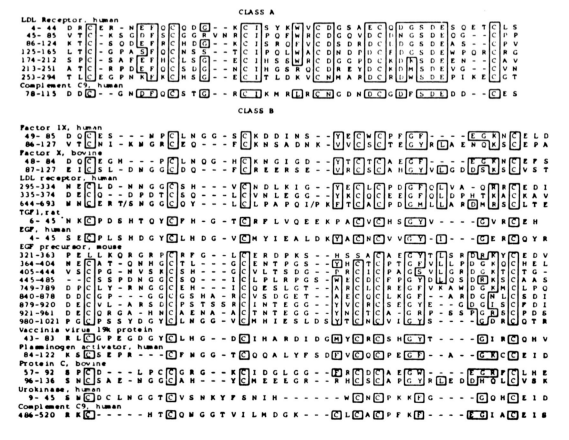

FIGURE 13.   Aligned sequences of cysteine-rich domains of C9 with cysteine-rich segments (see Stanley et al.[42]) of other proteins using six physical parameters.[55]

cysteine-rich domain is thought to be the LDL binding site in the LDL-receptor.[48] Recent studies[49] suggest that this domain exhibits also a functional role in C9, since suramin, an agent abrogating the LDL-receptor-apoprotein interaction,[50] completely inhibits C9 polymerization and suppresses C9 activity on C5b-8-bearing erythrocytes. This particular domain seems to be present also in C8α, reflecting a structural similarity between C8α and C9. Although specific anti-C9 or anti-C8α antibodies do not cross-react, antibodies to the peptide corresponding to the most conserved region of this cysteine-rich domain do.[51]

A second cysteine-rich domain of C9 shows high homology to domains present in epidermal growth factor receptor precursor, LDL-receptor, factor IX, X and protein C of the coagulation cascade, tissue plasminogen activator, urokinase, and other proteins including viral proteins (Figures 12, 13).[52,42] The function of this domain is not known in any of these proteins. In general, these high-cysteine domains are highly stable elements and may occur in proteins as stabilizing elements without other functional significance. Most of the cysteine-rich domains are encoded by individual exons.[48]

## D. A Molecular Model of C9

A battery of monoclonal antibodies to C9 has allowed the characterization of the structure of C9 in more detail.[23] The epitopes recognized by different antibodies were determined by immunoblotting using peptides of C9 generated by enzymatic or chemical proteolysis, as well as bacterially expressed, cloned cDNA fragments.[23] An example is shown in Figure 14, where trypsin- and thrombin-cleaved C9 has been analyzed using two different monoclonal antibodies. Since the exact cleavage points of the two proteolytic enzymes are known, the binding epitopes can be mapped. The overlapping fragments of C9 cleaved by enzymes or BNPS-skatole and expressed hybrid proteins are shown in Figure 14a. Figure 14b shows schematically where the monoclonal antibodies bind. The position of the enzyme cleavage, carbohydrate attachment, and epitope sites define some topological constraints for any model of C9, since

1. All monoclonal antibodies were initially screened with native monomeric C9
2. All enzymes must cleave sites exposed on native C9
3. N-linked oligosaccharide must remain exposed in monomeric and polymeric C9
4. The neoantigens and lipid binding sites must be buried in monomeric C9

It can therefore be deduced that surface structures are clustered in small regions like sections D and F (Figure 15). Monoclonal antibody M34 binds to the C9a portion of C9 and inhibits C9 polymerization,[53] supporting the importance of the high cysteine region of C9a in C9 polymerization and activity. Monoclonal BC5 binds only to the central portion of C9 close to the thrombin clevage site. BC5 binds only to poly C9 and not to monomeric C9, suggesting that drastic conformational changes occur in this part. Indeed, this central part may act as a hinge region during the restricted unfolding of C9 in the C9 polymerization process. M42 and M47 inhibit sucrose efflux when added from the outside, and the recognized epitopes are proposed to be close to the central pore of poly C9.[23,53]

## V. CONCLUSIONS AND PERSPECTIVES

The study of the molecular events during C9 polymerization proved rewarding not only to define better the mechanism of complement-mediated cytolysis but also to reveal a general principle by which cell membranes can be physically impaired. The principle of amphipathic membrane channel-forming complexes generated by the polymerization of lytically inactive, monomeric precursors seems not to be restricted to the complement system. Recently, it was demonstrated that cytotoxic lymphocytes (see Chapter 15) lyse target cells according

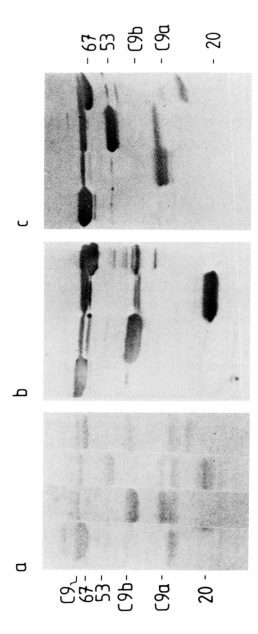

FIGURE 14.   Monoclonal antibody binding to proteolytic fragments of C9. Fragments of C9 were separated by SDS-PAGE and transferred to nitrocellulose. (Panel a) protein stain. (Panel B) immunostain using antibody M42. (Panel) immunostain using antibody M47. Each panel contains (left to right): untreated C9, α-thrombin cleaved C9, trypsin cleaved C9, and *Staphylococcus* V8 protease on C9.

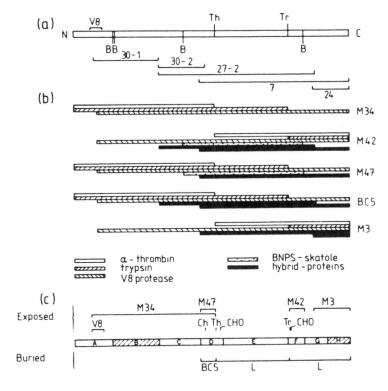

FIGURE 15. Topology of complement component C9. The proteolytic, BNPS-skatole and hybrid protein fragments used in this study are shown in (a). V8, *Staphylococcus* V8 protease; Th, α-thrombin; Tr, trypsin; B, BNPS-skatole cleavage sites. The collated results of Western blots are shown in (b). Each bar represents the size and position of a C9 fragment which binds to the monoclonal antibodies shown. Using these data, the epitopes for five monoclonal antibodies are shown in (c) together with the enzyme cleavage sites, domains containing lipid-interacting sites (L), and probable sites of N-linked oligosaccharide attachment (CHO). Brackets denote areas of the molecule which have been mapped. Exposed and buried refer to the accessibility of features in monomeric C9. (From Stanley, K. K. et al., *EMBO J.*, 4, 375, 1985. With permission.)

to this mechanism, utilizing a protein (perforin) which shares many structural and functional features with C9.

C9 is a mosaic protein, comprising functional or structural domains shared with other proteins. Studies showing the exact roles of these domains in C9 should eventually lead also to the understanding of their functions in other proteins. The genomic structure of C9 may also serve to study the exon-shuffling hypothesis, as proposed by Gilbert.[54] Studies of the structural and functional features of C9 may therefore contribute to the elucidation of other exciting principles of fundamental biological significance.

## NOTE ADDED IN PROOF

The reader is referred to the article of Stanley and Herz[56] for more recent data and references on the structure and function of C9.

## ACKNOWLEDGMENTS

We are grateful to Dr. Keith Stanley for allowing us to discuss some of his unpublished results (see Figures 11 and 13). We thank E. Burnier, Z. Freiwald, and R. Etges for their excellent assistance. J. Tschopp is supported by a grant from the Swiss National Science Foundation (No. 3.163-0.85) and E. R. Podack by USPH grants NIH AI 21999, CA 39201, and American Cancer Society Grant IM 396.

# REFERENCES

1. **Bordet, J.,** Les leucocytes et les propriétés actives du serum chez les vaccinés, *Ann. Inst. Pasteur,* 9, 462, 1895.
2. **Green, H. P., Barrow, P., and Goldberg, B.,** Effect of antibody and complement on permeability control in ascites tumor cells and erythrocytes, *J. Exp. Med.,* 110, 699, 1959.
3. **Borsos, T., Dourmashkin, R. R., and Humphrey, J. H.,** Lesions in erythrocyte membranes caused by immune hemolysis, *Nature,* 202, 251, 1964.
4. **Singer, S. J. and Nicholson, G. L.,** The fluid mosaic model of the structure of cell membranes, *Science,* 175, 720, 1972.
5. **Lachmann, P. J. and Thompson, R. A.,** Reactive lysis: the complement-mediated lysis of unsensitized cells. II. The characterization of activated reactor as C56 and the participation of C8 and C9, *J. Exp. Med.,* 131, 643, 1970.
6. **Lachmann, P. J., Munn, E. A., and Weissmann, G.,** Complement-mediated lysis of liposomes produced by the reactive lysis procedure, *Immunology,* 19, 983, 1970.
7. **Haxby, J. A., Kinsky, C. B., and Kinsky, S. C.,** Immune response of a liposomal model membrane, *Proc. Natl. Acad. Sci. U.S.A.,* 61, 300, 1968.
8. **Kinsky, S. C., Bonsen, P. P. M., Kinsky, C. B., Van Deenen, L. L. M., and Rosenthal, A. F.,** Preparation of immunologically responsive liposomes with phosphonyl and phosphinyl analogs of lecithin, *Biochim. Biophys. Acta,* 233, 815, 1971.
9. **Lachmann, P. J., Bowyer, D. E., Nical, P., Dawson, R. M. C., and Munn, E. A.,** Terminal stages of complement lysis, *Immunology,* 24, 135, 1973.
10. **Mayer, M. M.,** Mechanism of cytolysis by complement, *Proc. Natl. Acad. Sci. U.S.A.,* 69, 2954, 1972.
11. **Tschopp, J. and Podack, E. R.,** Membranolysis by the ninth component of human complement, *Biochem. Biophys. Res. Commun.,* 16, 1409, 1981.
12. **Bhakdi, S., Füssle, R., and Tranum-Jensen, J.,** *Staphylococcus* α-toxin. Oligomerization of hydrophilic monomers, *Proc. Natl. Acad. Sci. U.S.A.,* 78, 5475, 1981.
13. **Howard, P. and Buchley, J. T.,** Membrane glycoprotein receptor and hole-forming properties of a cytolytic protein toxin, *Biochemistry,* 21, 1662, 1982.
14. **Bhakdi, S., Roth, M., Sziegoleit, A., and Tranum-Jensen, J.,** Isolation and identification of two hemolytic forms of Streptolysin-O, *Infect., Immun.,* 46, 394, 1984.
15. **Lowrey, D. and Podack, E. R.,** Purification and characterization of N.perforin from *Nagleria fowleri* in UCLA-Proceedings: Membrane Mediated Cytotoxicity, Bonavida, B., Collies, R. J., Eds., Alan R. Liss, New York, in press.
16. **Biesecker, G. and Müller-Eberhard, H. J.,** The ninth component of human complement: purification and physicochemical characterization, *J. Immunol.,* 124, 1291, 1980.
17. **Bhakdi, S. and Tranum-Jensen, J.,** On the cause and nature of C9-related heterogeneity of terminal complement complexes generated on target erythrocytes through the action of whole serum, *J. Immunol.,* 133, 1453, 1984.
18. **Morgan, B. P., Daw, R. A., Siddle, K., Luzio, J. P., and Campbell, A. K.,** Immunoaffinity purification of human complement component C9 using monoclonal antibodies, *J. Immunol. Methods,* 64, 269, 1983.
19. **Tschopp, J., Engel, A., and Podack, E. R.,** Molecular weight of poly C9: 12 to 18 molecules form the transmembrane channel of complement, *J. Biol. Chem.,* 259, 1922, 1984.
20. **Tschopp, J.,** Circular polymerization of the membranolytic ninth component of complement: dependence on metal ions, *J. Biol. Chem.,* 259, 10569, 1984.
21. **Dankert, J. R., Shiver, J. W., and Esser, A. F.,** Ninth component of complement: self aggregation and interaction with lipids, *Biochemistry,* 24, 2754, 1985.
22. **Podack, E. R. and Tschopp, J.,** Polymerization of the ninth component of complement: formation of poly C9 with a tubular ultrastructure resembling the membrane attack complex of complement, *Proc. Natl. Acad. Sci. U.S.A.,* 79, 574, 1982.
23. **Stanley, K. K., Kocher, H. P., Luzio, J. P., Jackson, P., and Tschopp, J.,** The sequence and topology of human complement component C9, *EMBO J.,* 4, 375, 1985.

24. **Tschopp, J., Amiguet, P., and Schäfer, S.,** Increased hemolytic activity of the trypsin-cleaved ninth component of complement, *Mol. Immunol.*, 23, 57, 1986.

25. **Tschopp, J.,** unpublished data, 1985.

26. **DiScipio, R. G., Gehring, M. R., Podack, E. R., Kan, C. C., Hugli, T. E., and Fey, G. H.,** Nucleotide sequences of cDNA and derived amino acid sequence of human complement component C9, *Proc. Nat. Acad. Sci. U.S.A.*, 81, 7298, 1984.

27. **Dankert, J. R. and Esser, A. F.,** Proteolytic modification of human complement protein C9: loss of poly (C9) and circular lesion formation without impairment of function, *Proc. Natl. Acad. Sci. U.S.A.*, 82, 2128, 1985.

28. **Tschopp, J., Podack, E. R., and Müller-Eberhard, H. J.,** The membrane attack complex of complement: C5b-8 complex as accelerator of C9 polymerization, *J. Immunol.*, 134, 495, 1985.

29. **Sims, P. J.,** Complement protein C9 labeled with fluorescein isothiocyanate can be used to monitor C9 polymerization and formation of cytolytic membrane lesion, *Biochemistry*, 23, 3248, 1984.

30. **Podack, E. R. and Tschopp, J.,** Circular polymerization of the ninth component of complement-ring closure of the tubular complex confers resistance to detergent dissociation and to proteolytic degradation, *J. Biol. Chem.*, 257, 15204, 1982.

31. **Ware, C. F. and Kolb, W. P.,** Assembly of the functional membrane attack complex of human complement: formation of disulfide-linked C9 dimers, *Proc. Natl. Acad. Sci. U.S.A.*, 78, 6426, 1981.

32. **Yamamoto, K. I. and Migita, S.,** Mechanisms for the spontaneous formation of covalently linked polymers of the terminal membranolytic complement protein (C9), *J. Biol. Chem.*, 258, 7887, 1983.

33. **Yamamoto, K. I., Kawashima, T., and Shunsuka, M.,** Glutathione-catalyzed disulfide-linking of C9 in the membrane attack complex of complement, *J. Biol. Chem.*, 257, 8573, 1982.

34. **Tschopp, J., Müller-Eberhard, H. J., and Podack, E. R.,** Formation of transmembrane tubules by spontaneous polymerization of the hydrophilic complement protein C9, *Nature (London)*, 298, 534, 1982.

35. **Falk, R., Dalmasso, A. P., Kim, Y., Tsai, Ch. H., Scheinman, J. I., Gewurz, H., and Michael, A. F.,** Neoantigen of the polymerized ninth component of complement, *J. Clin. Invest.*, 72, 560, 1983.

36. **Mollnes, T. E., Lea, T., Harboe, M., and Tschopp, J.,** Monoclonal antibodies recognizing a neoantigen of poly (C9) detect the human terminal complement complex in tissue and plasma, *Scand. J. Immunol.*, 22, 183, 1985.

37. **Mayer, M., Micheals, D. W., Ramm, L. E., Withlow, M. B., Willoughby, J. B., and Shin, M. L.,** Membrane damage by complement, *Crit. Rev. Immunol.*, 2, 133, 1981.

38. **Young, J. D. E., Cohn, Z. A., and Podack, E. R.,** The ninth component of complement and the pore-forming protein (perforin 1) from cytotoxic T cells: structural, immunological, and functional similarities, *Science*, 233, 184, 1986.

39. **Amiguet, P., Brunner, S., and Tschopp, J.,** The membrane attack complex of complement: lipid insertion of tubular and non tubular poly C9, *Biochemistry*, 24, 7328, 1985.

40. **Ishida, B., Wisnieski, B. J., Lavine, C. H., and Esser, A. F.,** Photolabeling of a hydrophobic domain of the ninth component of human complement, *J. Biol. Chem.*, 257, 10551, 1982.

41. **Tschopp, J.,** Ultrastructure of the membrane attack complex of complement: heterogeneity of the complex caused by different degrees of C9 polymerization, *J. Biol. Chem.*, 259, 7857, 1984.

42. **Stanley, K. K., Page, M., Campbell, A. K., and Luzio, J. P.,** A mechanism for the insertion of complement component C9 into target membranes, *Mol. Immunol.*, in press.

43. **Esser, A. F., Dankert, J. R., Hensen, J. P., and Leung, K. P.,** Membrane insertion of C9 requires "non ordered" lipid bilayer, *Complement*, 2, 23, 1985.

44. **Boyle, M. D. P., Langone, J. J., and Borsos, T.,** Studies on the terminal stages of immune hemolysis. IV. Effect of metal salts, *J. Immunol.*, 122, 1209, 1979.

45. **Boyle, M. D. P., Langone, J. J., and Borsos, T.,** Studies on the terminal stages of immune hemolysis. III. Distinction between the insertion of C9 and the formation of a transmembrane channel, *J. Immunol.*, 120, 1721, 1978.

46. **Biesecker, G., Gerard, C., and Hugli, T. E.,** An amphiphilic structure of the ninth component of human complement. Evidence from analysis of fragments produced by thrombin, *J. Biol. Chem.*, 257, 2584, 1982.

47. **Hadding, U. and Müller-Eberhard, H. J.,** The ninth component of human complement: isolation, description and mode of action, *Immunology*, 16, 719, 1969.

48. **Südhof, T. C., Goldstein, J. L., Brown, M. S., and Russel, D. W.,** The LDL receptor gene: a mosaic of exons shared with different proteins, *Science*, 228, 815, 1985.

49. **Tschopp, J.,** unpublished

50. **Daniel, Th. O., Schneider, W. J., Goldstein, J. L., and Brown, M. S.,** Visualization of lipoprotein receptors by ligand blotting, *J. Biol. Chem.*, 258, 4606, 1983.

51. **Tschopp, J. and Mollnes, T. E.,** Antigenic cross-reactivity of C8α with the "cysteine-rich" domain shared by C9 and LDL-receptor, *Proc. Natl. Acad. Sci. U.S.A.*, in press.

52. **Doolittle, R. F.,** The genealogy of some recently evolved vertebrate proteins, *TIBS*, 10, 233, 1985.

53. **Morgan, B. P., Luzio, J. P., and Campbell, A. K.,** Inhibition of complement induced 14C sucrose release by intracellular and extracellular monoclonal antibodies to C9: evidence that C9 is a transmembrane protein, *Biochem. Biophys. Res. Commun.,* 118, 616, 1984.
54. **Gilbert, W.,** Why genes in pieces?, Nature, 271, 501, 1978.
55. **Zalkin, H., Argos, P., Narayana, S. V. L., Tiedeman, A. A., and Smith, J. M.,** Identification of a trp G-related glutamine amidine transfer domain in *Escherichia coli* GMP synthetase, J. Biol. Chem., 260, 3350, 1985.
56. **Stanley, K. K. and Herz, J.,** Topological mapping of complement component C9 by recombinant DNA techniques suggests a novel mechanism for its insertion into target membranes, *EMBO J.,* 6, p. 951, 1987.

Chapter 12

# PORE SIZE OF LESIONS INDUCED BY COMPLEMENT ON RED CELL MEMBRANES AND ITS RELATION TO C5b-8, C5b-9, AND POLY C9

**Agustin P. Dalmasso and Barbara A. Benson**

## TABLE OF CONTENTS

## I. INTRODUCTION

The membrane attack complex (MAC) of complement is composed of the terminal complement proteins C5b through C9. Two different general mechanisms may participate in the production of the cytolytic effect of the MAC on target membranes. One involves removal of lipids from the target membrane and is a consequence of the high affinity of the MAC for membrane lipids. The other mechanism is due to channel formation in the target membrane. It appears that the MAC can generate two different types of transmembrane channels. One is a "lipid channel" which is caused by the binding of membrane lipids to the components of the MAC, resulting in disorganization of the lipid bilayer, with channel formation at the interphase between the MAC-bound lipids and the lipid bilayer. The other type consists of tubular structures composed of polymers of C9 (poly C9) which penetrate the membrane and function as "protein channels". In addition to forming protein channels, because of the high affinity for membrane lipids, the poly C9 structure may also create lipid channels.

Both mechanisms of MAC-induced lysis may have significant roles under different circumstances, particularly with different target membranes. The complement-induced channels impair the permeability properties of the membrane and seem to play the major role in lysis of certain cell types like the erythrocyte. Because of the high intracellular colloid-osmotic pressure, water penetrates into the cell resulting in rapid cell swelling, secondary membrane rupture, and cell lysis.[1,2] On the other hand, removal of membrane lipids has been proposed as the mechanism of lysis for certain bacteria and viruses that do not have a sufficient colloid-osmotic gradient with the extracellular fluid to undergo osmotic lysis.[3] Lipid removal may also play a major role in lysis of nucleated cells, which are generally resistant to complement lysis and require large amounts of MAC for cell death. Removal of the MAC by exocytosis and endocytosis results in severe loss of membrane lipids, compromising the viability of the cell.[4] In addition, channel formation by membrane-bound MAC that escape endocytosis or exocytosis may contribute to the lysis of a cell that has been injured sublethally by the MAC-mediated removal of membrane lipids.

Knowledge about the pore size of the complement channels becomes particularly important in view of the different mechanisms involved in the production of membrane damage by complement. In this paper we will discuss different approaches that have been taken to establish the pore size of the complement lesion on red cell membranes, the available information in relation to the various components of the MAC, as well as the influence of other factors on the pore size of the complement lesion. Current interpretations of pore size estimates will be presented with regard to the possible mechanisms of production of complement lesions.

## II. APPROACHES TO INVESTIGATE THE PORE SIZE OF THE COMPLEMENT LESION

In these studies it is essential to exclude the possible influence of secondary membrane disruptions due to colloid-osmotic lysis. The initial studies were carried out with intact red cells that were treated with complement and protected from colloid-osmotic swelling with high concentrations of macromolecules such as bovine serum albumin (BSA) or Dextrans to equalize the osmotic pressure inside and outside the red cells.[1,2] Removal of the protective molecule allows swelling and lysis to occur and the extent of complement damage can be determined from the amount of hemoglobin released. From the effective diffusion diameter of the macromolecules that are able to provide osmotic protection it is possible to estimate the pore size of the complement lesion. This approach has been extended to the study of lesions in intact red cells treated with limiting amounts of complement and therefore expected to develop small lesions. Red cells are treated with complement in the presence of a protective

**Table 1**
**MOLECULES USED FOR ESTIMATING THE**
**FUNCTIONAL PORE SIZE OF COMPLEMENT**
**LESIONS**

| Marker molecule | d (nm)[a] | Marker molecule | d (nm) |
|---|---|---|---|
| Rb$^+$ (hydrated) | 0.46 | Dextran 10 | 4.7 |
| Inositol | 0.70 | Ovalbumin | 5.5 |
| Glucose | 0.72 | Hemoglobin | 6.2 |
| Sucrose | 0.88 | Dextran 20 | 6.4 |
| Raffinose | 1.14 | BSA | 7.2 |
| Cyanocobalamin | 1.7 | Dextran 40 | 8.5 |
| Inulin | 2.8 | Aldolase | 9.6 |
| Ribonuclease A | 3.6 | IgA | 11.4 |
| Carbonic anhydrase | 4.6 | Apoferritin | 12.2 |

[a]  d = effective diffusion diameter. The numbers given are twice the Stokes radii, without correction for the asymmetry of the molecules.

macromolecule, washed and suspended in 0.3 *M* of a monosaccharide or oligosaccharide solution. If the solute is unable to pass through the lesion, the cell remains osmotically protected; if the solute is small enoght to pass through the lesion, the cell will swell and lyse.[5] Again, the effective diffusion diameter of the solute is used to estimate the pore size. Experiments have also been performed by measuring the rate of influx of radiolabeled marker molecules into the complement-treated red cells in the presence of osmotic protection with large macromolecules.[6]

A second approach uses resealed red cell ghost membranes which retain the selective membrane permeability of the intact cell but contain only a small fraction of the original hemoglobin.[7] Generally, a mild degree of colloid-osmotic swelling after complement treatment is prevented with a low concentration of albumin in the buffer solution. Resealed membranes and intact erythrocytes are damaged by complement in an identical manner, as shown by the observation that under various conditions of complement treatment the release from membranes of small radioactive molecules, such as sucrose, was similar to the release of hemoglobin from red cells.[8] Pore size determination by molecular sieving is based on the use of a set of marker molecules of known effective diffusion diameters. The pore size is estimated to be between the diameter of the largest molecule that is able to diffuse through the lesion and the smallest molecule that can not pass through it. Measurements of either efflux or influx of radiolabeled molecules can be used. For efflux studies the marker molecules are trapped inside the membranes during the resealing process, followed by treatment with complement.[8-11] For influx studies, complement-treated membranes are suspended in solutions containing the radiolabeled marker molecule, and the rate of entrance into the membranes is then measured.[12,13] Enhancement of marker uptake inside the membranes can be achieved by enclosing, during resealing, antibodies against the marker of interest.[14] Since with moderate doses of complement, IgG is too large to pass through the pore, the antibody will bind the marker molecules that enter the membranes, preventing them from diffusing back out. Nonelectrolyte, spherical molecules are best suited for pore size estimation. Because Dextran molecules are highly asymmetric, proteins have often been used as probes for pores in the 3 to 12 nm diameter range. A list of the molecules that have been used to estimate the pore size of complement lesions is given in Table 1, with the corresponding effective diffusion diamters in nm.

The pore size of the complement lesion has also been studied with artificial membranes. Hapten-bearing liposomes with internal marker molecules have been treated with specific antibody and complement, and the release of the markers has been measured.[15,16] Dye penetration through the complement lesion has been ascertained by electron microscopy.[17] Transmembrane channels have been studied by measurement of electrical conductance across these complement-treated bilayers.[16,18-20]

## III. PORE SIZE HETEROGENEITY OF THE COMPLEMENT LESION

The first studies with osmotic protection of red cells indicated that the functional lesion had a diameter between 4.5 and 6.0 nm, since Dextran 20 or BSA but not Dextran 10 prevented cell lysis.[1,2] Although estimates based on the effective diffusion diameter could not be considered accurate because the Dextran molecules are very asymmetric, the observation was useful and essentially correct for sheep red cells treated with relatively large doses of complement. Further studies to define the pore size of the effective complement lesion demonstrated a high degree of heterogeneity, with diameters from ~0.6 to ~12.0 nm.[5,9] The most important variable responsible for this high degree of heterogeneity was the concentration of complement used to treat the membranes.[9,16]

Molecular sieving experiments from resealed membranes treated with whole human complement at moderate to high concentrations indicated a minimum lesion diameter of 4.0 to 5.5 nm and an upper limit of 11.0 nm with very large complement concentrations.[8-10] However, under conditions of limiting complement concentration, either with whole complement or with assembly of the MAC from purified components, the estimated size of the functional lesion was much lower and exhibited considerable heterogeneity, with pore size diameters down to ~0.6 nm.[5,9,11] With limiting amounts of complement, in particular low concentrations of C9, few lesions were formed.[9,11] Studies on the rate of marker influx through complement lesions formed with limiting complement indicated that even small molecules, sucrose or raffinose, do not diffuse freely through the channel.[6,12,13] Although from the kinetics of sucrose exchange the diameter of the effective lesion was calculated to be 2.3 nm, it was concluded that the functional lesion could be as small as 0.6 to 1.2 nm in diameter.[6] The presence of very small lesions 0.7 to 1.1 nm in diameter was confirmed using osmotic blockers of differing size.[5]

Studies with artificial membranes also showed that the complement lesion consists of discrete channels of varying size. Marker release from liposomes indicated a pore diameter of at least 3 nm, releasing glucose and inulin but not macromolecular proteins.[15,16] Conductance measurements on planar lipid bilayers showed the complement lesion to be 1.0 to 4.0 nm, with an average diameter of 2.4 nm.[16] Although the observed fluctuations in current and the increase in current with added C9 are indicative of lesions of varying size, it was postulated that they could in part be due to opening and closing of the channels.[19,20] Although this mechanism might apply to the smaller channels, it does not appear to be pertinent to the larger channels that might be related to poly C9 and are very stable, with lesions persisting up to 72 hr.[10,11,21]

## IV. RELATIONSHIP OF PORE SIZE TO THE LYTIC EFFECT OF C8, C9, AND POLY C9 IN THE MEMBRANE ATTACK COMPLEX

Complement channels can develop in biological membranes at three of the final steps of MAC assembly. Very small channels are formed upon binding of C8 to membrane associated C5b-7. Small channels develop with the binding of one C9 molecule to the C5b-8 complex. Larger channels are generated when additional molecules of C9 are bound to the C5b-8 complex or when C5b-9 complexes coalesce. Finally, the largest channels may be formed with generation of poly C9. The physicochemical nature of most types of complement channels may be the result of membrane lipid rearrangement in the vicinity of the MAC.[3]

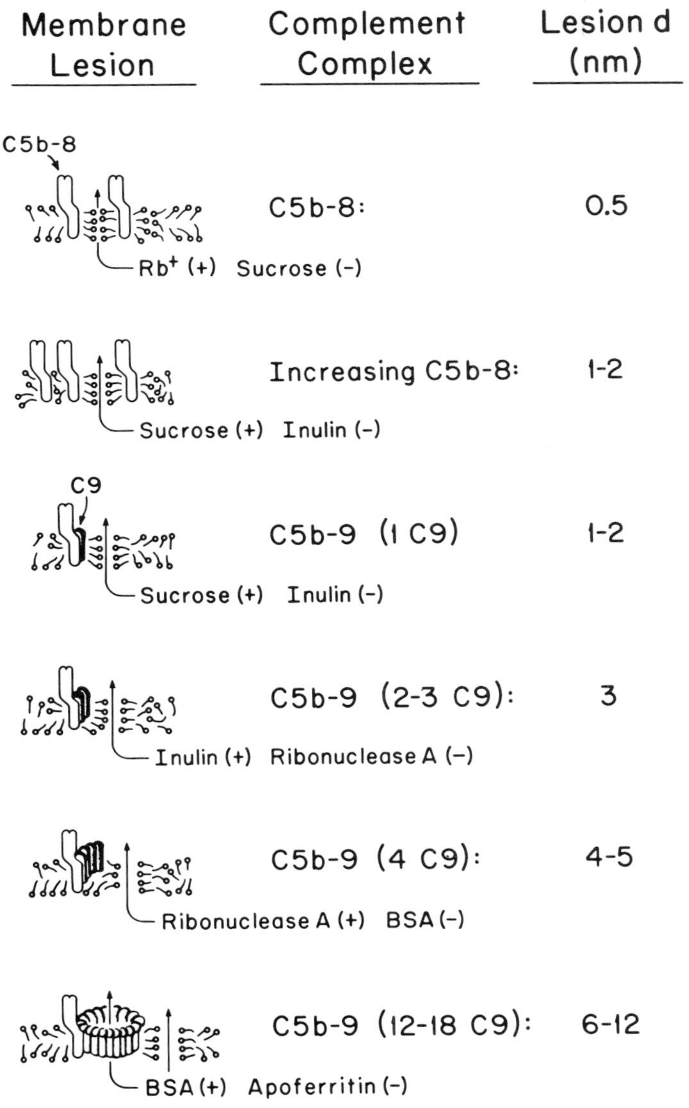

| Membrane Lesion | Complement Complex | Lesion d (nm) |
|---|---|---|
| C5b-8 Rb⁺ (+) Sucrose (−) | C5b-8: | 0.5 |
| Sucrose (+) Inulin (−) | Increasing C5b-8: | 1-2 |
| C9 Sucrose (+) Inulin (−) | C5b-9 (1 C9) | 1-2 |
| Inulin (+) Ribonuclease A (−) | C5b-9 (2-3 C9): | 3 |
| Ribonuclease A (+) BSA (−) | C5b-9 (4 C9): | 4-5 |
| BSA (+) Apoferritin (−) | C5b-9 (12-18 C9): | 6-12 |

FIGURE 1. Schematic representation of possible complement channel structure in red cell membranes generated by different complexes of the complement attack proteins. Results of molecular efflux studies were used to obtain estimates of lesion size.

Because of its high affinity for lipids, also poly C9 might be able to generate channels through rearrangement of membrane lipids. In addition, poly C9 might be able to form very large functional channels through the interior walls of the poly C9 protein tubule.[22] Figure 1 shows an interpretation of complement channel structure and size according to molecular sieving experiments in resealed red cell membrane ghosts treated with progressively larger complexes of the terminal complement proteins.

Assembly of the MAC begins with the generation of the C5b fragment and subsequent attachment of the C5b-7 complex to the cell membrane.[23] At this point there is little perturbation of the membrane lipid bilayer,[24] no effective lytic channel, and no ultrastructural lesion, except for a membrane-bound protein stalk.[25] Addition of C8 increases the lipid binding capacity of the complex,[24] and though no visible lesion is formed beyond a thickening on the protein stalk near the membrane,[25] there is movement of ions across the membrane shown by $Rb^+$ release.[26] Hemolysis proceeds very slowly, after a considerable delay.[27] It has been shown that some C5b-8 sites will form small lesions in 2 to 3 hr but require 4 to 5 times longer for small molecules, such as sucrose, to reach equilibrium.[28] The amount of cell-bound C8 required for an effective lytic lesion in the absence of C9 is large, and lysis is dependent on the number of C5b-7 sites available since only one molecule of C8 is bound to the complex.[29] Experiments with planar lipid bilayers indicate that the C5b-8 channels have an average diameter of 1.6 nm and open and close continuously.[19,20]

Addition of C9 results in stabilization of the channel, increase in the lipid binding capacity of the complex,[24] rapid red cell lysis, and the visible classical ultrastructural lesion associated with complement.[25] Kinetic evaluation of hemolysis caused by C5b-8 indicates the participation of multiple bound complexes is needed in contrast to C5b-9 mediated hemolysis where a few complexes containing one C9 molecule per complex is sufficient. While incorporation of one C9 molecule into the C5b-8 complex is sufficient to generate a lytic lesion, the effective size of the lesion has been shown to increase with the multiplicity of bound C9.[5,30-33] Dose response molecular sieving studies with increasing amounts of C9 indicate that the channel formed with one C9 molecule in the C5b-9 complex is 0.9 to 2 nm in diameter. Incorporation of 2 or 3 C9 molecules increases the size to 3 nm and binding of 4 molecules results in channels of at least 4 nm[30,31] (Figure 1). This is in accordance with the mathematical model of size heterogeneity that assumes progressively larger channels are formed as C9 molecules are added to the complex.[32] The calculated pore diameter when 3 C9 molecules are bound is 1.1 to 1.5 nm, significantly smaller than the 3 nm observed by molecular sieving; however, it is clear that C9 multiplicity is a factor in lesion heterogeneity. The C5b-9 channel is stable for long periods of time to the exchange of marker molecules, at least 3 hr and up to 72 hr with very slow loss of effective lesions.[10,11,21] However, patch conductance measurements of ion flux indicate that the C9 dependent channel flickers open and closed, and the values measured are time-averaged flux through multiple pores of varying sizes.[20] This observation could correlate the large estimated lesion size with the observed low rate of marker exchange through the lesion and may be a factor in the increase of marker flux with more bound C5b-9 complexes.[34]

By using C8, C9-depleted serum reconstituted with C8 and C9 at high C9 to C8 ratios it was possible to bind 12 to 16 molecules of C9 per complex.[22] However, addition of purified C9 to saturate existing C5b-8 complexes results in the binding of only 3 to 4 molecules of C9 in the MAC.[35] With excess purified C9, it was shown that sucrose-permeable and sucrose-impermeable ghosts have similar ratios of C9 to C8 of about 3.0, thus not all bound C9 form functional lesions.[29] In whole serum, where C9 is present in limited amounts with respect to C8, 2 to 3 molecules of C9 are bound in the MAC at low doses of serum. Cells treated under these conditions, when examined by electron microscopy, showed incomplete poly C9 rings and large areas of patchy protein deposition.[33] The C5b-9 pore in complexes containing an average of 3 C9 molecules is an asymmetrical channel with an inner diameter ranging from 3 to 6 nm.[25] At higher concentrations of serum, 6 to 9 molecules of C9 were bound to the C5b-8 complex; addition of C9 to low doses of serum allowed the formation of large-sized lesions, and the density of poly C9 rings increased.[33] The variations reported in the membrane bound C9 to C8 ratio appear to be dependent on the experimental conditions. Saturation of C5b-8 sites with purified C9 gives ratios of 3 to 4, while generation of the lesion in the presence of excess C9 in serum gives higher ratios of 6 to 16. High miltiplicity of C9 binding and release of the large marker molecules from target ghost membranes seem to occur with large doses of whole complement. This was interpreted as a requirement of tubular poly C9 to express the larger lesions. Recent studies with thrombin-cleaved C9 (C9$^n$), which is unable to form completely closed poly C9 tubules but remains hemolytically active, demonstrated that C9$^n$ is able to form lesions capable of releasing inulin (3 nm diameter).[36]

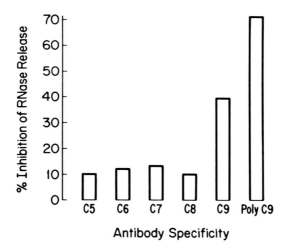

FIGURE 2. Inhibitory effect of antibodies to terminal complement components upon the efflux of ribonuclease (RNase) from resealed sheep red cell ghost membranes treated with human complement proteins. IgG factions from goat antisera to C5, C6, C7, C8, and C9 at 300 mg protein/mℓ were incubated with $2 \times 10^8$ complement-treated ghost membranes for 90 min at 37°C. The anti-poly C9 was monoclonal antibody to a neoantigen of poly C9 and was used as described before.[39] Other experimental conditions were as published in Reference 39.

The ability of C9[n] to form the largest lesions, 5 to 10 nm diameter, has not been investigated. The C9[n] is more efficient than native C9 in the release of small markers from ghost membranes, since half the number of membrane bound C9[n] compared to intact C9 is able to achieve the same degree of release.[36] More C9 is required to increase the lesion size, but tubular poly C9 formation does not seem essential for lesions in the 0.6 to 4 nm range.

Although all five terminal complement proteins, C5b, C6, C7, C8, and C9, are necessary to assemble a functional lesion on a cell membrane, under certain conditions purified C9 alone is able to spontaneously polymerize into circular structures resembling the classical complement lesion.[22,37] Poly C9 can be formed in liposomes, allowing the release of markers and dye penetration into the vesicle.[37] Studies with polyclonal antibodies to the terminal complement components indicate that only antibodies to determinants on C9 are able to inhibit the passage of marker molecules through an existing complement channel.[38] As shown in Figure 2, the release of ribonuclease A (3.6 nm diameter) from ghost membranes by C5b-9 complex assembled from purified components was not inhibited by antibodies to C5, C6, C7, or C8 but was significantly inhibited by antibodies to C9. Binding studies showed that antibodies to each terminal component bound efficiently to complement-treated membranes.[38] A monoclonal antibody that reacts with a neoantigen in poly C9 but not with native C9 also caused inhibition of ribonuclease efflux.[38] Other experiments with monoclonal antibodies to several different determinants on native C9 also showed inhibition of marker release by these antibodies, depending on whether they were present outside or inside the resealed membranes.[39] Thus C9 is an asymmetrical transmembrane protein and the one protein in the attack complement most closely associated with the lesion. The C5b-8 site on the membrane bilayer serves to bind the C9 molecule and accelerates the polymerization of C9 in the attack complex,[22,40] but does not seem to be an integral part of the poly C9 structure, since protein cross-linking experiments of the MAC produced no covalently linked complexes of C8 and C9.[41,42]

## V. PORE SIZE HETEROGENEITY AND THE MECHANISM OF COMPLEMENT MEMBRANE ATTACK

Any model to explain the effects of complement on membranes must take into consideration the pore size of the lesions induced by complement on red cells and other types of membranes. Of paramount importance is that the pore size of the lesion can span a diameter of ~0.6 nm to ~12.0 nm, an approximately 20-fold difference between the smallest and the largest lesion (Figure 1). This wide range is related primarily to the number of MAC per cell membrane and the C9 to C8 ratio. Pore size heterogeneity can be readily explained by a "leaky patch" model, as discussed by Esser[3,43] and Sims.[29] This model was based on the observation of an increasing affinity for phospholipids that the MAC expresses during the progression of its assembly[24] and on the disorganization of lipid bilayers that complement is capable of producing.[43] The strong interaction between MAC and membrane lipids would result in reorganization of the lipid bilayer and loss of the permeability barrier in areas surrounding the MAC. According to this mechanism, increases in lesion size are possible by expansion or overlapping of the disorganized areas. Binding of few C5b-8 complexes to the bilayer produces some disorganization of the bilayer, but does not yield a functional lesion. The presence of large numbers of C5b-8 complexes and the resulting overlap of their "spheres of influence" in a cooperative manner can generate small lesions. Addition of one C9 molecule to the complex increases the lipid-binding capacity of the complex, and, as more C9 molecules are incorporated, the area of lipid rearrangement increases, followed by larger effective lesions. Multiple bound MAC can also interact and result in overlapping areas of bilayer disorganization, giving larger lesions. With this model the effect of the target membrane on lesion size (see Section VI) could result from different binding affinities of the MAC for the different lipids present in the membrane. Thus a membrane comprised of a high percentage of phospholipids with a very high affinity for the MAC would have more bilayer disorganization and larger lesions than a membrane whose lipids react weakly with the MAC.

The high degree of pore size heterogeneity of the complement lesion is a major obstacle for accepting a protein channel, as for example in the "doughnut" model,[16] as the sole mechanism of complement mediated lysis. However, because complete tubular structures of poly C9 have been demonstrated to behave as functional channels,[37,44] it is possible that the larger complement lesions may be related to a protein channel. This would be in agreement with the observation that the upper limit of the pore size of complement lesions in red cell membranes correlates with the diameter of the lesions measured by electron microscopy.[9] It is known that these complement structures are due to poly C9.[22] On the other hand, C9 is the component of the MAC that is most intimately related to the functional lesion, as demonstrated by inhibition of marker molecule efflux from resealed ghost membranes with anti-C9 but not with antisera to the other MAC proteins.[38,39] The observation that inhibition of efflux of the relatively large marker molecules ribonuclease A and BSA (3.6 and 7.2 nm diameter, respectively) could be obtained with a monoclonal antibody to a neoantigen of poly C9 suggests that the poly C9 protein channel may be functional in complement-treated red cell membranes.

## VI. OTHER FACTORS AFFECTING THE PORE SIZE OF THE COMPLEMENT LESION

The heterogeneity of the complement lesion pore size does not depend exclusively on the number of membrane-bound MAC and the quantitative relationship among C5b-7, C8, and C9. The following additional factors may be able to affect the pore size of the complement lesion: the intracellular and extracellular cationic composition, the species of complement,

**Table 2**
**COMPARISON OF THE CAPACITY OF HUMAN AND**
**GUINEA PIG COMPLEMENT TO INDUCE EFFLUX OF**
**MARKER MOLECULES FROM RESEALED SHEEP RED**
**CELL GHOST MEMBRANES**

| | % Marker released with:[a] | | | |
|---|---|---|---|---|
| Marker molecule | 5% Human serum | 50% Human serum | 0.5% Guinea pig serum | 50% Guinea pig serum |
| Sucrose | 97.6 | 99.7 | 83.1 | 93.7 |
| Ribonuclease | 63.2 | 97.4 | 73.8 | 91.5 |
| Bovine serum albumin | 10.9 | 90.9 | 1.5 | 8.4 |
| IgA | 6.9 | 50.8 | 0 | 7.8 |
| Apoferritin | 4.2 | 4.2 | ND | ND |

[a] Percent marker release was measured after complement treatment for 90 min at 37°C. Experimental conditions are given in Reference 8. ND, not done.

the species of the red cell membranes, and the fluidity of the lipid bilayer of the target cell membrane.

The pore size of the lesion induced by C5b-9 on resealed red cell membranes containing high potassium concentration (HK) was found to be enlarged when extracellular $K^+$ was substituted for $Na^+$.[45] It was known that a proportion of the HK red cells that remain unlysed after treatment with limited concentrations of complement in extracellular $Na^+$ are lysed upon further incubation in extracellular $K^+$.[46,47] This observation implied that the $K^+$ effect could not be mediated by an enhancement in the uptake of the terminal complement proteins, which has recently been confirmed by directly measuring the uptake of radiolabeled components.[45] The enhancing effect of extracellular $K^+$ upon lysis of HK red cells can be abrogated with extracellular $Li^+$ at concentrations as low as $6 \times 10^{-5} M$.[47] This action of $Li^+$ is most probably mediated through an effect on the pore of the C9 dependent lesion. It is not known why, in contrast to HK red cells, red cells containing a low $K^+$ concentration are only minimally affected by changes in the extracellular cationic composition.[46,48]

Measurement of the complement lesion under the electron microscope gave distinctly different values depending on the species of complement used to treat the cell. Both guinea pig and rabbit complement produced, on sheep red cell membranes, lesions with an internal diameter of 8.0 to 8.8 nm, whereas larger lesions of about 10.3 nm were obtained with human complement.[49] Under conditions of limiting complement, the observed lesion size by molecular sieving or osmotic protection did not seem to differ with species of complement. However, with large doses of serum, the maximum lesion size on sheep red cell membranes was dependent on the source of complement (Table 2). While a large dose of human complement resulted in lesions up to 11 nm in diameter, allowing the release of IgA, similar doses of guinea pig complement produced lesions only 7 nm in diameter.[9] These results correlated with previous measurements of the ultrastructural lesions. It is not known if the formation of lesions of different functional size by human or guinea pig complement is caused by differences in the binding of C9 to the 5b-8 complex or is dependent on other properties of the bound C5b-9 complex.

The species of the target membrane was also found to affect the lesion size.[50] Release of markers from resealed erythrocyte ghosts of different species, rabbit and human, by sheep complement indicated two distinctly different patterns of lesion size. Under the conditions used, few small lesions were formed with either target membrane, since release of marker

## Table 3
## EFFECT OF THE TARGET MEMBRANE ON THE
## EFFLUX OF MARKER MOLECULES FROM
## COMPLEMENT TREATED RESEALED RED CELL
## GHOST MEMBRANES[a]

| | % Marker released with: | | | |
| | Rabbit membranes | | Human membranes | |
| Marker molecule | 10% Serum | 50% Serum | 10% Serum | 50% Serum |
| --- | --- | --- | --- | --- |
| Sucrose | 95.7 | 96.6 | 98.1 | 99.5 |
| Ribonuclease | 90.8 | 94.9 | 93.7 | 97.3 |
| Bovine serum albumin | 45.6 | 85.3 | 6.0 | 7.5 |
| IgA | 17.5 | 50.7 | 2.3 | 2.6 |
| Apoferritin | 7.1 | 5.4 | ND | ND |

[a]  Resealed ghost membranes were prepared from rabbit or human red cells and used
at $2 \times 10^8$/m$\ell$. They were reacted with sheep complement via the alternative
pathway in the presence of 8 m$M$ EGTA and 2 m$M$ MgCl$_2$ for 90 min at 37°C.
Other methodological details are given in Reference 8. ND, not done.

molecules of small size and intermediate size was almost complete, irrespective of the dose
of sheep complement. However, there were significant differences in the release of the large
marker molecules (Table 3). Human membranes did not allow the formation of lesions larger
than 7 nm even at high doses of serum, whereas in rabbit membranes lesions greater than
7 nm with a maximum diameter of 11 nm were readily formed. Therefore, while effective
lesion size may be dependent on the number of C9 molecules bound per C5b-8 complex,
other factors can affect the observed distribution of lesion size. Possibly the ability of C9
molecule to insert themselves into the membrane bilayer is the limiting factor since this
would allow both the source of complement and the target membrane to affect lesion
formation.

Treatment of red cell membranes with complement, particularly the terminal proteins C8
and C9, results in significant changes in the lipid organization, with a reduction in membrane
fluidity.[51] This decrease in fluidity was still observed when limited cross-linking of the
membrane proteins was carried out with glutaraldehyde, prior to complement treatment.[52]
However, higher doses of glutaraldehyde made the membrane lipid bilayer more rigid, and
no further fludity change could be observed upon interaction with complement. Under these
conditions there was no reduction in the release of marker molecules. In fact, the release
of the large carbohydrates inulin and Dextran 20 was enhanced in the more rigid membranes,
even though the number of bound MAC was similar to untreated membranes.[53] The lesions
formed by the same dose of complement were larger in membranes with a more rigid bilayer
than in the more fluid untreated membranes.

## VII. CONCLUSIONS

As the result of studies from several laboratories, the following conclusions can be made
regarding the pore size of the lesion induced by complement on red cell membranes:

1.   Under defined conditions of complement treatment the lesions that develop have discrete pore size.
2.   By varying the conditions of complement treatment, lesions with pore diameters of

~0.6 nm to ~12.0 nm have been described, which represent approximately a 20-fold difference between the larger and smaller lesions. This is of major relevance in considering models for the mechanism of membrane damage by complement.

3.  Very small lesions may develop with large amounts of bound C5b-8, but not with C5b-7.

4.  The pore size of the lesion increases with increasing multiplicity of bound C9 per C5b-8 complex or with increasing numbers of bound MAC per membrane.

5.  Physically, C9 is intimately related to the complement channel, as shown by the observation that anti-C9, but not antisera to C5, C6, C7, or C8, inhibits the efflux of marker molecules through the complement lesion from resealed ghost membranes.

6.  C9 is inserted in the membrane as a transmembrane protein and forms polymers containing up to 16 molecules of C9 (poly C9). However, polymerized C9 forming incomplete tubules is sufficient for generation of small- to large-size channels.

7.  Although completely polymerized tubular poly C9 can function as a channel in model membrane system, its biological role remains unclear.

8.  The pore size is affected by the intracellular and extracellular cationic composition. In particular red cells with a high $K^+$ content develop much larger channels in $K^+$ than in $Na^+$ media.

9.  The pore size of the complement lesion can be affected by the species of complement. Thus, the maximum pore size produced on sheep red cell membranes has a diameter of 11 nm with human complement, but only 7 nm with guinea pig complement.

10. The pore size is also affected by the species of origin of the target red cell membrane. With sheep complement, the maximum pore size has a diameter of 11 nm with rabbit membranes and only 7 nm with human membranes.

11. Changes in fluidity of the red cell membrane lipid bilayer affected the pore size of the lesion, such that larger lesions appeared in membranes with a more rigid bilayer.

## VIII. ACKNOWLEDGMENTS

We wish to thank Lori Geiser for typing the manuscript. The studies that were carried out in the authors' laboratory were supported by funds from the Veterans Administration.

## REFERENCES

1.  **Green, H. P., Barrow, P., and Goldberg, B. G.,** Effect of antibody and complement on permeability control in ascites tumor cells and erythrocytes, *J. Exp. Med.*, 110, 699, 1959.

2.  **Sears, D. A., Weed, R. J., and Swisher, S. N.,** Differences in the mechanism of in vitro immune hemolysis related to antibody specificity, *J. Clin. Invest.*, 43, 975, 1964.

3.  **Esser, A. F.,** Interactions between complement proteins and biological and model membranes, in *Biological Membranes*, Chapman, D., Ed., Academic Press, New York, 1982, 277.

4.  **Morgan, B. P., Campbell, A. K., Luzio, J. P., and Hallett, M. B.,** Recovery of polymorphonuclear leucocytes from complement attack, *Biochem. Soc. Trans.*, 12, 779, 1984.

5.  **Boyle, M. D. P., Gee, A. P., and Borsos, T.,** Studies on the terminal stages of immune hemolysis. VI. Osmotic blockers of differing Stokes' radii detect complement-induced transmembrane channels of differing size, *J. Immunol.*, 123, 77, 1979.

6.  **Li, C. K. N. and Levine, R. P.,** Molecular transport via the functional complement lesion, *Mol. Immunol.*, 17, 1465, 1980.

7.  **Schwoch, G. and Passow, H.,** Preparation and properties of human erythrocyte ghosts, *Mol. Cell. Biochem.*, 2, 197, 1973.

8.  **Giavedoni, E. B., Chow, Y. M., and Dalmasso, A. P.,** The functional size of the primary complement lesion in resealed erythrocyte membrane ghosts, *J. Immunol.*, 122, 240, 1979.

9. **Dalmasso, A. P. and Benson, B. A.,** Lesions of different functional size produced by human and guinea pig complement in sheep red cell membranes, *J. Immunol.,* 127, 2214, 1981.

10. **Ramm, L. E. and Mayer, M. M.,** Life-span and size of the trans-membrane channel formed by large doses of complement, *J. Immunol.,* 124, 2281, 1980.

11. **Ramm, L. E., Whitlow, M. B., and Mayer, M. M.,** Size distribution and stability of the trans-membrane channels formed by complement complex C5b-9, *Mol. Immunol.,* 20, 155, 1983.

12. **Sims, P. J. and Lauf, P. K.,** Steady-state analysis of tracer exchange across the C5b-9 complement lesion in a biological membrane, *Proc. Natl. Acad. Sci. USA,* 75, 5669, 1978.

13. **Sims, P. J. and Lauf, P. K.,** Analysis of soluble diffusion across the C5b-9 membrane lesion of complement: evidence that individual C5b-9 complexes do not function as discrete, uniform pores, *J. Immunol.,* 125, 2617, 1980.

14. **Simone, C. P. and Henkart, P.,** Inhibition of marker influx into complement-treated resealed erythrocyte ghosts by anti-C5, *J. Immunol.,* 128, 1168, 1982.

15. **Katoaka, T., Williamson, J. R., and Kinsky, S. C.,** Release of macromolecule markers (enzymes) from liposomes treated with antibody and complement, *Biochim. Biophys. Acta,* 298, 158, 1973.

16. **Mayer, M. M., Michaels, D. W., Ramm, L. E., Whitlow, M. B., Willoughby, J. B., and Shin, M. L.,** Membrane damage by complement, *CRC Crit. Rev. Immunol.,* 2, 133, 1981.

17. **Bhakdi, S. and Tranum-Jensen, J.,** Molecular nature of the complement lesion, *Proc. Natl. Acad. Sci. USA,* 75, 5655, 1978.

18. **Wobschall, D. and McKeon, C.,** Step conductance increases in bilayer membranes induced by antibody-antigen-complement action, *Biochim. Biophys. Acta,* 413, 317, 1975.

19. **Michaels, D. W., Abramovitz, A. S., Hammer, C. H., and Mayer, M. M.,** Increased ion permeability of planar lipid bilayer membranes after treatment with C5b-9 cytolytic attack mechanism of complement, *Proc. Natl. Acad. Sci. USA,* 73, 2852, 1976.

20. **Jackson, M. B., Stephens, C. L., and Lecar, H.,** Single channel currents induced by complement in antibody-coated cell membranes, *Proc. Natl. Acad. Sci. USA,* 78, 6421, 1981.

21. **Boyle, M. D. P., Gee, A. P., and Borsos, T.,** Heterogeneity in the size and stability of transmembrane channels produced by whole complement, *Clin. Immunol. Immunopathol.,* 20, 287, 1981.

22. **Podack, E. R., Tschopp, J., and Müller-Eberhard, H. J.,** Molecular organization of C9 within the membrane attack complex of complement. Induction of circular C9 polymerization by the C5b-8 assembly, *J. Exp. Med.,* 156, 268, 1982.

23. **Müller-Eberhard, H. J.,** The membrane attack complex, *Springer Semin. Immunopathol.,* 7, 93, 1984.

24. **Podack, E. R., Biesecker, G., and Müller-Eberhard, H. J.,** Membrane attack complex of complement: generation of high-affinity phospholipid binding sites by fusion of five hydrophilic plasma proteins, *Proc. Natl. Acad. Sci. USA,* 76, 897, 1979.

25. **Tschopp, J.,** Ultrastructure of membrane attack complex of complement. Heterogeneity of the complex caused by different degree of C9 polymerization, *J. Biol. Chem.,* 259, 7857, 1984.

26. **Gee, A. P., Boyle, M. D. P., and Borsos, T.,** Distinction between C8-mediated and C8/C9-mediated hemolysis on the basis of independent $^{86}$Rb and hemoglobin release, *J. Immunol.,* 124, 1905, 1980.

27. **Stolfi, R. L.,** Immune lytic transformation: a state of irreversible damage generated as a result of the reaction of the eighth component in the guinea pig complement system, *J. Immunol.,* 100, 46, 1968.

28. **Ramm, L. E., Whitlow, M. B., and Mayer, M. M.,** Size of the transmembrane channels produced by complement proteins C5b-8, *J. Immunol.,* 129, 1143, 1982.

29. **Sims, P. J.,** Complement pores in erythrocyte membranes. Analysis of C8/C9 binding required for functional membrane damage, *Biochim. Biophys. Acta,* 732, 541, 1983.

30. **Ramm, L. E., Whitlow, M. B., and Mayer, M. M.,** Transmembrane channel formation by complement: functional analysis of the number of C5b6, C7, C8, and C9 molecules required for a single channel, *Proc. Natl. Acad. Sci. USA,* 79, 4751, 1982.

31. **Ramm, L. E., Whitlow, M. B., and Mayer, M. M.,** The relationship between channel size and the number of C9 molecules in the C5b-9 complex, *J. Immunol.,* 134, 2594, 1985.

32. **DeLisi, C., Boyle, M., and Borsos, T.,** Analysis of the colloid osmotic step of complement-mediated immune hemolysis, *J. Immunol.,* 125, 2055, 1980.

33. **Bhakdi, S. and Tranum-Jensen, J.,** On the cause and nature of C9-related heterogeneity of terminal complement complexes generated on target erythrocytes through the action of whole serum, *J. Immunol.,* 133, 1453, 1984.

34. **Sims, P. J.,** Permeability characteristics of complement-damaged membranes: Evaluation of the membrane leak generated by the complement proteins C5b-9, *Proc. Natl. Acad. Sci. USA,* 78, 1838, 1981.

35. **Stewart, J. L., Monahan, J. B., Brickner, A., and Sodetz, J. M.,** Measurement of the ratio of the eighth and ninth components of human complement on complement-lysed membranes, *Biochemistry,* 23, 4016, 1984.

36. **Dankert, J. R. and Esser, A. F.,** Proteolytic modification of human complement protein C9: Loss of poly(C9) and circular lesion formation without impairment of function, *Proc. Natl. Acad. Sci. USA,* 82, 2128, 1985.
37. **Tschopp, J., Müller-Eberhard, H. J., and Podack, E. R.,** Formation of transmembrane tubules by spontaneous polymerization of the hydrophilic complement protein C9, *Nature (London),* 298, 534, 1982.
38. **Dalmasso, A. P., Benson, B. A., and Falk, R. J.,** Complement channels in membranes: inhibition with a monoclonal antibody to a neoantigen of polymerized C9, *Biochem. Biophys. Res. Comm.,* 125, 1013, 1984.
39. **Morgan, B. P., Luzio, J. P., and Campbell, A. K.,** Inhibition of complement-induced [$^{14}$C] sucrose release by intracellular and extracellular monoclonal antibodies to C9: evidence that C9 is a transmembrane protein, *Biochem. Biophys. Res. Comm.,* 118, 616, 1984.
40. **Tschopp, J., Podack, E. R., and Müller-Eberhard, H. J.,** The membrane attack complex of complement: C5b-8 complex as accelerator of C9 polymerization, *J. Immunol.,* 134, 495, 1985.
41. **Yamamoto, K. I. and Migita, S.,** Evidence for polymeric assembly of C9 within the membrane attack complex of complement, *J. Immunol.,* 129, 2335, 1982.
42. **Monahan, J. B., Stewart, J. L., and Sodetz, J. M.,** Studies of the association of the eighth and ninth components of human complement within the membrane-bound cytolytic complex, *J. Biol. Chem.,* 258, 5056, 1983.
43. **Esser, A. F., Kolb, W. P., Podack, E. R., and Müller-Eberhard, H. J.,** Molecular reorganization of lipid bilayers by complement: A possible mechanism for membranolysis, *Proc. Natl. Acad. Sci. U.S.A.,* 76, 1410, 1979.
44. **Zalman, L. S. and Müller-Eberhard, H. J.,** Comparison of channels formed by poly C9, C5b-8 and the membrane attack complex using the liposome swelling assay, *Fed. Proc.,* 44, 551, 1985.
45. **Sims, P. J. and Wiedmer, T.,** The influence of electrochemical gradients of Na$^+$ and K$^+$ upon the membrane binding and pore forming activity of the terminal complement proteins, *J. Membrane Biol.,* 78, 169, 1984.
46. **de Bracco, M. M. E. and Dalmasso, A. P.,** Effect of the cationic environment on immune haemolysis of high potassium and low potassium sheep erythrocytes, *Immunology,* 17, 559, 1969.
47. **Dalmasso, A. P., Lelchuk, R., Giavedoni, E. B., and de Isola, E. D.,** The modifications of the final stages of the complement reaction by alkali metal cations, *J. Immunol.,* 115, 63, 1975.
48. **Dalmasso, A. P., Giavedoni, E. B., Lelchuk, R., and de Bracco, M. M. E.,** Role of intracellular and extracellular cationic composition in immune lysis of mammalian erythrocytes, *J. Immunol.,* 111, 527, 1973.
49. **Humphrey, J. H. and Dourmashkin, R. R.,** The lesions in cell membranes caused by complement, *Adv. Immunol.,* 11, 75, 1969.
50. **Benson, B. A. and Dalmasso, A. P.,** Development of distinct patterns of complement lesion size in different target membranes, *Fed. Proc.,* 40, 965, 1981.
51. **Mason, R. P., Giavedoni, E. B., and Dalmasso, A. P.,** Complement-induced decrease in membrane mobility: introducing a more sensitive index of spin-label motion, *Biochemistry,* 16, 1196, 1977.
52. **Giavedoni, E. B., Mason, R. P., and Dalmasso, A. P.,** Complement-induced modifications in membrane fluidity: Studies with resealed and glutaraldehyde-treated erythrocyte membrane ghosts, *J. Immunol.,* 120, 2003, 1978.
53. **Giavedoni, E. B., Chow, Y. M., and Dalmasso, A. P.,** Complement lysis of resealed red cell membrane ghosts pretreated with glutaraldehyde, *J. Immunol.,* 122, 1643, 1979.

Chapter 13

# PORE SIZE AND FUNCTIONAL PROPERTIES OF DEFINED MAC AND POLY C9 COMPLEXES: RECONSTITUTION INTO MODEL LIPID MEMBRANES

**John Ding-E Young, Zanvil A. Cohn, and Eckhard R. Podack**

## TABLE OF CONTENTS

# I. INTRODUCTION

The membrane attack complex (MAC) of complement is formed by the assembly of the five terminal components of complement in the target cell membrane which results in membrane damage and cytolysis. Ultrastructural studies have shown that membranes damaged by the MAC show tubular membrane lesions of approximately 100 Å in internal diameter.[1-4] These observations are consistent with the doughnut channel model for complement-mediated killing proposed earlier by Mayer.[5] The assembly of these membrane-attack components involves an initial insertion of C5b-7 into membranes,[6] followed by the subsequent binding of C8 and C9 to form the tubular lesions.[7,8]

C9 appears to be responsible largely for the formation of the tubular structure associated with the MAC.[4,9,10] Polymerization of C9 into circular lesions occurs after prolonged incubation of the monomer at temperature exceeding 37°C.[11,12]

A transmembrane tubule with an internal diameter of 100 Å and a length of 160 Å, as reported for the MAC and the polymerized C9 (poly C9), would be expected to have unique molecular sieving properties that would be consistent with the colloid-osmotic type of killing suggested previously for the MAC. Moreover, it remains to be established that one single protein species in the MAC (that is, poly C9) may produce functional lesions of the type previously thought to be associated with the whole complement cascade.

High-impedance planar lipid bilayers provide a unique opportunity to examine the molecular sieving properties of channel-forming proteins.[13] This is possible due to the high resistance of these membranes, which allows the precise measurements of small current fluctuations associated with single functional molecules. We have reconstituted human poly C9 into model lipid bilayers (phospholipid vesicles and planar lipid bilayers) and measured directly the ionic current driven through poly C9 molecules. Our results imply that large channels are formed by poly C9 that resemble closely those formed by cytolytic proteins isolated from cytotoxic T lymphocytes and NK cells.

# II. POLYMERIZATION OF C9 AND INCORPORATION INTO BILAYERS

Purified monomeric C9 can be polymerized spontaneously by prolonged incubation of C9 with lipid at 37°C. C9 also polymerizes in the presence of $Zn^{2+}$, which drastically reduces the amount of time required for its polymerization. Examination of this material by negative contrast electron microscopy reveals the characteristic appearance of ring and tubular structures of poly C9 (Figure 1b). C9 can also be incorporated and polymerized in lipid vesicles (Figure 1a to c). In addition to complete circular lesions, a number of incomplete and linear polymers are also visualized.

To obtain a homogeneous population of poly C9 for single channel measurements, rate zonal centrifugation is used to enrich for circular poly C9.[14] This preparation of poly C9 is resistant to dissociation by SDS and reducing agents and on SDS-PAGE, migrates with an apparent $M_r$ of $1.1 \times 10^6$.

Voltage-clamped planar bilayers are prepared from monolayers of soybean phospholipids.[15-17] Usually only bilayers with a baseline conductance ($g$, expressed in S, 1 S = A/V) that does exceed 10 pS are used for functional reconstitution of poly C9 channels. C9 that has been polymerized (in solution or lipid vesicles) can be transferred to planar bilayers. The incorporation of poly C9 into planar bilayers requires the use of detergents (possibly for protein micelle formation). Direct addition of poly C9 to bilayers in the absence of detergent does not result in any measurable channel incorporation.

Figure 2 shows typical conductance measurements with poly C9.[24] Monomeric C9 does not result in any conductance change, even after prolonged incubation with the bilayer at room temperature (Figure 2a). Incorporation of poly C9, however, results in immediate

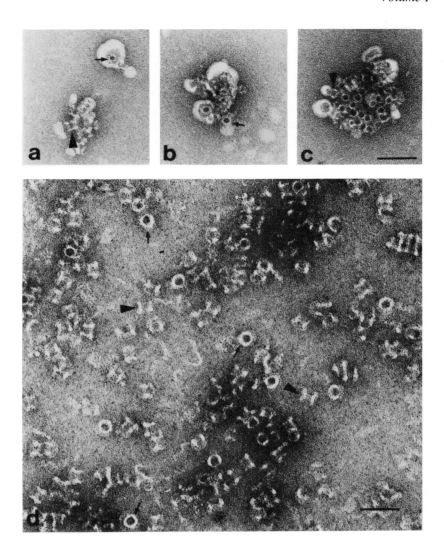

FIGURE 1.    Ultrastructure of poly C9 used in conductance measurements. (a-c) assembly of poly C9 in lipid vesicles. (d) C9 polymerized in solution. Poly C9 is visualized as a stain-filled tubule with an internal diameter of 10 to 11 nm (top views being imaged as rings, *black arrows*) and a length of 16 nm (side views, *black arrowheads*). Scale bars: 80 nm (a to c); 57 nm (d).

current increase, which occurs as a progressive summation of discrete current steps. The steps are heterogeneous in size, showing no decay or closing as a function of time. Poly C9-vesicles can also be incorporated into planar bilayers by means of a fusion protocol that allows the fusion of proteoliposomes with the planar bilayer in the absence of any detergent (Figure 2b). Exposure of bilayers to poly C9-vesicles without these manipulations (i.e., previous solubilization with detergent or fusion of proteoliposomes with bilayer) does not result in any conductance increase.

The simultaneous polymerization of C9 and channel formation needs to be demonstrated in order to assess the function of C9 polymerization. We recently succeeded in polymerizing C9 in the planar bilayer, by using $Zn^{2+}$ as the catalyst. Addition of $Zn^{2+}$ to monomeric C9 at 25 to 30°C results in immediate current increase, which can be resolved as a summation of discrete current steps.

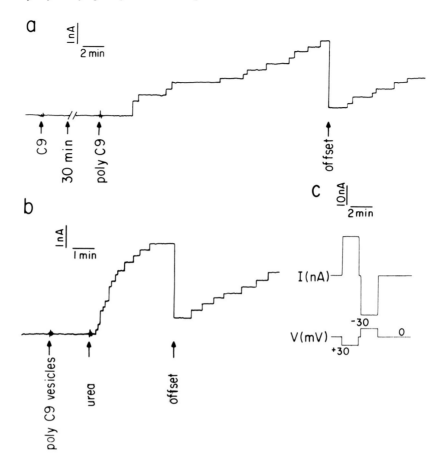

FIGURE 2.    Channel formation produced by poly C9. (a) Planar bilayer prepared in 0.1 *M* NaCl and clamped at +30 mV was exposed to monomeric C9 (15 μg/mℓ) and poly C9-vesicles (3.5 μg/mℓ, in 0.1% Triton X-100). (b) Planar bilayer bathed in 0.1 *M* NaCl and 10 m*M* CaCl$_2$ was exposed to poly C9-vesicles (14 μg protein:42 μg lipid in total membrane buffer of 4 mℓ), followed by an osmotic stress with urea to 300 m*M*. A burst of fusion occurred, with simultaneous channel incorporation. (c) Effect of voltage (V) polarity on membrane current (I) associated with poly C9. The voltage was switched from +30 to −30 mV, as indicated. Note that the magnitude of the current remains unaltered. (Young, J. D.-E., Cohn, Z. A., and Podack, E. R., *Science*, 233, 184, 1986. With permission.)

The reconstituted poly C9 channels do not sense voltage polarity, as indicated by the observation that the conductances attained with equal voltage pulses but of opposite polarities are symmetrical (Figure 2c). Moreover, the channels associated with poly C9 are highly resistant to closing by an increase of transmembrane electrical field. The current-voltage relationship (described in more detail elsewhere in this volume) shows a linear curve with little deviation from linearity occuring only at voltages that exceed 100 mV. It can be concluded that poly C9 forms stable, voltage-insensitive membrane channels, remaining preferentially in the open state, an attribute that would be consistent with the expected cytolytic function associated with the MAC.

The large current steps shown in Figure 2 would suggest an ion flow of at least 10$^8$ ions/s/molecule. To visualize the current fluctuations associated with individual molecules of poly C9, the amount of protein used for the conductance measurements is lowered until only single channels are recorded (Figure 3).[24] Channels are induced to close and to fluctuate

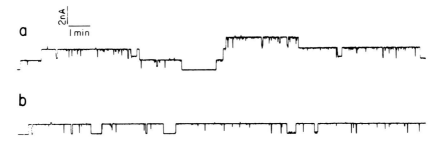

FIGURE 3. Single-channel fluctuations of poly C9. Planar bilayer prepared in 0.1 *M* NaCl and clamped at +120 mV was exposed to poly C9 at ng levels in the presence of 0.1% Triton X-100. (From Young, J. D.-E., Cohn, Z. A., and Podack, E. R., *Science*, 233, 184, 1986. With permission.)

between open and closed states only at voltages exceeding 100 mV (Figure 3). Several intermediate states have been identified, in addition to the fully open and closed states. The magnitude of the single channel current increases proportionally with an increase of membrane voltage, suggesting that the poly C9 channel has a hollow, water-filled tubular structure.

Histograms of single poly C9 channel conductance using a variety of preparations allows us to infer that in 0.1 *M* NaCl, poly C9 has a conductance that ranges 1 to 6 nS. By modelling the poly C9 channel as a cylindrical structure filled with an aqueous solution of the same specific conductance as the external solution, the size of the pore can be estimated from the magnitude of each discrete conductance step by the relationship:

$$g_o = \sigma \pi \ r^2/l$$

in which $\sigma$ is the specific conductance of the aqueous phase and "r" and "l" are the radius and length of the pore, respectively. This calculation yields functional diameters of 60 to 80 Å, which are comparable to the minimal functional diameters of 40 Å[18] and 55 Å[19] previously estimated for the MAC.

As expected for a channel of this size, poly C9 shows little ion selectivity. The channel is freely permeable to all monovalent ions tested and even to divalent ions ($Ca^{2+}$, $Mg^{2+}$, $Zn^{2+}$), albeit at a lower rate. Electrolyte and macromolecule sieving properties can also be examined with poly C9-vesicles, where bulk transfer of solutes across membranes is measured. Poly C9-channels are permeable to lucifer yellow (mol. wt. 457) and sucrose (mol. wt. 342) and to glucosamine (Stokes diameter of 8 Å).

The MAC has also been reconstituted into planar lipid bilayers. The single channel currents associated with the MAC are comparable to those produced by poly C9. The open channel lifetime, however, is significantly shorter than that observed for poly C9. C8 also conducts in the bilayer. However, the channels formed by C8 are several-fold smaller than the poly C9 channels and have a much shorter open channel lifetime.

## III. CONCLUSION

Planar lipid bilayers have previously been used to demonstrate that the association of antigen, antibody, and complement results in increased membrane permeability.[20,21] These results were substantiated (1) by the finding that the membrane permeability increase was produced by the association of the individual components of the MAC and was observed only when C8 and C9 were present,[22] and (2) by single channel recordings of the antigen-antibody induced whole serum complement complexes.[23] However, little was known about the molecular nature or components of the membrane lesion, since all previously published experiments involved multi-molecular reactions. Our demonstration that one single species of protein is capable of producing functional membrane lesions may provide new insight into the molecular nature of the functional transmembrane channel formed by the MAC.

Poly C9 channels are large aqueous channels lacking ion selectvity and are virtually insensitive to the normal transmembrane field found across biological membranes. It is easy to conceive cell killing by means of transmembrane channels that have these properties. Once inserted into the target membranes, it is expected that poly C9 channels would not be affected by membrane potential and by other modulatory factors and would remain permanently open, allowing leakage of water, ions, and macromolecules across the membrane.

The multiple sizes of poly C9 channels suggests that poly C9 may behave as a functional channel even before complete polymerization has occurred. It is possible that poly C9 may be lytic to cells prior to complete polymerization into the EM-visible tubular lesions.

In vivo, C5b-8 would probably provide an attachment site for C9 on the target membrane and promote rapid polymerization of bound C9. In the absence of C5b-8, for example, spontaneous polymerization of C9 may occur but at a low efficiency. The need for C5b-8 may be bypassed by raising the temperature of incubation or by including $Zn^{2+}$ in the C9 polymerization buffer. Another function suggested for C5b-8 is the formation of functional channels at the C8 stage.[22] However, as pointed out, the C8 channels show different unit conductances, open-close kinetics, and voltage-current relationships from those described here for poly C9.

Cell killing by insertion of membrane channels is not unique to the complement system. Pore-formation has also been described for protozoan parasites and recently for the cytotoxic T lymphocytes and NK cells. Moreover, C9 shares functional and structural homology with the lymphocyte pore-forming protein (perforin 1). Proteins with similar killing function and mechanism may have emerged from the same ancestral protein during evolution in order to carry out the separate but closely related functions of humoral and cellular immune responses.

## IV. ACKNOWLEDGMENTS

We thank the excellent technical assistance of M. A. DiNome and S. S. Ko. This work was supported in part by grants from the Cancer Research Institute and the Lucille P. Markey Charitable Trust to John Ding-E Young; by grants CA30198 and AI070127 from NIH to Zanvil A. Cohn; and by NIH grants AI18525 and CA34524 and by the American Cancer Society grant IM396 to Eckhard R. Podack. John Ding-E Young is a Lucille P. Markey Scholar; Eckhard R. Podack is an established investigator of the American Heart Association.

## REFERENCES

1. **Humphrey, J. H. and Dourmashkin, R. R.,** The lesions in cell membranes caused by complement, *Adv. Immunol.,* 11, 75, 1969.
2. **Bhakdi, S., Bjerrum, O. J., Rother, U., Knufermann, H., and Wallach, D. F. H.,** Immunochemical analysis of membrane-bound complement detection of the terminal complement complex and its similarity to "intrinsic" erythrocyte membrane proteins, *Biochim. Biophys. Acta,* 406, 21, 1975.
3. **Biesecker, G., Podack, E. R., Halverson, C. A., and Muller-Eberhard, H. J.,** C5b-9 dimer: isolation from complement lysed cells and ultrastructural identification with complement-depedent membrane lesions, *J. Exp. Med.,* 149, 448, 1979.
4. **Podack, E. R., Esser, A. F., Biesecker, G., and Muller-Eberhard, H. J.,** Membrane attack complex of complement. A structural analysis of its assembly, *J. Exp. Med.,* 151, 301, 1980.
5. **Mayer, M. M.,** Mechanism of cytolysis by complement, *Proc. Natl. Acad. Sci. U.S.A.,* 69, 2954, 1972.

6. **Hammer, C. H., Nicholson, A., and Mayer, M. M.,** On the mechanism of cytolysis by complement: Evidence on insertion of C5b and C7 subunits of the C5b, 6, 7 complex into phospholipid bilayer of erythrocyte membranes, *Proc. Natl. Acad. Sci. U.S.A.,* 72, 5076, 1975.

7. **Podack, E. R., Stoffel, W., Esser, A. F., and Muller-Eberhard, H. J.,** Membrane attack complex of complement: distribution of subunits between the hydrocarbon phase of target membranes and water, *Proc. Natl. Acad. Sci. U.S.A.,* 78, 4544, 1981.

8. **Hu, V. W., Esser, A. F., Podack, E. R., and Wisnieski, B. J.,** The membrane attack mechanism of complement: photolabeling reveals insertion of terminal proteins into target membrane, *J. Immunol.,* 127, 380, 1981.

9. **Dourmashkin, R. R.,** The structural events associated with the attachment of complement components to cell membranes in reactive lysis, *Immunology,* 35, 205, 1978.

10. **Podack, E. R., Tschopp, J., and Muller-Eberhard, H. J.,** Molecular organization of C9 within the membrane attack complex of complement, *J. Exp. Med.,* 156, 268, 1982.

11. **Podack, E. R. and Tschopp, J.,** Polymerization of the ninth component of complement (C9): formation of poly (C9) with tubular ultrastructure resembling the membrane attack complex of complement, *Proc. Natl. Acad. Sci. U.S.A.,* 79, 574, 1982.

12. **Tschopp, J., Muller-Eberhard, H. J., and Podack, E. R.,** Formation of transmembrane tubules by spontaneous polymerization of the hydrophilic complement protein C9, *Nature,* 298, 534, 1982.

13. **Montal, M. and Mueller, P.,** Formation of bimolecular membranes from lipid monolayers and a study of their electrical properties, *Proc. Natl. Acad. Sci. U.S.A.,* 69, 3561, 1972.

14. **Podack, E. R. and Tschopp, J.,** Circular polymerization of the ninth component of complement, *J. Biol. Chem.,* 257, 15204, 1982.

15. **Young, J. D.-E, Young, T. M, Lu, L. P., Unkeless, J. C., and Cohn, Z. A.,** Characterization of a membrane pore-forming protein from *Entamoeba histolytica, J. Exp. Med.,* 156, 1677, 1982.

16. **Young, J. D.-E, Blake, M., Mauro, A., and Cohn, Z. A.,** Properties of the major outer membrane protein of *Neisseria gonorrhoeae* incorporated into model lipid membranes, *Proc. Natl. Acad. Sci. U.S.A.,* 80, 3831, 1983.

17. **Young, J.D.-E, Unkeless, J. C., Young, T. M., Mauro, A., and Cohn, Z. A.,** Role for mouse macrophage IgG Fc receptor as ligand-dependent ion channel, *Nature,* 306, 186, 1983.

18. **Giavedoni, E. B., Chow, Y. M., and Dalmasso, A. P.,** The functional size of the primary complement lesion in resealed erythrocyte membrane ghosts, *J. Immunol.,* 122, 240, 1979.

19. **Ramm, L. E. and Mayer, M. M.,** Life-span and size of the transmembrane channel formed by large doses of complement, *J. Immunol.,* 124, 2281, 1980.

20. **Barfort, P., Arquilla, E. R., and Vogelhut, P. O.,** Resistance changes in lipid bilayers: immunological applications, *Science,* 160, 1119, 1968.

21. **Wobschall, D. and McKeon, C.,** Step conductance increases in bilayer membranes induced by antibody-antigen-complement action, *Biochim. Biophys. Acta,* 413, 317, 1975.

22. **Michaels, D. W., Abramovitz, A. S., Hammer, C. H., and Mayer, M. M.,** Increased ion permeability of planar lipid bilayer membranes after treatment with the C5b-9 cytolytic attack mechanism of complement, *Proc. Natl. Acad. Sci. U.S.A.,* 73, 2852, 1976.

23. **Jackson, M. B., Stephens, C. L., and Lecar, H.,** Single channel currents induced by complement in antibody-coated cell membranes, *Proc. Natl. Acad. Sci. U.S.A.,* 78, 6421, 1981.

24. **Young, J. D.-E., Cohn, Z. A., and Podack, E. R.,** The ninth component of complement and the pore-forming protein (perforin-1) from cytotoxic T cells: structural, immunological, and functional similarities, *Science,* 233, 184, 1986.

Chapter 14

# MECHANISMS OF THE CELLULAR DEFENSE RESPONSE OF NUCLEATED CELLS TO MEMBRANE ATTACK BY COMPLEMENT

**by Moon L. Shin and David F. Carney**

## TABLE OF CONTENTS

# I. OVERVIEW

Formation of complement (C) channels by activation and insertion of the terminal C components, C5-C9, into the plasma membrane (PM) of a variety of mammalian cells and microorganisms will result in altered ion flux across the PM that can lead to colloid osmotic deregulation and eventual cytolysis. Membrane attack by C5b-9 against nucleated cells (NC), in particular, has been of interest for a number of years, due in part to the fact that NC are relatively resistant to lysis mediated by C5b-9, when compared to erythrocytes. The ability of NC to survive limited C attack may be due to a variety of factors endogenous to NC, most of which are probably directly or indirectly associated with the complex metabolic activities associated with NC. The actual mechanisms responsible for the relative resistance of NC to lysis by C have been studied in detail and are believed to not only involve factors that influence the efficiency of formation of C5b-9 channels in the PM, but also the ability of these C channels in the PM to mediate cytolysis. Several factors influence efficient formation of C channels that not only include characteristics of the target cell, such as the lipid composition of the PM[1-5] and regulatory proteins on the cell surface,[6-9] but also include characteristics of the antigen or antibody responsible for C activation,[10-14] regulatory factors in the serum,[15-17] and the species of C.[9,18-21] The possible role of factors which influence the efficiency of formation of C channels on NC with respect to the lytic susceptibility of NC to C has been reviewed in detail[22] and will be mentioned only briefly in this chapter. Emphasis will be placed, instead, on some of the more recent work that has dealt with the metabolic compensatory mechanisms unique to NC that promote cell survival following the formation of C channels in the PM.

# II. HISTORICAL PERSPECTIVE

The earliest reports describing that NC could be lysed by immune serum, or more specifically antibody and complement, were derived from studies that centered around the field of tumor immunotherapy.[23-26] Although the in vitro cytotoxic properties of so-called "anti-tumor serum" date back to the 1930s,[23,24] it was not until 1953 that C was first implicated as the required cytotoxic factor in anti-tumor serum[27] by showing that C could lyse tumor cells in vitro, as well as in vivo, when supplemented in the presence of specific antibody. Besides cancer immunotherapy, NC killing by complement had also gained popularity in the 1950s and 1960s from the standpoint that the cytotoxic properties of C could be used as an indicator in in vitro cytotoxic assays to screen NC for the presence of antibody bound to the cell surface. This assay, referred to as the "cytotoxicity test", is still in use to examine for the presence of antigenic markers on the surface of tumor cells and normal cells, the latter for purposes such as HL-A histocompatibility testing. This assay is also useful for screening patient and donor serum for the presence of antibodies against specific determinants on the surface of NC. Unfortunately, there have been inherent difficulties and inconsistencies regarding the use of complement in tumor cell killing or cytotoxicity testing due to the relative resistance observed for many of the NC to C-mediated cytolysis. This in turn has led to an extensive search into the reasons for the inefficiency of C to lyse NC.

# III. THE ROLE OF ANTIGENIC EXPRESSION IN THE EFFICIENCY OF C ATTACK

The resistance of NC against C-mediated cytolysis was initially blamed primarily on the qualitative or quantitative lack of antigen expression on the cell surface, which would result in inefficient C activation.[10,28,29] However, several subsequent studies concluded that the lytic susceptibility of NC in the presence of antibody and C did not necessarily correlate with antigen expression on the cell surface.[14,22,30-34] In the same respect, several NC that were resistant to lysis by C were shown to activate C efficiently in the presence of antibody, as demonstrated by fixation of large amounts of C1,[14,31] as well as C3 and C4,[32,35] and C8[32] to their cell surfaces (Table 1). These initial important observations made it clear that the inefficiency of C to lyse NC was not necessarily due to the inefficiency of C activation (reviewed in detail in Reference 22). It was therefore proposed that other factors independent of C activation must also be involved in the resistance of NC to C-mediated cytolysis.

## IV. ALTERING THE RESISTANCE OF NUCLEATED CELLS BY METABOLIC MODULATION

The observation that the extent of lysis of NC by C did not necessarily correlate with the extent of C activation or fixation prompted investigation by various approaches into the possibility that metabolic properties unique to NC might influence the ability of C5b-9 to lyse NC.[32,35-37] One extensive series of studies examined the effects of several metabolic modulators on the lytic efficiency of C.[22,33,38-49] It was observed in these studies that metabolic inhibitors, such as puromycin and actinomycin D rendered human lymphoid cells more sensitive to killing by C,[33,38] and also that these agents plus mitomycin, adriamycin, 5-fluorouracil, and others increased the sensitivity of guinea pig hepatoma cells to lysis by C.[40,42,43] In contrast, an increase in resistance was observed after guinea pig hepatoma cells were treated with various anabolic hormones, such as hydrocortisone, insulin, and epinephrine[44,46] or 3′5′ cyclic AMP[45,46,48] — the latter similarly effective in rat mast cells and mouse thymocytes.[39,41]

While the data derived with these metabolic modulating agents suggest that the resistance of NC to cytolysis by C can be associated with metabolic activities, there are inherent complications associated with this interpretation. For example, most of the agents used could affect many metabolic pathways and end-products, and it is therefore difficult to ascertain specific site(s) of action. However, in spite of this nonspecificity, a correlation has been made between the effect of these drugs on the resistance of cells to C-mediated cytolysis and lipid metabolism.[22,47,50,51] Various drugs and hormones that increased the sensitivity of guinea pig hepatoma cells to lysis by C also interfered with the ability of the cell to synthesize specific complex lipids.[47,50,51] The action of these agents on lipid metabolism was reversible, in that removal of the agent led to an increase in cell survival, as well as an increase in lipid synthesis. In the same respect, some agents that increased the resistance of cells to lysis by C also enhanced lipid synthesis.[47,51] An important corollary to this association between lipid synthesis and resistance to lysis by C can be derived from the fact that modulation of the lipid composition of the membrane lipid bilayer will alter the susceptibility of liposomes,[1] microorganisms,[2] erythrocytes,[1] and NC[3-5] to C-mediated lysis. The conclusions from these latter studies point out that the lipid composition of the PM has an important influence on the efficiency of C attack by affecting the efficiency of C channel formation.

It is important to note in the context of this discussion that lysis of cells by C can be separated into two distinct phases. The first phase pertains to the requirement for activation of C with subsequent formation of functional C channels in the PM. The second phase involves the ability of C channels in the PM to mediate cytolysis.[37,52,53] There is reason to believe that C channels in the PM of NC, unlike erythrocytes, need not necessarily lead to cytolysis, and that NC are capable of surviving limited C attack due to a metabolic defense response mechanism that interferes with the ability of C channels in the PM to mediate cytolysis — to be discussed in greater detail in the following sections. Therefore, it is difficult in most cases to establish whether metabolic modulation by various drugs and hormones alter the lytic susceptibility of NC to C by affecting formation of C channels and/ or by altering the lytic efficiency of C channels in the PM.

# Table 1

## COMPARISON OF THE QUANTITY OF C4 AND C3 ON Ab-SENSITIZED LINE-1 HEPATOMA CELLS WITH THE AMOUNT OF CYTOLYSIS AFTER ADDITION OF GUINEA PIG (GPC) AND HUMAN (HuC) COMPLEMENT

| Cell treatment[a] | % Trypan blue positive cells[b] | Molecules C4 per cell × ($10^{-5}$)[c] | Molecules C3 per cell × ($10^{-5}$)[c] |
|---|---|---|---|
| 1. Line-1 + anti-Forssman 1/5 + GPC 1/8 | 61 ± 4 | 11.1 ± 2.5 | 7.4 ± 0.74 |
| 2. Line-1 + anti-Forssman 1/300 + GPC 1/8 | 3 ± 3 | 1.9 ± 1.1 | 1.65 ± 0.8 |
| 3. Line-1 + anti-line-1 1/30 + GPC 1/8 | 0 | <0.27 ± 0.03 | 0.48 ± 0.37 |
| 4. Line-1 + VBS + GPC 1/8 | 0 | 0.5 ± 0.5 | 0.27 ± 0.16 |
| 5. Line-1 + anti-Forssman 1/5 + HuC 1/8 | 95 ± 1.5 | 10.0 ± 2.4 | 2.6 ± 0.56 |
| 6. Line-1 + anti-Forssman 1/800 + HuC | 56 ± 0.6 | 3.2 ± 0.84 | 3.7 ± 1.0 |
| 7. Line-1 + anti-line-1 1/30 + HuC 1/8 | 65 ± 2 | 6.3 ± 0.73 | 3.8 ± 0.53 |
| 8. Line-1 + VBS + HuC 1/8 | 0 | 0.24 ± 0.24 | 1.53 ± 0.5 |

[a]  C1 fixing sites generated per cell with dilutions of antibody: anti-Forssman diluted 1:5; 0.56 × $10^5$ + 0.03, anti-Forssman diluted 1/300; 0.011 × $10^5$ + 0.002, anti-line-1 diluted 1/30; 0.171 × $10^5$ + 0.05.

[b]  Percent Trypan blue positive cells = [1 − (% nonstained in experiments/% nonstained in cell control)] × 100.

[c]  Number of molecules/cell calculated from an estimated mol wt of 230,000 for Hu and GPC4 and 185,000 for Hu and GPC3. Calculations made after subtracting in each experiment the amount of C4 or C3 in additional control tubes receiving VBS and C 1:8 alone (no cells).

From Ohanian, S. H. and Borsos, T., *J. Immunol.*, 114, 1292, 1975. With permission.

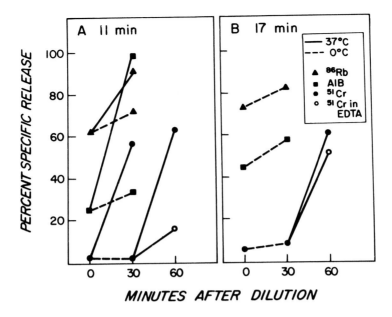

FIGURE 1. Prevention of $^{51}$Cr release by EDTA for P815 cells damaged by Ab + C in albumin. P815 cells were incubated with Ab (1/100 final dilution) and C in 13% albumin at 37°C for either 11 min (A) or 17 min (B). Cell suspensions were next cooled to 0°C, then either diluted 5-fold with ice-cold medium and samples immediately or maintained at 0°C (broken line) or 37°C (solid line) for 30 min. $^{86}$Rb release (▲), $^{14}$C-aminoisobutyric acid (AIB) release (■), $^{51}$Cr release after dilution with medium (●), and $^{51}$Cr release after dilution with EDTA solution (○) were determined. Addition of EDTA to prevent further membrane damage by C also prevented $^{51}$Cr release when the extent of C attack was limited (A). However, $^{51}$Cr release could not be prevented if the membrane damage by C was more extensive (B). (From Burakoff, S. J., Martz, E., and Benacerraf, B., *Clin. Immunol. Immunopathol.*, 4, 108, 1975. With permission.)

## V. LYTIC EFFICIENCY OF C CHANNELS ON NUCLEATED CELLS

To gain a better understanding of the cellular events that are involved in the resistance of NC to C-mediated lysis, a number of studies have examined changes in cells that occur after formation of functional C channels in the PM. In an early series of experiments designed to examine and compare the lytic efficiency of C channels in the PM of NC and erythrocytes, osmotic blocking was used to delay lysis by C in order to observe early pre-lytic changes induced by C channels.[36] The results of these experiments indicated that when osmotic lysis of mouse mastocytoma cells was prevented with extracellular albumin, NC could survive C attack if the extent of C damage was limited and C activation was stopped prior to removal of the osmotic protection (Figures 1 and 2). From these results, the authors concluded that surviving cells did not lyse due either to (1) inherent properties of the primary membrane lesions produced by C that promote leakiness but not lysis, or (2) the possibility that NC are capable of effective "repair" of limited membrane damage produced by C. The possibility that a similar situation might also be produced in erythrocytes, however, can be ruled out based on the well-established single-hit theory for lysis of erythrocytes by C, whereby one C channel is sufficient to lyse an erythrocyte,[54-57] and also on evidence that C channels are indeed relatively stable in the PM of erythrocytes, with a half-life of several hr at 37°C.[58,59]

In another assay system designed to examine the lytic efficiency of C channels in the PM of NC, a limited number of C channels were formed on guinea pig hepatoma cells by incubating antibody coated cells briefly with C, prior to washing to removing excess C.[37] These cells, designated T* and analogous to E*,[52,53] require further incubation at 37°C to

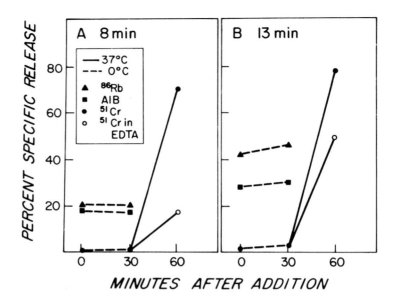

FIGURE 2.   Failure of EDTA to prevent $^{51}$Cr loss from P815 cells damaged without osmotic protection. P815 cells were incubated with Ab (1/100 final dilution) and C without albumin at 37°C for either 8 min (A) or 13 min (B). Cell suspensions were next cooled to 0°C, then either diluted 5-fold with ice-cold medium and sampled immediately or maintained at 0°C (broken line) or 37°C (solid line) for 30 min. $^{86}$Rb release (▲), $^{14}$C-aminoisobutyric acid (AIB) release (■), $^{51}$Cr release after dilution with medium (●), and $^{51}$Cr release after dilution with EDTA solution (○) were determined. The addition of EDTA to prevent further membrane damage by C prevented $^{51}$Cr release only if the extent of membrane damage was mild, as shown in (A), where only 20% $^{86}$Rb release was observed vs. 45% $^{86}$Rb release as in (B). (From Burakoff, S. J., Martz, E., and Benacerraf, B., *Clin. Immunol. Immunopathol.*, 4, 108, 1975. With permission.)

convert T* to dead cells, as determined by vital dye uptake. The effect of 3'5' cAMP, which was known to render cells more resistant to lysis by C,[39,41] on the conversion of T* to dead cells was assessed to determine if metabolic modulation with this agent could influence the lytic efficiency of C channels in the PM.[45] Cyclic AMP appeared to suppress the process of cell death itself in this experiment, since removal of cAMP after 30 min to 3 hr resulted in conversion of some of the protected cells to dead cells. However, the number of T* that converted to dead cells after removal of cAMP reduced in proportion with the length of time of exposure to cAMP. Other cyclic nucleotides, such as 3'5' cyclic guanine, cytosine, thymidine, and uridine monophosphates, were all ineffective, as were 2'3' cyclic adenosine, guanine, and uridine monophosphates. It was concluded from these experiments that metabolic activities stimulated by cAMP are involved in active repair of membrane damage mediated by C5b-9.

Another important finding that helped to clarify the issue pertaining to the lytic efficiency of C channels in the PM of NC was the observation that release of $^{86}$Rb$^+$ trapped within NC could occur following limited C attack without subsequent cytolysis, even in the absence of osmotic protection.[36] The implications of this finding, which were later confirmed by others,[60] are important with respect to the striking contrast with erythrocytes, since C channels cannot exist in the PM of erythrocytes without leading to lysis unless osmotically protected, in view of the single-hit characteristics for C-mediated lysis of erythrocytes.[54-57] The monitoring of membrane potential has also been employed for studying the C channels in the PM, where membrane potentials across the PM have been observed during C attack against neuroblastoma-glioma hybrid cells and primary mouse and rat muscle cells.[61] In this study, a decrease in membrane potential and parallel decrease in electrical resistance were observed a few minutes after adding either lytic or sublytic doses of C, both changes of which were reversible only after addition of the sublytic dose of C. Reversible depolarization of membrane potential has also been observed following limited treatment of human platelets with C5b-9.[62]

## VI. SINGLE-HIT VS. MULTI-HIT CHARACTERISTICS OF NUCLEATED CELL LYSIS BY C

There have been several observations that could be construed as possible indications that the cytocidal action of C attack against NC may not be a one-hit process, as is the case for erythrocytes.[60,61,63] The first direct evidence demonstrating that lysis of NC by C exhibited multi-hit characteristics was shown in a set of experiments that were designed to investigate and compare the susceptibility of nucleated cells and erythrocytes to C attack based on the number of C channels required for lysis, thus bypassing the complications associated with the initiating events of C activation and C channel formation.[64] This was accomplished by exposing erythrocytes and human lymphocytic and histiocytic cell lines coated with excess antibody to excess C6-deficient rabbit serum reconstituted with varying dilutions of C6 and measuring end-point cell lysis. Since C6 was the only limiting factor, cell lysis could be directly compared to the number of C5b-9 complexes formed, with one molecule of C6 per C5b-9. The results revealed that the NC remained viable in the presence of a limited number of $^{86}Rb^+$-releasing C channels and required multiple C channels for cytolysis, in contrast to the single channel requirement for erythrocytes (Figure 3). Thus, it became clear that the resistance of NC to lysis by C could be explained in part by the inefficiency of C channels to mediate cytolysis after formation in the PM.

## VII. ELIMINATION OF C CHANNELS FROM THE SURFACE OF NUCLEATED CELLS

For NC to survive in the presence of a limited number of C channels in the PM, these cells must be able to counteract the altered osmotic state by either sufficiently increasing the rate of ion efflux or reducing the rate of influx. For example, if $Na^+/K^+$ ATPases in the PM of NC were greater in number and/or activity than those on erythrocytes, efficient ion efflux could correct a mild osmotic imbalance created by a limited number of C channels in the PM of NC. However, no evidence to date has been able to associate the resistance of NC to C-mediated lysis with compensation by ion redistribution, although ouabain-sensitive repolarization has been observed in human platelets following limited treatment with C5b-9.[62] In fact, evidence against the role of $Na^+/K^+$ ATPases in the resistance of a human histiocytic cell line to lysis by C was derived from experiments in which ouabain was used to inhibit 95% of the $Na^+/K^+$ ATPase activity without subsequently affecting the lytic susceptibility to C.[65] An alternative way that NC might be able to survive C attack is by reducing the rate of influx through C channels in the PM. To accomplish this, C channels in the PM would have to be functionally destroyed or removed from the cell surface at a sufficient rate to overcome the lethal ion shifts mediated by C channels. Experimental evidence in favor of this defense mechanism has shown that PM-bound antigens, antibodies, and C4 on the cell surface can be eliminated from the cell surface of nucleated cells.[66-73] The first direct evidence showing that C5b-9 channels were functionally unstable on the surface of NC was derived from intracellular marker release experiments.[74] In these experiments, radiolabeled markers were loaded into human histiocytic tumor cells prior to forming a limited number of C channels in the PM. Aliquots of these cells, suspended in medium containing radiolabeled marker at a concentration equal to the intracellular level to keep the intracellular concentration of marker constant, were incubated at different temperatures. At

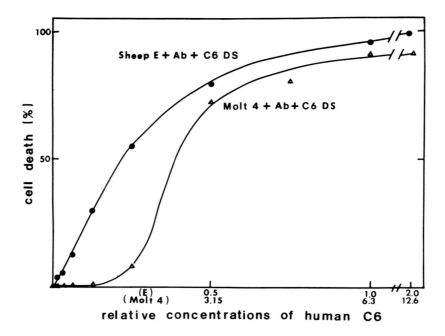

FIGURE 3.    C6 dose response of nucleated cell or erythrocyte lysis. Molt 4 cells coated with IgG antibody were incubated for 90 min at 37°C with excess C6-deficient rabbit serum (1:4 final dilution) and limiting concentrations of human C6. Cell death was measured by vital dye uptake. A sigmoidal dose-response curve was obtained with nucleated cells (△) in contrast to the monotonic characteristics of a parallel experiment with antibody-sensitized erythrocytes (●). The relative C6 concentration of 1.0 = 63 units of hemolytic activity and 323 mg of protein. (From Koski, C. L., Ramm, L. E., Hammer, C. H., Mayer, M. M., and Shin, M. L., *Proc. Natl. Acad. Sci. USA*, 80, 3816, 1983. With permission.)

various time points, the marker present in the medium was removed, and life-span of the channels was estimated by measuring marker release through the remaining channels. The results from these experiments revealed that the functional activity of C channels in the PM decreased at a rate that was temperature dependent, with a relatively short half-life of one minute at 37°C (Figure 4), in contrast to the stable nature of C channels on erythrocytes (Table 2). The stability of C5b-9 has also been assessed on the surface of human polymorphonuclear leukocytes by incubating cells bearing C5b-9 for various time intervals at various temperatures and then determining the capacity of radiolabeled anti-C9 to bind to the remaining C5b-9 on the cell surface at 0°C.[75] The half-life for C5b-9 on the surface of these cells was determined to be 3.5 min.

To further investigate the multichannel requirement for lysis of NC by C, the functional activity of the terminal C intermediates, C5b-7 and C5b-8, was examined after formation in the plasma membrane of Ehrlich ascites tumor cells, a mouse carcinoma cell line.[76] The rationale for this approach was based on the fact that the various terminal C complexes formed in lipid bilayers are quantitatively and qualitatively different with respect to certain physical characteristics, such as channel size and depth of penetration within the membrane.[58,59,77-81] Therefore, if the metabolic processes in NC that are involved in the elimination of terminal C complexes are influenced by one or more of these physical characteristics, the elimination rate of each of the various terminal C complexes might also be different. To determine the stability of terminal C complexes in the PM of Ehrlich cells, cells bearing a limited number of C5b-7, C5b-8, or C5b-8 in the presence of a sublytic number of C5b-9 (C5b-8,9$^{lim}$) were incubated at 37°C for various time intervals before converting the

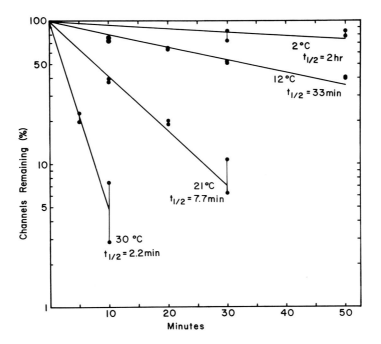

FIGURE 4.   Rate of C channel loss from the surface of U937 cells at various temperatures. Results are displayed as semi-logarithmic plots. After channel formation and washing, one portion of the cell suspension was incubated for 3 hr at 2°C and assayed for released $^{14}$C-aminoisobutyric acid ($^{14}$C-AIB). A second portion was incubated at either 2, 12, 21, or 30°C with extracellular $^{14}$C-AIB for the time intervals indicated. At each interval, the cells were washed to remove the extracellular $^{14}$C-AIB, incubated for 3 hr at 2°C, and assayed for released $^{14}$C-AIB. (From Ramm, L. E., Whitlow, M. B., Koski, C. L., Shin, M. L., and Mayer, M. M., *J. Immunol.*, 131, 1411, 1983. With permission).

## Table 2
## TESTS OF CHANNEL STABILITY ON ERYTHROCYTES MEMBRANES

|  |  |  | Marker release assay[a] | |
|  |  |  | --- | --- |
| Experiment no. | GPS (μl/mℓ) | Marker tested | Immediate assay (%) | Assay after 3 hr delay at 37°C (%) |
| 1 | 4.5 | Raffinose | 39 + 2.3 | 40 + 2.8 |
| 2 | 5.5 | Raffinose | 36 + 1.6 | 39 + 4.4 |
| 3 | 4.0 | Raffinose | 15.2 + 2.8 | 17.5 + 1.2 |
|  |  | Alanine | 25.7 + 3.0 | 27.1 + 0.9 |
| 4 | 4.0 | Raffinose | 17.2 + 2.4 | 15.0 + 1.3 |
|  |  | Alanine | 22.6 + 2.5 | 19.5 + 1.1 |

[a]   Incubation for 180 min at 37°C.

From Ramm, L. E., Whitlow, M. B., and Mayer, M. M., *Mol. Immunol.*, 20, 155, 1983. With permission.

remaining complexes to lytic C5b-9, where the degree of lysis would correspond directly to the number of complexes remaining. The minimum time necessary to form an optimum number of terminal C complexes in the PM was determined by kinetic analysis of lytic C5b-9 formation, where 70% of the maximum number of C channels were formed within 15 min at 37°C. The results of these comparative studies, summarized in Figure 5a, revealed that 30% of the C5b-7 complexes in the PM of Ehrlich cells disappeared during the first 15 min, and thereafter the remaining complexes retained their functional activity for up to 60 min. C5b-8 complexes disappeared at a more rapid rate, with only 25% of the complexes remaining functional after 60 min. C5b-8,9$^{lim}$ in the PM of Ehrlich cells disappeared even more rapidly than C5b-8 complexes alone, and only 10% of these complexes remained functional after 60 min. In the latter case, excess C9 added to TAC8,9$^{lim}$ would most likely convert the remaining C5b-8 sites to C5b-9 because C9 will not bind to the preformed C5b-9 complexes at 37°C.[82] Disappearance was observed to be a temperature-dependent process, since these complexes did not disappear when the cells were maintained at 0°C. In contrast to the instability of terminal C complexes on Ehrlich cells, C5b-7 or C5b-8 on sheep erythrocytes remained fully functional at 37°C for up to 60 min. The initial half-lives for the various terminal C complexes were 31 min for C5b-7, 20 min for C5b-8, and 10 min for C5b-8,9$^{lim}$ (Figure 5b). From this data, we postulated that differences in the functional properties of the terminal C complexes, especially channel size, might be responsible for differences in the rate of disappearance, based on the finding that terminal C complexes with the larger known functional pore sizes disappeared more rapidly than those with a smaller pore size. Also of interest was the finding that C5b-8 complexes disappeared faster when C5b-9 complexes were also present, suggesting that the presence of one terminal C complex in the PM can influence the disappearance rate of another. Disappearance of C5b-8 complexes has also been observed after formation in the PM of human polymorphonuclear leukocytes.[75]

## VIII. THE ROLE OF Ca$^{2+}$ IN ELIMINATION OF TERMINAL C COMPLEXES

The differences in the rates of disappearance of terminal C complexes suggest that these complexes in some way influence the metabolic processes that are responsible for their disappearance. To examine the mechanisms responsible for the different rates of disappearance for the various terminal C complexes, we first postulated[76] that Ca$^{2+}$ flux through these complexes might have an important influence on the rate of disappearance. The idea linking Ca$^{2+}$ flux with the rate of disappearance was based not only on correlations between the known pore size of these complexes (hence the amount of ion flux) and the disappearance rates, but also on the known involvement of Ca$^{2+}$ in many metabolic processes, including membrane mobilization, which might be responsible for removal of terminal C complexes from the cell surface.[83-89] To examine the influence of Ca$^{2+}$ flux on disappearance of terminal C complexes on Ehrlich cells, the disappearance rate has been measured in the presence of various concentrations of extracellular Ca$^{2+}$, [Ca$^{2+}$]$_o$.[90] The results of these studies indicated that the [Ca$^{2+}$]$_o$ influenced the rate of disappearance to a greater extent when terminal C complexes with larger pore diameters were present by prolonging the disappearance rate as the [Ca$^{2+}$]$_o$ was sufficiently lowered. The effect of [Ca$^{2+}$]$_o$ was most pronounced for C5b-8,9$^{lim}$, which disappeared with a T$_{1/2}$ of 5.5 min when suspended in buffer containing 1.5 m$M$ Ca$^{2+}$, as compared with a T$_{1/2}$ of 10 min in the presence of 0.15 m$M$ Ca$^{2+}$ (Figure 6). In addition, virtually no C5b-8,9$^{lim}$ complexes remained after 20 min in the presence of 1.5 m$M$ Ca$^{2+}$, whereas 5% of these complexes still remained functional after 60 min at 0.15 m$M$ Ca$^{2+}$. The [Ca$^{2+}$]$_o$ had less of an effect on C5b-8 alone, and least with C5b-7 (Figure 7). The addition of EGTA to chelate Ca$^{2+}$ has also been shown to prolong elimination of C5b-9 from the surface of human polymorphonuclear leucocytes.[91]

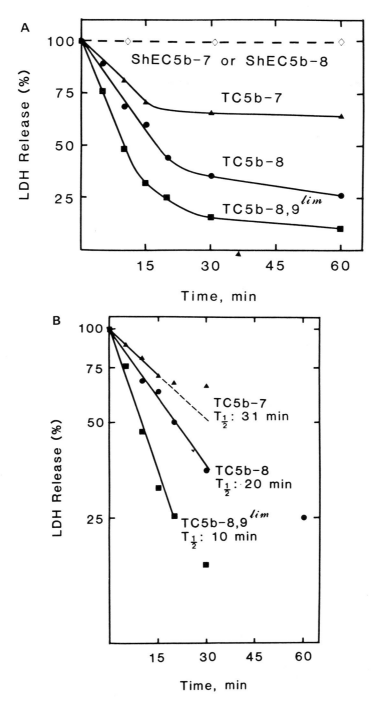

FIGURE 5. Stability of terminal C complexes in the plasma membrane of Ehrlich cells or sheep erythrocytes. TAC7 and ShEAC7 or TAC8 and ShEAC8 (antibody-coated tumor cells or sheep erythrocytes bearing a limited number of C5b-7 or C5b-8 sites, respectively) and TAC8 containing a sublytic dose of C9 were placed at 37°C. At various time intervals, excess C8 and C9 or C9 only were added to an aliquot of cells, which were then incubated for 90 min at 37°C. LDH or hemoglobin release was measured in the supernatants. (A) C5b-7 (▲), C5b-8 (●), and C5b-8 with a sublytic number of C5b-9 complexes (■) disappeared progressively with time from the surface of EATC. C5b-7 or C5b-8 complexes on ShE remained functionally stable (—). (B) the results in A expressed on a semilogarithmic plot. The initial T1/2 for C5b-7 complexes is 31 min (▲), 20 min for C5b-8 (●), and 10 min for C5b-8 in the presence of a sublytic number of C5b-9 (■). (From Carney, D. F., Koski, C. L., and Shin, M. L., *J. Immunol.*, 134, 1804, 1985. With permission.)

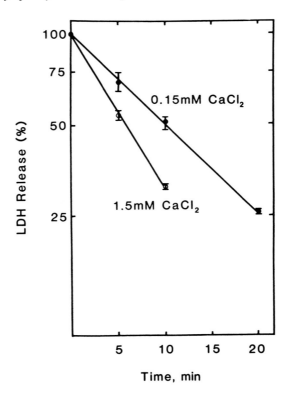

FIGURE 6.    Effect of $[Ca^{2+}]_o$ on the initial rate of disappearance of C5b-8,9$^{lim}$ in the plasma membrane of Ehrlich cells. TAC8 plus a sublytic dose of C9 at 0°C were suspended in buffer containing 1.5 or 0.15 m$M$ CaCl$_2$. Aliquots of cells were placed at 37°C and at various time intervals, excess C9 was added and further incubated for 90 min at 37°C. LDH was measured in the supernatants. The LDH released from TAC8,9$^{lim}$ after the addition of excess C9 at time 0 was considered as 100%. The initial T$_2^1$ for C5b-8,9$^{lim}$ in the presence of 1.5 m$M$ Ca$^{2+}$ was 5.6 min (○) and 10 min for 0.15 m$M$ (●). These data represent the mean ± SD of the mean of duplicate determinations from at least two experiments. (From Carney, D. F., Hammer, C. H., and Shin, M. L., *J. Immunol.*, 137, 263, 1986. With permission.)

The role of $Ca^{2+}$ on disappearance of terminal C complexes was further investigated in a related set of experiments designed to examine the effect of terminal C complexes on the cellular $Ca^{2+}$ concentrations, $[Ca^{2+}]_i$.[90] In these experiments, Quin 2 loaded Ehrlich cells were monitored in a spectrofluorometer after the addition of human serum deficient in either C8 (C8D-HS) or C9 (C9D-HS) with or without C9 to form C5b-7 or C5b-8 or C5b-8 with a sublytic number of C5b-9, respectively. In the presence of C9D-HS at a dose comparable to that used in assays to determine the functional disappearance of C5b-8, the $[Ca^{2+}]_i$ increased from a baseline of 140 n$M$ to a maximum of 167 n$M$ (or 19% increase) at 7 min after serum addition (Figure 8). Doubling the dose of C9D-HS resulted in a maximum increase in the $[Ca^{2+}]_i$ at 7 min to 231 n$M$ (or an increase of 65%). At this dose of C9D-HS, the $[Ca^{2+}]_i$ sharply declined after reaching a maximum increase at 7 min, but still remained elevated above baseline after 15 min. It is of interest that the $[Ca^{2+}]_i$ declines rapidly after reaching a maximum at 7 min after addition of the higher dose of C9D-HS, although the number of C5b-8 sites on the cell surface is still increasing at this time.[76] This decline is most likely due to accelerated redistribution of cellular free $Ca^{2+}$, rather than elimination of C5b-8, by sequestration into organelles,[92-94] and/or increased $Ca^{2+}$ efflux[94,95] at a rate dependent on the $[Ca^{2+}]_i$.[96] An increase in the $[Ca^{2+}]_i$ could not be detected in the presence of C5b-7 complexes in the PM, even after the addition of enough C8D-HS to yield a final concentration as high as 1/6.

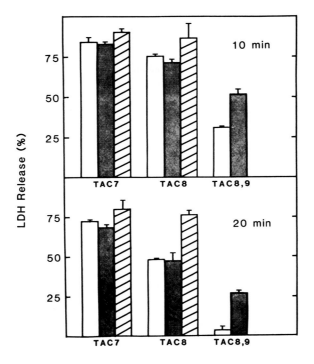

FIGURE 7. Effect of $[Ca^{2+}]_o$ on the stability of terminal C complexes in the plasma membrane of Ehrlich cells. TAC7, TAC8, or TAC8 plus a sublytic dose of C9 at 0°C were suspended in buffer containing 1.5 (open bar), 0.15 (shaded bar), or 0.015 m$M$ CaCl$_2$ (cross-hatched bar). Aliquots of cells were placed at 37°C. Excess C8 and C9 or C9 only were added to the suspensions at various time intervals and the cells were further incubated for 90 min at 37°C. LDH was measured in the supernatants and the LDH released after converting the intermediates to C5b-9 at time 0 was considered as 100%. The $[Ca^{2+}]_o$ influenced the disappearance of C5b-8,9$^{lim}$ more than C5b-8, whereas C5b-7 was least affected. These data represent the mean ± SD of the mean of duplicate determinations from at least two experiments. (From Carney, D. F., Hammer, C. H., and Shin, M. L., *J. Immunol.*, 137, 263, 1986. With permission.)

To determine the influence of C5b-9 channels on the $[Ca^{2+}]_i$, a large number of C5b-8 sites were formed with a 1/30 dilution of C9D-HS prior to adding low doses of C9 to yield C5b-9 channels with small pore sizes[97-99] to prevent leakage of Quin 2. At a C9 input of 3, 6, or 12 ng, the $[Ca^{2+}]_i$ increased to a maximum of 45, 75, and 275% over baseline, respectively, compared to a 32% increase over baseline for TAC8 recorded immediately prior to C9 addition (Figure 9). The disproportionate increase in the $[Ca^{2+}]_i$ that was observed after addition of between 6 and 12 ng of C9 may be due to an increase in channel size as C9 input increases,[97-99] in addition to an increase in the number of C5b-9 complexes. Also of interest was the observation that the greater the rise in the $[Ca^{2+}]_i$, the more rapid the decline toward the TAC8 baseline after the peak was reached, perhaps due to very rapid elimination of C5b-9,[74-76] as well as accelerated cellular Ca$^{2+}$ redistribution, as discussed above. These data strongly suggests that Ca$^{2+}$ influx through terminal C complexes plays an important role in the elimination of these complexes from the cell surface of NC.

Ca$^{2+}$-coupled receptor-ligand interactions are commonly associated with increases in the $[Ca^{2+}]_i$ via stimulated release of Ca$^{2+}$ from intracellular stores and/or the opening of Ca$^{2+}$ channels in the PM,[100-102] and it is possible that the insertion of terminal C complexes into the PM might indirectly contribute to raising the $[Ca^{2+}]_i$ by also stimulating similar metabolic pathways. Metabolic stimulation via membrane perturbation by terminal C complexes in the PM is theoretically possible based on the observation that reorientation of bilayer lipids

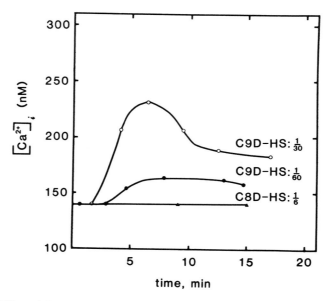

FIGURE 8.   Effect of C5b-8 and C5b-7 complexes in the plasma membrane of Ehrlich cells on the $[Ca^{2+}]_i$. Quin 2 loaded TA were monitored in a spectrofluorometer for changes in the $[Ca^{2+}]_i$ after addition of C9D-HS or C8D-HS to form C5b-8 or C5b-7 complexes in the PM, respectively. Increases in the $[Ca^{2+}]_i$ were observed in the presence of a dose of C9D-HS comparable to that used in functional disappearance experiments (●), with a proportionate increase in the $[Ca^{2+}]_i$ as the dose of C9D-HS was doubled (○). No increase in the $[Ca^{2+}]_i$ was observed in the presence of C8D-HS even at very high doses (▲). The data for each experimental condition are representative of tracings from at least two experiments. (From Carney, D. F., Hammer, C. H., and Shin, M. L., *J. Immunol.*, 137, 263, 1986. With permission.)

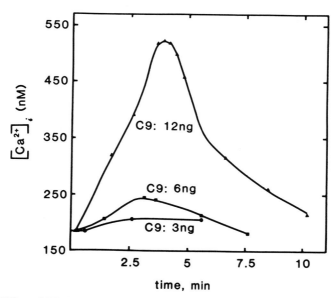

FIGURE 9.   Effect of C5b-8 in the presence of a sublytic number of C5b-9 in the plasma membrane of Ehrlich cells on the $[Ca^{2+}]_i$. Quin 2 loaded TA bearing an excess number of C5b-8 complexes were monitored for changes in the $[Ca^{2+}]_i$ in a spectrofluorometer after the addition of various sublytic doses of C9. The $[Ca^{2+}]_i$ increased disproportionately with the C9 dose to a maximum over baseline of 45% with 3 ng C9 (●), 75% with 6 ng C9 (■), and 275% with 12 ng C9 (▲), while increasing 32% in the presence of C9D-HS immediately prior to C9 addition. The data for each experimental condition are representative of tracings from at least two experiments. (From Carney, D. F., Hammer, C. H., and Shin, M. L., *J. Immunol.*, 137, 263, 1986. With permission.)

occurs following insertion of these complexes into lipid membranes,[103] which could have a direct modulatory effect on lipid-dependent enzymes and other proteins associated with the PM.[104,105]

## IX. FATE OF TERMINAL C COMPLEXES ON THE SURFACE OF NUCLEATED CELLS

It is well established, at least in the cell lines studied thus far, that C channels are far less stable in the PM of NC than in erythrocytes. While loss of PM-bound immunoglobulin,[67-73] and C3 and C4[73] from the surface of NC has been described, due perhaps to shedding[67,69,70] or enzymatic degradation,[68,71,72] no direct evidence exists for shedding or degradation of all or part of PM-associated C5b-9. It is unlikely that shedding or degradation could account for the rapid elimination of terminal C complexes since surface markers such as IgG, C3, and C4, are lost relatively slowly by this process. Another possibility is that extrusion of portions of the PM that contain C5b-9, such as would occur via blebbing, might result in removal of C5b-9 from the cell surface. This appears, at least in part, to account for the loss of C5b-9 from the surface of human polymorphonuclear leukocytes, which has been described to involve capping of C5b-9 prior to removal by vesiculation of PM into the medium.[106] However, it is also likely that removal of C channels on the surface of NC occurs primarily by endocytosis, based on the high degree of endocytic activity in NC.

There are several reasons to suspect that endocytosis may be one of the most important mechanisms for elimination of C channels from the surface of NC, and thus cell survival. For example, macrophages and fibroblasts endocytose the equivalent of their entire cell surface in 30 min and 2 hr, respectively,[107] which demonstrates the tremendous capacity for PM removal by this pathway. In addition, endocytosis of receptors, especially after ligand attachment, is often a very rapid process, with a receptor half-life on the cell surface after ligand binding of as little as 2 to 5 min.[108] Also, both receptor-mediated as well as fluid phase endocytosis appear to be regulated in part by $Ca^{2+}$,[83-89] which correlates with the effect of $Ca^{2+}$ on elimination of terminal C complexes.[90] Direct evidence showing that terminal C complexes can be removed from the cell surface of NC by endocytosis has been obtained by immuno-electron microscopic examination with the use of colloidal gold as a tracer for C5b-8.[76] Specific binding of colloidal gold to C5b-8 at 0°C was followed by warming of the cells to 37°C for various time intervals prior to fixation to trace the fate of the particles. The gold particles were seen in membrane invaginations and endocytic vesicles near the cell surface after 7 min at 37°C, and were associated mostly with multivesicular bodies after 30 min, correlating well with the functional kinetic data for disappearance of C5b-8 (Figure 10).

## X. SUMMARY

Two essential requirements are necessary for lysis of NC by C. First, C5b-9 channels must be formed in the PM, and second, the effects of C channels must override the compensatory mechanisms that NC might employ to survive. In contrast, lysis of erythrocytes requires only the presence of C channels and is inevitable even when only one C channel is present in the PM. The inefficiency of C channels in the PM of NC to mediate cytolysis appears to be due to the relative instability of these channels in the PM. C5b-9 channels, as well as terminal C intermediates, have been shown to be eliminated from the cell surface after formation in the PM of several NC types, by a variety of methods. Disappearance of terminal C complexes is to a large extent probably due to rapid endocytosis, considering the extensive endocytic capacity of most NC. However, elimination of terminal C complexes via shedding or blebbing probably also occurs to some extent, depending on

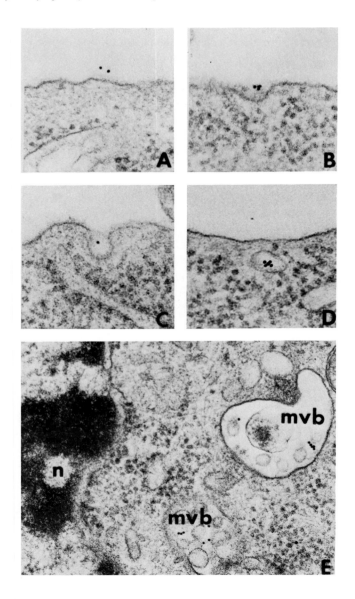

FIGURE 10.   The fate of C5b-8 complexes on the cell surface of Ehrlich cells studied by immuno-electron microscopy. TAC8 treated with goat anti-C5 IgG at 0°C were incubated with colloidal gold particles conjugated to rabbit anti-goat IgG at 0°C. Cells were fixed immediately or after incubation at 37°C for 7 min or 30 min. Colloidal gold particles were exclusively associated with the membrane surface when the cells were maintained at 0°C (A), and were frequently seen in areas of membrane invagination (B and C) or occasionally in intracellular vesicles near the cell surface (D) after 7 min at 37°C. After incubation at 37°C for 30 min, colloidal gold particles were most frequently seen in intracellular multivesicular bodies (E). (n, nucleus; mvb, multivesciular body). (From Carney, D. F., Koski, C. L., and Shin, M. L., *J. Immunol.,* 134, 1804, 1984. With permission.)

the characteristics of the target cell, as well as the extent of C-mediated damage. The rate of elimination of terminal C complexes apparently depends on characteristics of the complex present in the PM, and seems to correlate directly with the known functional pore size of the complex. It appears that a $Ca^{2+}$ signal mediated by terminal C complexes in the PM may be involved in the elimination of these complexes, in that quantitative changes in the

$[Ca^{2+}]_o$ and probably the $[Ca^{2+}]_i$ influence the rate of elimination. It is expected that many metabolic activities may potentially be stimulated by terminal C complexes in the PM of NC, that in many cases may be mediated through an increase in the $[Ca^{2+}]_i$. Arachidonic acid metabolism,[109-111] enhanced membrane lipid transmethylation,[112] lipid synthesis,[47,113] and superoxide production[114] can be enhanced following C channel formation in the PM of NC and may have important implications in the cellular response to immune related phenomena. Future studies on the interaction of the terminal C complexes with NC will be required to further define the role of C5b-9 as a modulator of metabolic activities associated with NC.

# REFERENCES

1. **Shin, M. L., Paznekas, W. A., and Mayer, M. M.,** On the mechanism of membrane damage by complement. The effect of length and unsaturation of the acyl chains in liposomal bilayers and the effect of cholesterol concentration in sheep erythrocyte and liposomal membranes, *J. Immunol.*, 120, 1996, 1978.
2. **Dahl, J. S., Dahl, C. E., and Levine, R. P.,** Role of fatty acyl composition and membrane fluidity in the resistance of *Acholeplasma Laidlawii* to complement-mediated killing, *J. Immunol.*, 123, 104, 1979.
3. **Yoo, T. J., Chin, H. C., Spector, A. A., Whitaker, R. J., Denning, C. M., and Lee, N. F.,** Effect of fatty acid modifications of cultured hepatoma cells on susceptibility to complement-mediated cytolysis, *Cancer Res.*, 40, 1084, 1980.
4. **Schlager, S. I. and Ohanian, S. H.,** Tumor cell lipid composition and sensitivity to humoral immune killing. II. Influence of plasma membrane and intracellular lipid and fatty acid content, *J. Immunol.*, 125, 508, 1980.
5. **Ohanian, S. H., Schlager, S. I., and Saha, S.,** Effect of lipids, structural precursors of lipids and fatty acids on complement-mediated killing of antibody sensitized nucleated cells, *Mol. Immunol.*, 19, 535, 1982.
6. **Fearon, D. T.,** Regulation by membrane sialic acid of β-1H-dependent decay-dissociation of amplification of C3 convertase of the alternative complement pathway, *Proc. Natl. Acad. Sci. USA*, 75, 1971, 1978.
7. **Fearon, D. T.,** Regulation of the amplification C3 convertase of human complement by an inhibitory protein isolated from human erythrocyte membrane, *Proc. Natl. Acad. Sci. USA*, 76, 5867, 1979.
8. **Nicholson-Weller, A., Burge, J., and Austen, F.,** Purification from guinea pig erythrocyte stroma of a decay-accelerating factor for the classical C3 convertase, C4b,2a, *J. Immunol.*, 127, 2035, 1981.
9. **Shin, M. L., Hansch, G., Hu, V. W., and Nicholson-Weller, A.,** Membrane factors responsible for homologous species restriction of complement-mediated lysis: evidence for a factor other than DAF operating at the stage of C8 and C9, *J. Immunol.*, 136, 1777, 1986.
10. **Moller, E. and Moller, G.,** Quantitative studies on the sensitivity of normal and neoplastic mouse cells to the cytotoxic action of isoantibodies, *J. Exp. Med.*, 115, 527, 1962.
11. **Linscott, W. D.,** An antigen density effect on the hemolytic efficiency of complement, *J. Immunol.*, 104, 1307, 1970.
12. **Ferrone, S., Cooper, N. R., Pellegrino, M. A., and Reisfeld, R. A.,** Interaction of histocompatibility (HL-A) antibodies and complement with synchronized human lymphoid cells in continuous culture, *J. Exp. Med.*, 137, 55, 1973.
13. **Edidin, M. and Henney, C. S.,** Effect of capping H-2 antigens on the susceptibility of target cells to humoral and T-cell mediated lysis, *Nature*, 246, 47, 1973.
14. **Evans, C. H., Ohanian, S. H., and Cooney, A. M.,** Tumor specific and forssman antigens of guinea pig hepatoma cells: Comparison of tumor cells grown *in vivo* and *in vitro*, *Int. J. Cancer*, 15, 512, 1975.
15. **Tamura, N. and Nelson, R. A., Jr.,** Three naturally occurring inhibitors of complement in guinea pig and rabbit serum, *J. Immunol.*, 99, 582, 1967.
16. **Lachman, P. J. and Muller-Eberhard, H. J.,** The demonstration in human serum of "conglutinogen activating factor" and its effect on the third component of complement, *J. Immunol.*, 100, 691, 1968.
17. **Ruddy, S. and Austen, K. F.,** C3b inactivator of man. II. Fragments produced by C3b inactivator cleavage of cell-bound or fluid phase C3b, *J. Immunol.*, 107, 742, 1971.
18. **Walford, R. L., Gallagher, R., and Sjaarda, J. R.,** Serological typing of human lymphocytes with immune serum obtained after homografting, *Science*, 144, 868, 1964.
19. **Walford, R. L., Latta, H., and Troup, G. M.,** The reaction between human lymphocytes and allogeneic antisera: A serologic and electron microscopic study, *Ann. N.Y. Acad. Sci.*, 129, 490, 1966.

20. **Haughton, G. and McGehee, M. P.,** Cytolysis of mouse lymph node cells by alloantibody: a comparison of guinea pig and rabbit complements, *Immunology,* 16, 447, 1969.
21. **Hansch, G. M., Hammer, C. H., Vanguri, P., and Shin, M. L.,** Homologous species restriction in lysis of erythrocytes by terminal complement proteins, *Proc. Natl. Acad. Sci. USA,* 78, 5118, 1981.
22. **Ohanian, S. H. and Schlager, S. I.,** Humoral immune killing of nucleated cell: mechanisms of complement-mediated attack and target cell defense, *CRC Crit. Rev. Immunol.,* 1, 165, 1981.
23. **Lumsden, T.,** Tumor immunity: the effects of the eu- and pseudo-globulin fractions of anti-cancer sera on tissue cultures, *J. Pathol. Bacteriol.,* 34, 349, 1931.
24. **Lumsden, T.,** On cytotoxins lethal to nucleated mammalian cells normal and malignant, *Am. J. Cancer,* 31, 430, 1937.
25. **Flax, M. H.,** The action of anti-Ehrlich ascites tumor antibody, *Cancer Res.,* 16, 774, 1956.
26. **Wissler, R. W. and Flax, M. H.,** Cytotoxic effects of antitumor serum, *Ann. N.Y. Acad. Sci.,* 69, 773, 1957.
27. **Kalfayan, B. and Kidd, J. G.,** Structural changes produced in brown-pearce carcinoma cells by means of a specific antibody and complement, *J. Exp. Med.,* 97, 145, 1953.
28. **Ferrone, S., Cooper, N. R., Pellegrino, M. A., Reisfeld, R. A.,** The lymphocytotoxic reaction: The mechanism of rabbit complement action, *J. Immunol.,* 107, 939, 1971.
29. **Young-Rodenchuk, J. M. and Gyenes, L.,** Differences in the sensitivity of tumor cells and normal lymphocytes toward lysis by alloantibodies and guinea pig or rabbit complement, *Transplantation,* 20, 20, 1975.
30. **Lerner, R. A., Oldstone, M. B. A., and Cooper, N. R.,** Cell cycle-dependent immune lysis of moloney virus-transformed lymphocytes: Presence of viral antigen, accessibility to antibody, and complement activation, *Proc. Natl. Acad. Sci. USA,* 68, 2584, 1971.
31. **Ohanian, S. H., Borsos, T., and Rapp, H. J.,** Lysis of tumor cells by antibody and complement. I. Lack of correlation between antigen content and lytic susceptibility, *J. Natl. Cancer Inst.,* 50, 1313, 1973.
32. **Pellegrino, M. A., Ferrone, S,. Cooper, N. R., Dierich, M. P., and Reisfeld, R. A.,** Variation in susceptibility of a human lymphoid cell line to immune lysis during the cell cycle, *J. Exp. Med.,* 140, 578, 1974.
33. **Ferrone, S., Pellegrino, M. A., Dierich, M. P., and Reisfeld, R. A.,** Effect of inhibitors of macromolecular synthesis on HLA antibody mediated lysis of cultured lymphoblasts, Tissue antigens, 4, 275, 1974.
34. **Liang, W. and Cohen, E. P.,** Complement sensitivity of somatic hybrids of a complement-resistant murine leukemia cell line, *J. Natl. Cancer Inst.,* 55, 309, 1975.
35. **Ohanian, S. H. and Borsos, T.,** Lysis of tumor cells by antibody and complement. II. Lack of correlations between amount of C4 and C3 fixed and cell lysis, *J. Immunol.,* 114, 1292, 1975.
36. **Burakoff, S. J., Martz, E., and Benacerraf, B.,** Is the primary complement lesion insufficient for lysis? Failure of cells damaged under osmotic protection to lyse in EDTA or at low temperature after removal of osmotic protection, *Clin. Immunol. Immunopathol.,* 4, 108, 1975.
37. **Boyle, M. D. P., Ohanian, S. H., and Borsos, T.,** Studies on the terminal stages of antibody-complement-mediated killing of a tumor cell. I. Evidence for the existence of an Intermediate, T*, *J. Immunol.,* 116, 1272, 1976.
38. **Miyasima, T., Hirata, A. A., and Terasaki, P. I.,** Escape from sensitization to HLA antibodies, *Tissue Antigens,* 2, 64, 1972.
39. **Ebbesen, P. and Arnus, K. M.,** Enhancement of the dye-exclusion cytotoxic test by insulin and inhibition by cyclic adenosine 3:5-monophosphate and theophylline, *Transplantation,* 16, 476, 1973.
40. **Segerling, M. S., Ohanian, S. H., and Borsos, T.,** Effect of metabolic inhibitors on killing of tumor cells by antibody and complement, *J. Natl. Canc. Inst.,* 53, 1411, 1974.
41. **Kaliner, M. and Austen, K. F.,** Adenosine 3'5'-Monophosphate: Inhibition of complement-mediated cell lysis, *Science,* 183, 659, 1974.
42. **Segerling, M. S., Ohanian, S. H., and Borsos, T.,** Chemotherapeutic drugs increase killing of tumor cells by antibody and complement, *Science,* 188, 55, 1975.
43. **Segerling, M. S., Ohanian, S. H., and Borsos, T.,** Enhancing effect by metabolic inhibitors on the killing of tumor cells by antibody and complement, *Cancer Res.,* 35, 3195, 1975.
44. **Schlager, S. I., Ohanian, S. H., and Borsos, T.,** Inhibition of antibody-complement-mediated killing of tumor cells by hormones, *Cancer Res.,* 36, 3672, 1976.
45. **Boyle, M. D. P., Ohanian, S. H., and Borsos, T.,** Studies on the terminal stages of antibody-complement-mediated killing of a tumor cell. II. Inhibition of transformation of T* to dead cells by 3'5' cAMP, *J. Immunol.,* 116, 1276, 1976.
46. **Boyle, M. D. P., Ohanian, S. H., and Borsos, T.,** Studies on the terminal stages of antibody-complement-mediated killing of a tumor cell. III. Effect of membrane active agents, *J. Immunol.,* 117, 106, 1976.
47. **Schlager, S. I., Ohanian, S. H., and Borsos, T.,** Correlation between the ability of tumor cells to resist humoral immune attack and their ability to synthesize lipid, *J. Immunol.,* 120, 463, 1978.

48. **Lo, T. N. and Boyle, M. D. P.,** Relationship between the intracellular cyclic adenosine 3':5'-monophosphate level of tumor cells and their sensitivity to killing by antibody and complement, *Cancer Res.,* 39, 3156, 1979.

49. **Ramm, L. E., Whitlow, M. B., and Mayer, M. M.,** Complement lysis of nucleated cells: Effect of temperature and puromycin on the number of channels required for cytolysis, *Mol. Immunol.,* 21, 1015, 1984.

50. **Schlager, S. I. and Ohanian, S. H.,** A role for fatty acid composition of complex cellular lipids in the susceptibility of tumor cells to humoral immune killing, *J. Immunol.,* 123, 146, 1979.

51. **Schlager, S. I. and Ohanian, S. H.,** Tumor cell lipid composition and sensitivity to humoral immune killing. II. Influence of plasma membrane and intracellular lipid and fatty acid content, *J. Immunol.,* 125, 508, 1980.

52. **Mayer, M. M. and Levine, L. J.,** Kinetic studies on immune hemolysis. III. Description of terminal process which follows the $Ca^{++}$ and $Mg^{++}$ reaction steps in the action of complement on sensitized erythrocytes, *J. Immunol.,* 72, 511, 1954.

53. **Kabat, E. A. and Mayer, M. M.,** *Experimental Immunology,* Charles C Thomas, Springfield, Ill., 1961, 176.

54. **Mayer, M. M.,** Development of the One-Hit Theory of Immune Hemolysis, in *Immunochemical Approaches to Problems in Microbiology,* Heidelberger, M. and Plescia, D. J., Eds., Rutgers University Press, New Brunswick, N. J., 1961, 268.

55. **Borsos, T., Rapp, H. J., and Mayer, M. M.,** Studies on the second component of complement. I. The reaction between EAC'1,4 and C'2: evidence on the single site mechanism of immune hemolysis and determination of C'2 on a molecular basis, *J. Immunol.,* 87, 310, 1961.

56. **Hingson, D. J., Massengill, R. K., and Mayer, M. M.,** The kinetics of release of $^{86}$rubidium and hemoglobin from erythrocytes damaged by antibody and complement, *Immunochemistry,* 6, 295, 1969.

57. **Hoffman, L. C.,** Statistical evaluation of reaction mechanisms in immune hemolysis. II. The kinetics of release of $^{86}$rubidium and hemoglobin from erythrocytes damaged by antibody and complement, *Immunochemistry,* 6, 309, 1969.

58. **Ramm, L. E. and Mayer, M. M.,** Life-span and size of the transmembrane channel formed by large doses of complement, *J. Immunol.,* 124, 2281, 1980.

59. **Ramm, L. E., Whitlow, M. B., and Mayer, M. M.,** Size distribution and stability of the trans-membrane channels formed by complement complex C5b-9, *Mol. Immunol.,* 20, 155, 1983.

60. **Boyle, M. D., Ohanian, S. H., and Borsos, T.,** Lysis of tumor cells by antibody and complement. VII. Complement-dependent $^{86}$Rb release — a nonlethal event?, *J. Immunol.,* 117, 1346, 1976.

61. **Stephens, C. L. and Henkart, P. A.,** Electrical measurements of complement-mediated membrane damage in cultured nerve and muscle cells, *J. Immunol.,* 122, 455, 1979.

62. **Wiedmer, T. and Sims, P. J.,** Effect of complement proteins C5b-9 on blood platelets, *J. Biol. Chem.,* 260, 8014, 1985.

63. **Reske-Kunz, A. B., Scheid, M. P., Abbott, J., Metakis, L. J., Polley, M. J., and Boyse, E. A.,** Action of complement in the lysis of mouse sarcoma cells sensitized with H-2 alloantibody, *Transplantation,* 28, 149, 1979.

64. **Koski, C. L., Ramm, L. E., Hammer, C. H., Mayer, M. M., and Shin, M. L.,** Cytolysis of nucleated cells by complement: Cell death displays multi-hit characteristics, *Proc. Natl. Acad. Sci. USA,* 80, 3816, 1983.

65. **Ramm, L. E., Whitlow, M. B., and Mayer, M. M.,** Complement lysis of nucleated cells: Effect of temperature and puromycin on the number of channels required for cytolysis, *Mol. Immunol.,* 21, 1015, 1984.

66. **Old, L. J., Stockert, E., Boyse, E. A., and Kim, J. H.,** Antigenic modulation. Loss of TL antigen from cells exposed to TL antibody. Study of the phenomenon in vitro, *J. Exp. Med.,* 127, 523, 1968.

67. **Chang, S., Stockert, E., Boyse, E. A., Hammerling, U., and Old, L. J.,** Spontaneous release of cytotoxic alloantibody from viable cells sensitized in excess antibody, *Immunology,* 21, 829, 1971.

68. **Keisari, Y. and Witz, I. P.,** Degradation of immunoglobulins by lysosomal enzymes of tumors. I. Demonstration of the phenomenon using mouse tumors, *Immunochemistry,* 10, 565, 1973.

69. **Witz, I. P., Kinamon, S., Ran, M., and Klein, G.,** Tumor-bound immunoglobulins. The *in vitro* fixation on radioiodine-labeled anti-immunoglobulin reagents by tumor cells, *Clin. Exp. Immunol.,* 16, 321, 1974.

70. **Ran, M., Fish, R., Witz, I. P., and Klein, G.,** Tumor bound immunoglobulins. The *in vitro* disappearance of immunoglobulins from the surface of coated tumor cells, and some properties of released components, *Clin. Exp. Immunol.,* 16, 335, 1974.

71. **Fish, F., Witz, I. P., and Klein, G.,** Tumor bound immunoglobulins. The fate of immunoglobulin disappearing from the surface of coated tumor cells, *Clin. Exp. Immunol.,* 16, 355, 1974.

72. **Dauphinee, M. J., Talal, N., and Witz, I. P.,** Generation of noncomplement-fixing, blocking factors by lysosomal extract treatment of cytotoxic antitumor antibodies, J. Immunol., 113, 948, 1974.

73. **Segerling, M., Ohanian, S. H., and Borsos, T.,** The persistence of immunoglobulin, C4 and C3 bound to guinea pig tumor cells, *J. Natl. Cancer Inst.,* 57, 145, 1976.

74. **Ramm, L. E., Whitlow, M. B., Koski, C. L., Shin, M. L., and Mayer, M. M.,** Elimination of complement channels from the plasma membranes of U937, a nucleated mammalian cell line: Temperature dependence of the elimination rate, *J. Immunol.,* 131, 1411, 1983.

75. **Morgan, B. P., Campbell, A. K., Luzio, J. P., and Hallett, M. B.,** Recovery of polymorphonuclear leucocytes from complement attack, *Biochem. Soc. Trans.,* 12, 779, 1984.

76. **Carney, D. F., Koski, C. L., and Shin, M. L.,** Elimination of terminal complement intermediates from the plasma membrane of nucleated cells: The rate of disappearance differs for cells carrying C5b-7 or C5b-8 or a mixture of C5b-8 with a limited number of C5b-9, *J. Immunol.,* 134, 1804, 1985.

77. **Podack, E. R., Biesecker, G., and Muller-Eberhard, H. J.,** Membrane attack complex of complement: generation of high-affinity phospholipid binding sites by fusion of five hydrophilic plasma proteins, *Proc. Natl. Acad. Sci. USA,* 76, 897, 1979.

78. **Podack, E. R., Esser, A. F., Biesecker, G., and Muller-Eberhard, H. J.,** Membrane attack complex of complement. A structural analysis of its assembly, *J. Exp. Med.,* 151, 301, 1980.

79. **Hu, V. W., Esser, A. F., Podack, E. R., and Wisnieski, B. J.,** The membrane attack mechanism of complement: photolabeling reveals insertion of terminal proteins into target membrane, *J. Immunol.,* 127, 380, 1981.

80. **Ramm, L. E., Whitlow, M. B., and Mayer, M. M.,** Size of transmembrane channels produced by complement proteins C5b-8, *J. Immunol.,* 129, 1143, 1982.

81. **Ramm, L. E., Michaels, D. W., Whitlow, M. B., and Mayer, M. M.,** On the size heterogeneity and molecular composition of the trans-membrane channels produced by complement, in, *Biological Response Mediators and Modulators,* August, J. T., Ed., Academic Press, New York, 1983, 117.

82. **Bhakdi, S. and Tranum-Jensen, J.,** On the cause and nature of C9-related heterogeneity of C5b-9 complexes generated on erythrocyte membranes through the action of whole human serum, *J. Immunol.,* 133, 1453, 1984.

83. **Ceccarelli, B. and Hurlbut, W. P.,** $Ca^{2+}$-dependent recycling of synaptic vesicles at the frog neuromuscular junction, *J. Cell Biol.,* 87, 297, 1980.

84. **Prusch, R. D.,** Endocytic sucrose uptake in *Amoeba proteus* induced with the calcium ionophore A23187, *Science,* 209, 691, 1980.

85. **Goldstone, A. D., Koenig, H., and Lu, C. Y.,** Androgenic stimulation of endocytosis, amino acid, and hexose transport in mouse kidney cortex involves increased calcium fluxes, *Biochim. Biophys. Acta.,* 762, 366, 1983.

86. **Goldstone, H. D., Koenig, H., Lu, C. Y., and Trout, J. J.,** β-adrenergic stimulation evokes a rapid, $Ca^{2+}$ dependent stimulation of endocytosis, hexose, and amino acid transport associated with increased $Ca^{2+}$ fluxes in mouse kidney cortex, *Biochem. Biophys. Res. Comm.,* 114, 913, 1983.

87. **Tupper, J. T. and Bodine, P. V.,** Calcium effects on epidermal growth factor receptor-mediated endocytosis in normal and SV40-transformed human fibroblasts, *J. Cell. Physiol.,* 115, 159, 1983.

88. **Korc, M., Matrisian, L. M., and Magun, B. E.,** Cytosolic calcium regulates epidermal growth factor endocytosis in rat pancreas and cultured fibroblasts, *Proc. Natl. Acad. Sci. USA,* 81, 461, 1984.

89. **Truneh, A., Marshal, Z., and Leserman, L. D.,** A calmodulin antagonist increases the apparent rate of endocytosis of liposomes bound to MHC molecules via monoclonal antibodies, *Exp. Cell Res.,* 155, 50, 1984.

90. **Carney, D. F., Hammer, C. H., and Shin, M. L.,** Elimination of terminal complement complexes in the plasma membrane of nucleated cells: Influence of extracellular $Ca^{2+}$ and association with cellular $Ca^{2+}$, *J. Immunol.,* 137, 263, 1986.

91. **Morgan, B. P. and Campbell, A. K.,** The recovery of human polymorphonuclear leucocytes from sublytic complement attack is mediated by changes in intracellular free calcium, *Biochem. J.,* 231, 205, 1985.

92. **Cittadini, A., Scarpa, A., and Chance, B.,** Calcium transport in intact Ehrlich ascites tumor cells, *Biochim. Biophys. Acta,* 291, 246, 1973.

93. **Hines, R. N. and Wenner, C. E.,** The role of $P_i$ in glycolytic inhibition of calcium ion uptake in ELD ascites tumor cells, *Biochim. Biophys. Acta,* 465, 391, 1977.

94. **Cittadini, A., Bossi, D., Rosi, G., Wolf, F., and Terranova, T.,** Calcium metabolism in Ehrlich ascites tumor cells, *Biochim. Biophys. Acta,* 469, 345, 1977.

95. **Cittadini, A., Dani, A. M., Wolf, F., Bossi, D., and Calviello, G.,** Calcium permiability of Ehrlich ascites tumor cell plasma membrane in vivo, *Biochim. Biophys. Acta,* 686, 27, 1982.

96. **Carafoli, E. and Crompton, M.,** The regulation of intracellular calcium, *Curr. Top. Memb. Trans.,* 10, 151, 1978.

97. **Boyle, M. D. P., Gee, A. P., and Borsos, T.,** Studies on the terminal stages of immune hemolysis. VI. Osmotic blockers of differing stokes' radii detect complement-induced transmembrane channels of differing size, *J. Immunol.,* 123, 77, 1979.

98. **Ramm, L. E., Whitlow, M. B., and Mayer, M. M.,** Transmembrane channel formation by complement: functional analysis of the number of C5b-6, C7, C8, and C9 molecules required for a single channel, *Proc. Natl. Acad. Sci. USA*, 79, 4751, 1982.

99. **Ramm, L. E., Whitlow, M. B., and Mayer, M. M.,** The relationship between channel size and the number of C9 molecules in the C5b-9 complex, *J. Immunol.*, 134, 2594, 1985.

100. **Exton, J. H.,** Molecular mechanisms involved in α-adrenergic responses, *Mol. and Cell. Endocrinol.*, 23, 233, 1981.

101. **Cauvin, C., Loutzenhiser, R., and Van Breeman, C.,** Mechanisms of calcium antagonist-induced vasodilation, *Ann. Rev. Pharm. Tox.*, 23, 373, 1983.

102. **Fain, J. N.,** Activation of plasma membrane phosphotidylinositol turnover by hormones, *Vitam. Horm.*, 41, 117, 1984.

103. **Esser, A. F., Kolb, W. P., Podack, E. R., and Muller-Eberhard, H. J.,** Molecular reorganization of lipid bilayers by complement: A possible mechanism for membranolysis, *Proc. Natl. Acad. Sci. USA*, 76, 1410, 1979.

104. **Farias, R. N., Bloj, B., Morero, R. D., Sineriz, F., and Trucco, R. E.,** Regulation of allosteric membrane-bound enzymes through changes in membrane lipid composition, *Biochim. Biophys. Acta*, 415, 231, 1975.

105. **Sandermann, H.,** Regulation of membrane enzymes by lipids, *Biochim. Biophys. Acta*, 515, 209, 1978.

106. **Campbell, A. K. and Morgan, B. P.,** Monoclonal antibodies demonstrate protection of polymorphonuclear leukocytes against complement attack, *Nature*, 317, 164, 1985.

107. **Steinman, R. M., Brodie, S. E., and Cohn, Z. A.,** Membrane flow during pinocytosis. A stereologic analysis, *J. Cell Biol.*, 68, 665, 1976.

108. **Steinman, R. M., Mellman, I. S., Muller, W. A., and Cohn, Z. A.,** Endocytosis and the recycling of plasma membrane, *J. Cell Biol.*, 96, 1, 1983.

109. **Imagawa, D. K., Osifchin, N. E., Paznekas, W. A., Shin, M. L., and Mayer, M. M.,** Consequences of cell membrane attack by complement: Release of arachidonate and formation of inflammatory mediators, *Proc. Natl. Acad. Sci. USA*, 80, 6647, 1983.

110. **Betz, M. and Hansch, G. M.,** Release of arachidonic acid: a new function of the late complement components, *Immunobiology*, 166, 473, 1984.

111. **Hansch, G. M., Seitz, M., Martinotti, G., Betz, M., Rauterberg, E. W., and Gemsa, D.,** Macrophages release arachidonic acid, prostaglandin E₂, and thromboxane in response to late complement components, *J. Immunol.*, 133, 2145, 1984.

112. **Hansch, G. M., Betz, M., and Shin, M. L.,** Cytolysis of nucleated cells by complement: Inhibition of membrane-transmethylation enhances cell death by C5b-9, *J. Immunolol.*, 132, 1440, 1984.

113. **Gutter, F.,** Phospholipid sythesis in HeLa cells exposed to immunoglobulin G and complement, *Biochem. J.*, 128, 953, 1972.

114. **Roberts, P. A., Morgan, B. P., and Campbell, A. K.,** 2-chloroadenosine inhibits complement-induced reactive oxygen metabolite production and recovery of human polymorphonuclear leucocytes attacked by complement, *Biochem. Biophys. Res. Comm.*, 126, 962, 1985.

*Index*

# INDEX